2006–2009 Clinical Practice Guidelines for Midwifery & Women's Health

Nell L. Tharpe, MS, CNM, CRNFA

Midwife Publications, Inc.

East Boothbay, Maine

Adjunct Faculty

Midwifery Institute

Philadelphia University

Philadelphia, Pennsylvania

JONES AND BARTLETT PUBLISHERS

Sudbury, Massachusetts

BOSTON   TORONTO   LONDON   SINGAPORE

World Headquarters

Jones and Bartlett Publishers
40 Tall Pine Drive
Sudbury, MA 01776
978-443-5000
info@jbpub.com
www.jbpub.com

Jones and Bartlett Publishers
Canada
6339 Ormindale Way
Mississauga, Ontario L5V 1J2
Canada

Jones and Bartlett Publishers
International
Barb House, Barb Mews
London W6 7PA
UK

Jones and Bartlett's books and products are available through most bookstores and online booksellers. To contact Jones and Bartlett Publishers directly, call 800-832-0034, fax 978-443-8000, or visit our website, www.jbpub.com.

Substantial discounts on bulk quantities of Jones and Bartlett's publications are available to corporations, professional associations, and other qualified organizations. For details and specific discount information, contact the special sales department at Jones and Bartlett via the above contact information, or send an email to specialsales@jbpub.com.

Library of Congress Cataloging-in-Publication Data

Tharpe, Nell, 1956-
    Clinical practice guidelines for midwifery and women's health / Nell L. Tharpe. — 2006–2009 ed.
        p. ; cm.
    Includes bibliographical references and index.
    ISBN 0-7637-3822-0 (pbk. : alk. paper)
    1. Midwifery—Standards. 2. Maternity nursing—Standards. 3. Gynecologic nursing--Standards. I. Title.
    [DNLM: 1. Midwifery. 2. Genital Diseases, Female. 3. Pregnancy
Complications. 4. Women's Health.   WQ 165 T367c 2006]
RG950.T476 2006
618.2—dc22

                                        2005031570

6048

Production Credits
Acquisitions Editor: Kevin Sullivan
Production Director: Amy Rose
Associate Editor: Amy Sibley
Production Editor: Carolyn F. Rogers
Marketing Manager: Emily Ekle
Manufacturing and Inventory Coordinator: Amy Bacus
Composition: Paw Print Media
Cover Design: Timothy Dziewit
Cover Illustration: isa maria
Printing and Binding: Courier Stoughton
Cover Printing: Courier Stoughton

Printed in the United States of America
09 08 07 06 05   10 9 8 7 6 5 4 3 2 1

This edition is dedicated to my family. They taught me the importance of the classic midwifery practices of validation, active listening, and belief in each person's individual abilities.

Deep thanks go to all of the families who have honored me by allowing me to provide service to them.

Special thanks go to the midwives I have had the pleasure to know and work with, the educators who have guided my growth, and my colleagues from all walks of life who have mentored me.

Contents

Preface   xi

Chapter 1   Exemplary Midwifery Practice   1

Women First   3

How to Use This Book   3

The Purpose of Clinical Practice Guidelines   4

Documenting Midwifery Care   5

Developing a Collaborative Practice Network   5

Health Care As a Continuum   7

Cultural Diversity   8

Developmental Considerations   8

Risk Management   9

Summary   11

References   11

Chapter 2   Documentation of Midwifery and Women's Health Care   13

Standards for Documentation   14

Documentation as Communication: Skills and Techniques   14

Evaluation and Management Criteria   19

Documentation as Risk Management   19

Documenting Culturally Competent Care   20

Informed Consent   20

Components of Common Medical Records   21

Summary   28

References   28

Chapter 3   Care of the Woman During Pregnancy   29

Diagnosis of Pregnancy   30

Initial Evaluation of the Pregnant Woman   32

Evaluation of Health Risks in the Pregnant Woman   34

Ongoing Care of the Pregnant Woman   36

Care of the Pregnant Woman with Backache   39

Care of the Pregnant Woman with Constipation   41

Care of the Pregnant Woman with Dyspnea   43

Care of the Pregnant Woman with Edema   44

Care of the Pregnant Woman with Epistaxis   46

Care of the Pregnant Woman with Heartburn   47

Care of the Pregnant Woman with Hemorrhoids   48

Care of the Pregnant Woman with Insomnia   49

Care of the Pregnant Woman with Leg Cramps   51

Care of the Pregnant Woman with Nausea and Vomiting   52

Care of the Pregnant Woman with Pica   54

Care of the Pregnant Woman with Round Ligament Pain   55

Care of the Pregnant Woman with Varicose Veins   57

References   58

Chapter 4   Care of the Pregnant Woman with Prenatal Variations   61

Care of the Pregnant Woman with Iron Deficiency Anemia   62

Care of the Pregnant Woman with Fetal Demise   64

Care of the Pregnant Woman Exposed to Fifth's Disease   66

Care of the Pregnant Woman with Gestational Diabetes   68

Care of the Pregnant Woman with Hepatitis   72

Care of the Pregnant Woman with Herpes Simplex Virus   74

Care of the Pregnant Woman who is HIV Positive   76

Inadequate Weight Gain   79

Hypertensive Disorders in Pregnancy   81

Pruritic Urticarial Papules and Plaques of Pregnancy (PUPPP)   86

Care of the Woman who is Rh Negative   88

Size–Date Discrepancy   90

Toxoplasmosis   93

Urinary Tract Infection in Pregnancy   95

First Trimester Vaginal Bleeding   98

Bibliography   101

References   102

Chapter 5   Care of the Woman During Labor and Birthing   105

Initial Midwifery Evaluation of the Laboring Woman   106

Care of the Woman in First-Stage Labor   109

Care of the Woman in Second-Stage Labor   113

Care of the Woman in Third-Stage Labor   116

Amnioinfusion   120

Assisting with Cesarean Section   122

Caring for the Woman Undergoing Cesarean Birth   125

Caring for the Woman with Umbilical Cord Prolapse   128

Care of the Woman with Failure to Progress in Labor   130

Care of the Woman with Group B Strep   133

Care of the Woman undergoing Induction or Augmentation of Labor   136

Care of the Woman with Meconium-Stained Amniotic Fluid   139

Caring for the Woman with Multiple Pregnancy   142

Caring for the Woman with a Nonvertex Presentation   146

Caring for the Woman with Postpartum Hemorrhage   150

Postterm Pregnancy   153

Caring for the Woman with Pregnancy-Induced Hypertension in Labor   156

Care of the Woman with Preterm Labor   159

Care of the Woman with Prolonged Latent Phase Labor   163

Care of the Woman with Premature Rupture of the Membranes   165

Care of the Woman with Shoulder Dystocia   169

Care of the Woman Undergoing Vacuum-Assisted Birth   172

Care of the Woman During Vaginal Birth After Cesarean   174

References   177

Chapter 6   Care of the Mother and Baby After Birth   181

Postpartum Care, Week 1   181

Postpartum Care, Weeks 1–6   184

Postpartum Depression   187

Endometritis   190

Hemorrhoids   193

Mastitis   195

Newborn Resuscitation   197

Initial Examination and Evaluation of the Newborn   201

Care of the Infant Undergoing Circumcision   204

Assessment of the Newborn for Deviations from Normal   207

Well-Baby Care   210

References   213

Bibliography   214

Chapter 7   **Care of the Woman with Reproductive Health Needs:**
Care of the Well Woman   **215**

The Well-Woman Exam   216

Preconception Evaluation   220

Smoking Cessation   222

Fertility Awareness   225

Barrier Methods of Birth Control   227

Emergency Contraception   229

Hormonal Contraceptives: Pills, Patches, Rings, and Injections 232

The Intrauterine Device   236

Norplant Contraceptive Implant   239

Unplanned Pregnancy   241

Caring for Women as They Age   245

Hormone Replacement Therapy   249

Screening for Osteoporosis   253

Evaluation and Treatment of Women with
Perimenopausal Symptoms   256

References   259

Bibliography   261

Chapter 8   **Care of the Woman with Reproductive Health Needs:**
Reproductive Health Problems   **263**

Abnormal Mammogram   263

Abnormal Pap Smear   266

Amenorrhea   270

Bacterial Vaginosis   272

Breast Mass   275

Chlamydia   278

Colposcopy   281

Dysfunctional Uterine Bleeding   284

Dysmenorrhea   287

Endometrial Biopsy   290

Evaluation of Postmenopausal Bleeding   292

Endometriosis   295

Fibroid Uterus   297

Gonorrhea   300

Human Immunodeficiency Virus   303

Hepatitis   307

Human Papillomavirus   310

Herpes Simplex Virus   313

Genital Candidiasis   316

Nipple Discharge   318

Pediculosis   321

Pelvic Pain, Acute   323

Pelvic Pain, Chronic   325

Pelvic Inflammatory Disease   328

Premenstrual Syndrome   331

Syphilis   334

References   337

Bibliography   339

Chapter 9   **Primary Care in Women's Health**   **341**

Care of the Woman with Cardiovascular Problems   341

Care of the Woman with Dermatologic Disorders   346

Care of the Woman with Endocrine Disorders   352

Care of the Woman with Gastrointestinal Disorders   357

Care of the Woman with Mental Health Disorders   361

Care of the Woman with Musculoskeletal Problems   367

Care of the Woman with Respiratory Disorders   370

Care of the Woman with Urinary Tract Problems   375

References   380

Bibliography   381

Appendix: Calcium, Magnesium, and Iron Food Lists   382

Index   **383**

Preface

Disclaimer

The *2006–2009 Clinical Practice Guidelines for Midwifery & Women's Health* provided here represent a compilation of current practices that includes evidence-based, traditional, and empiric care from a wide variety of sources. The *Clinical Practice Guidelines for Midwifery & Women's Health* are used voluntarily and assume that the practicing women's health professional will temper them with sound clinical judgment, knowledge of patient or client preferences, national and local standards, and attention to sound risk management principles.

The *Clinical Practice Guidelines for Midwifery & Women's Health* are not all-inclusive, and there may be additional safe and reasonable practices that are not included. By accepting the *Clinical Practice Guidelines for Midwifery & Women's Health*, midwives and other women's health professionals are not restricted to their exclusive use.

Both the American College of Nurse-Midwives (ACNM) and the Midwives Alliance of North America (MANA) recommend that midwives utilize written policies and/or practice guidelines. The *Clinical Practice Guidelines for Midwifery & Women's Health* have grown out of a need for a concise reference guide to meet that recommendation.

The *Clinical Practice Guidelines for Midwifery & Women's Health* reflect current practice, and provide support and guidance for day-to-day clinical practice with diverse populations. Regional differences in practice styles occur; therefore, the guidelines are broadly based and designed to reflect current practice and literature as much as possible.

The *Clinical Practice Guidelines for Midwifery & Women's Health* are designed to be kept where you practice: a copy in your exam room(s), one copy for your birth setting, and another by the phone at home. These guidelines may be customized further with dated and initialed written additions, deletions, use of a highlighter, and so on. This is a working practice tool that should reflect your practice.

Midwives are blessed with a passion for their work. It is their patience and perseverance, which a laboring woman so appreciates, that has helped midwifery to grow. It is my hope that this book will make your professional practice simpler and more rewarding. This text is updated every three years. Comments and suggestions are always appreciated, with references and resources whenever possible.

This book is written for all the midwives, wherever they practice, and the women, children, and families that they care for.

Exemplary Midwifery Practice

Exemplary midwifery practice is woman oriented and focuses on excellence in the processes of providing care, improving maternal and child health and professionalism as a means of promoting the midwifery model of care.

Exemplary midwifery practice, according to Kennedy (2000), encompasses several key concepts. These concepts include the basic philosophy of midwifery and its active expression through the individual midwife's clinical practice. Each midwife's philosophy of care is reflected in her choice and use of healing modalities, the quality of her caring for and about women, and her support for midwifery as a profession. The midwife's underlying philosophy is brought to life through her clinical practice and professional involvement in midwifery. Throughout this book the driving philosophy is that of the American College of Nurse-Midwives.

Optimal midwifery care occurs when the midwife is able to support the physiologic processes of birth and well-woman care, while at the same time remaining vigilant for the unexpected (Kennedy, 2000). Remaining attuned to small details that might subtly indicate a significant change in maternal, fetal, or the well-woman's status provides the midwife with the opportunity for early identification of problems and prompt initiation of treatment geared toward improving outcomes. Midwifery encourages care that is individualized for each woman and each birth. Patience with the birth process is a hallmark of midwifery care. Midwives' compassionate and attentive care reinforces women's belief in their ability to give birth and care for themselves. By utilizing interventions and technology only when necessary, midwives bridge the chasm between medicine and traditional healing.

Exemplary midwives demonstrate professional integrity, honesty, compassion, and understanding. They are able to communicate effectively, remain open-minded and flexible, and are able to provide care in a nonjudgmental manner. When these attributes are coupled with excellent clinical skills they result in attentive and thorough assessments, excellent screening and preventive health counseling processes, and patience with the process of labor and birth.

Finally, midwives provide personalized care that is tailored to the individual and her present circumstances. Regardless of clinical practice setting or educational background, midwives endeavor to create an environment that engenders mutual

Box 1-1   Philosophy of the American College of Nurse-Midwives

We, the midwives of the American College of Nurse-Midwives, affirm the power and strength of women and the importance of their health in the well-being of families, communities, and nations. We believe in the basic human rights of all persons, recognizing that women often incur an undue burden of risk when these rights are violated.

We believe every person has a right to:

- Equitable, ethical, and accessible quality health care that promotes healing and health
- Health care that respects human dignity, individuality, and diversity among groups
- Complete and accurate information to make informed health care decisions
- Self-determination and active participation in health care decisions
- Involvement of a woman's designated family members, to the extent desired, in all health care experiences

We believe the best model of health care for a woman and her family:

- Promotes a continuous and compassionate partnership
- Acknowledges a person's life experiences and knowledge
- Includes individualized methods of care and healing guided by the best evidence available
- Involves therapeutic use of human presence and skillful communication

We honor the normalcy of women's life cycle events. We believe in:

- Watchful waiting and nonintervention in normal processes
- Appropriate use of interventions and technology for current or potential health problems
- Consultation, collaboration, and referral with other members of the health care team as needed to provide optimal health care

We affirm that midwifery care incorporates these qualities and that women's health care needs are well served through midwifery care.

Finally, we value formal education, lifelong individual learning, and the development and application of research to guide ethical and competent midwifery practice. These beliefs and values provide the foundation for commitment to individual and collective leadership at the community, state, national, and international level to improve the health of women and their families worldwide (American College of Nurse-Midwives [ACNM], 2004).

respect and focuses primarily on meeting the needs of the woman, or mother and family. Recognition of individual variation is tempered by a thorough grounding in both normal and pathologic processes. This broad scope provides the midwife with a clear view of the continuum of health and allows more accurate assessment and personalization of care.

The midwife whose ideal is to provide exemplary midwifery care must actively create a balance between her professional life as a midwife and the needs and demands of her personal life. Time off to refresh and rejuvenate is as necessary to quality practice as is ongoing professional education. Personal relationships nourish the midwife and provide emotional sustenance. Each midwife must remain attentive to her own needs in order to bring her best to midwifery.

Midwives strive to provide exemplary midwifery and women's health care. This demands the development of excellent clinical skills and the determination and persistence to couple them with sound clinical judgment. Each midwife is called upon, time and again, to make critical decisions and to act upon them in a way that is appropriate for the setting in which she practices, yet she must demonstrate respect and honor for the uniqueness of each woman and family in her care.

Women First

Midwifery and women's health is first and foremost about caring for women. Every woman deserves to receive care that is safe, satisfying, and fosters her ability to care for herself. Such care, to be effective, must address women's own cultural and developmental needs. As midwives care for women in our country's diverse communities, the ability to listen, and to integrate women's concerns into the care provided, is essential. The goal should be to provide care that meets the woman's expressed needs, is directed by the woman, and is not limited by the midwife's personal or professional philosophy of care.

Midwives and other women's health professionals practice within a health care system that is increasingly complex. Health care can be viewed as a continuum that ranges from alternative health practices, through holistic and general medical care, to highly specialized medical care. Often women do not have a frame of reference that allows them to formulate questions about the issues that concern them. Many clients may need guidance to obtain necessary health care. Women look to their care provider to provide direction that is consistent with their perceived needs and internal beliefs. Teasing out the health concerns that are important to women requires skill in active listening, sensitivity to cultural issues, and knowledge of common health practices, procedures, and preferences.

Meeting women's health needs requires considering all options for care or treatment and necessitates a broad-based and well-grounded network of collaborative relationships.

How to Use This Book

To provide optimum women's health care in today's busy environment the use of a systematic approach to organization is essential. This type of approach is central to providing care that is comprehensive and is least likely to result in clients "slipping through the cracks."

Clinical Practice Guidelines for Midwifery & Women's Health utilizes a format that is recognized throughout the health care continuum. By using this consistent format these guidelines foster a systematic and reliable mechanism for client assessment, problem identification, and treatment or referral. Clear identification of documentation essentials and practice pitfalls act as reminders to the busy professional. While the term *midwife* is used frequently throughout this book, the content and recommendations are equally relevant for other women's health professionals.

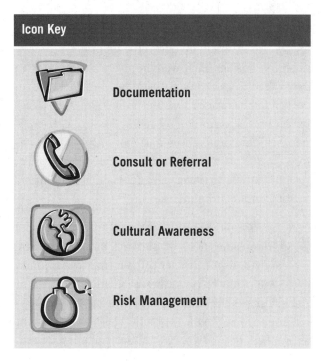

Icon Key

Documentation

Consult or Referral

Cultural Awareness

Risk Management

Symbols are used to indicate key areas that require particular attention. The purpose of the symbols is to heighten awareness, stimulate critical thinking in areas that are potentially problematic, and ensure comprehensive record keeping and communication. Safe midwifery and women's health practice includes not only providing quality care to the women we serve, but also practicing in a manner that protects the midwife from undue risk, whether it be from infectious disease, fear of persecution, or professional liability.

Documentation of care is the basic building block that supports midwifery practice. Documentation skills allow the midwife or other women's health professional to review the care provided at a later date.

Collaborative practice connects midwives to additional health professionals who provide ongoing or specialty care that is not within the midwife's scope of practice. Women's health care forms a continuum that extends from home birth and alternative care, through general medical and community-based medicine and midwifery, to high-tech tertiary care and specialty services.

Cultural awareness is essential for quality care of women in our multicultural world. We need to consider each woman as an individual who exists, not in our practice settings, but in her own corner of the world. Cultural influences may affect birth choices, birth control methods, sexual orientation, self-care preferences, and more. Cultural awareness includes consideration of the client's race, religion, ethnic heritage, age, generation, geographic factors, and cultural mores.

Risk management includes the thoughtful consideration of factors that potentially increase risk to the mother or baby, the well woman, or to the midwife providing care. Identification of risk factors is the first step in reducing their potential impact on midwifery practice. Risk management as applied to midwifery practice includes careful documentation of care provided. Integral components of the midwifery risk management plan include active listening to each woman as an individual, clearly stated expectations for your role as a midwife, and the woman's role when receiving care.

Evidence-based practice is the catchword of the day. Goode (2000) offers a multidisciplinary practice model that addresses nine key factors to consider when evaluating current research for clinical application:

- Pathophysiology
- Retrospective or concurrent record review
- Risk management data
- Local, national, and international standards
- Infection control data
- Patient or client preferences
- Clinical expertise
- Benchmarking data
- Cost effectiveness analysis

By integrating all of these factors into the evaluation of current research the midwife can validate her or his clinical decision making using an evidence-based practice model that also fits the midwifery model of care. Clinical expertise comes with time and attention to practice. The new practitioner or novice must maintain a heightened awareness of her or his limitations in order to set safe boundaries for practice.

The Purpose of Clinical Practice Guidelines

Clinical practice guidelines are used to direct and define parameters for care. This may be influenced by the accepted standards of the midwife's or women's health provider's professional organization(s). State laws, both statutes and regulations, may affect the scope of practice, as may hospital bylaws, birth center rules and regulations, health insurance contracts, and liability insurance policies.

Each individual midwife must define her or his scope of practice based on philosophy of midwifery practice, educational preparation, experience, skill level, and the individual practice setting. A midwife's scope of practice may vary from one practice location to another and may change throughout her career.

Each client who comes to a midwife for care has the right to information regarding the midwife's scope of practice, usual practice location(s), and provisions for access to medical or obstetrical care should this become necessary. Development of working relationships with area health care providers can be a valuable asset in fostering continuity of care.

Documenting Midwifery Care

If documentation is the key to validating quality care, then documentation skills are essential to midwifery practice. Careful and complete documentation serves as your legal record of events that have occurred. Standardizing the documentation *format* can free the midwife up to concentrate on the *content* of the documentation or note.

Optimally, records should provide the reader with a clear view of the client's presentation, the midwife's evaluation process, and the implementation and results of treatment or recommendations. Meticulous documentation also allows other professionals to follow the course of care provided and gain insight into the client's response. Client health records are an essential communication tool in a group practice and during consultation or referral.

For those midwives or students who seek to improve documentation skills, additional recommendations for documentation are addressed in detail in Chapter 2.

Developing a Collaborative Practice Network

 Midwives do not practice in isolation. Every midwife, regardless of practice location, needs a network of contacts to help provide ongoing care and services. The collaborative practice model allows for a wide variety of professional relationships that range from informal to highly structured arrangements.

Collaborative practice means that a working relationship is formed between the attending midwife and the physician or other health care provider. Midwives function as an integral part of the health care system. Not all services are appropriate for all women. Midwives have a responsibility to provide access to services as indicated by the individual woman's health, preferences, and the midwife's scope of practice. The primary goal of the collaborative relationship is accessing the best care for each client as needed.

The American College of Nurse-Midwives (ACNM) joint statement with the American College of Obstetricians and Gynecologists (ACOG) clearly states: "When obstetrician-gynecologists and certified nurse-midwives/certified midwives collaborate, they should concur on a clear mechanism for consultation, collaboration, and referral based on the individual needs of the patient" (ACNM, 2002).

Consultation or Referral?

Consultations and referrals provide for continuity of care when problems develop or when additional expertise is required. Consultations may range from informal conversations to problem-oriented evaluation of the client by the consultant. When midwives consult with OB/GYN physicians they need to remember that the physician practices a different specialty and may not have a similar approach to the problem as the midwife.

Development of professional relationships with physicians and other health care providers in your area begins with you. Make arrangements to meet and introduce yourself. Show consideration of the provider's schedule; for example, arrange a breakfast meeting or offer to bring lunch to the office. Make good eye contact, shake hands firmly, and present yourself as a competent, skilled, professional colleague. Your goal is to initiate a relationship, so that when you have a client who needs care, your credibility has been established. It is not required that you agree on philosophy of care or management styles, but it is important that you establish a good working relationship. It is also good practice to nurture your relationship with the office staff, for those times you may need them to interrupt during office hours.

Determining in advance what type of consult is indicated will affect what information you will provide. Present the consultation request in terms that direct the care you are seeking for your client. If you do not provide this direction, the physician will likely manage your client as she or he would her or his usual patients

The American Medical Association Evaluation and Management Services Guidelines states "A consultation is a type of service provided by a physician whose opinion or advice regarding evaluation and/or management of a specific problem is requested by another physician or other appropriate source" (AMA, 2004).

Forms of consultation that the midwife may use include the following types.

Informational "Just letting you know that Mrs. B is here in labor. She is a G3, P2002 at term, and is at 5 cms after one hour of labor. I expect an uneventful birth shortly." In this instance you have already established a professional relationship with a defined collaborating individual that includes notification in specific circumstances or as indicated according to your professional judgment. This may also include proactive consultation to provide information when there is potential for an emergency that may require additional support or expertise.

Request for Information or Opinion "Ms. K has atypical glandular cells on her most recent Pap smear. I've never seen this before. What do you recommend for her follow-up?" In this instance you are looking for information to guide your client's care when you have reached the limits of your scope of practice or when you work in a collaborative practice setting where you tailor the care you provide to both the client and the practice setting.

Request for Evaluation "I'm sending Mrs. S to you for evaluation of her enlarged uterus. She is a 47-year-old G2, P2002, who has had severe menorrhagia for the past five months. Her pelvic ultrasound is consistent with large uterine fibroids. We have discussed potential treatments, and she is interested in exploring endometrial ablation to treat her menorrhagia." In this instance the client has a problem that requires evaluation and treatment that is not within your scope of practice. Clearly stating previous discussions, client preferences, and your expectations for care can influence the care provided to the client. The expectation is that the client will return to you for care once the problem has resolved or been treated.

Transfer of Care "Mrs. R. has cervical cancer. I am transferring her to you for care of this problem." In this instance the client has a problem that necessitates ongoing physician management. Transfer of care means that the client is released from midwifery care, and the consultant is expected to assume responsibility for her medical care.

Emergency "Ms. P. has a postpartum hemorrhage. I believe she has retained placental parts. Her EBL is currently at 1000 ml. Please come to L & D immediately." In this instance the nature of the problem requires immediate action on the part of the consultant. Expectations for immediate physician evaluation of a client must be clearly stated.

For those midwives who practice in the out-of-hospital setting, calling the OB/GYN or pediatrician on-call may be preferable to simply calling 911 or the emergency room. If you have an established working relationship, a direct admission to the maternity unit may be possible.

Other Collaborative Practice Relationships
Primary care providers commonly care for midwifery clients in the event of a general medical problem such as hypertension, diabetes, or heart disease. Although some midwives have expanded their practice to include primary care services, this is often limited to treatment of acute conditions such as back pain, upper respiratory infections, and the like.

Every practitioner caring for women, regardless of their scope of practice, should develop a network of care providers that may include physicians, chiropractors, naturopaths, acupuncturists, dieticians, mental health professionals, social service personnel, clergy, support and self-help groups, local emergency services, homeless shelters, addiction centers, and so on. This network provides the mechanism by which midwives may address the varied needs of the women who come to them for care.

Key to providing woman-oriented care is to connect women with the services they require and may not know how to access. This may include a combination of mainstream medical care, alternative or complementary modalities, and nonmedical services. The role of the midwife is to listen to women, clarify their needs, and facilitate meeting those needs in a caring and nonjudgmental manner. Your individual philosophy of midwifery care should direct, but not drive, the care you provide.

Clear discussion of the parameters of midwifery practice, the practice location(s), practice limitations or boundaries required by collaborative relationships, practice agreements, and clinical options of midwifery care (including privileges) goes a long way toward evaluating whether a particular midwifery practice is appropriate for the individual client.

Women may come from settings where there is very limited access or availability of health care and accept whatever care is provided. Other women may have a strong need to direct their health care and mandate their active participation in all health-related decisions. Most women fall somewhere between these two examples.

Health Care As a Continuum

Health care can be thought of as a continuum that runs from alternative or self-care to general medical care to specialty and technologically sophisticated care. One example of this concept is the continuum of birth locations; they range from the client's home to freestanding or hospital based-birth centers, to small community hospitals and larger community hospitals, and finally to regional perinatal referral centers.

In an ideal world clients would be able to move back and forth along the continuum as best met their needs. From within a supportive health care system and environment, clients would have access to the full range of services and providers necessary for their care, including true collaborative practice based on meeting the needs of the client. Few health care professionals practice in such an ideal setting. No matter where we stand ourselves on the continuum, it remains imperative that we understand the range of services that are available for our clients.

The women who come to us for care, our clients, do not live in the health care world, and their awareness of what services are available may be influenced by issues of access, impact of advertising, social and cultural beliefs, the experiences of their friends or relatives, and the ever-present television and movie world. Unless we have an idea of the options out there, we will be less able to listen and hear what women are saying to us and less able to address their concerns in language they can understand.

Clients who are oriented toward alternative care may be influenced toward medical care, when necessary, in a trusting relationship with their midwife or health care provider. Clients who are comfortable and familiar with highly interventive care may be influenced toward self-care and noninterventionist care when it is recommended in an environment of trust and ready access to medical care if necessary.

Midwifery care is traditionally based on providing care that begins from noninterventionist care and includes interventions only as necessary or indicated. Deciding what interventions are "necessary" and when they are "indicated" defines our individual practice as midwives.

Cultural Diversity

 The world is fast becoming an international society. No matter where we practice, it is likely that each of us will provide care to women who come from different countries or cultures from ourselves or from locations other than where we obtained our basic midwifery education and training.

Awareness and sensitivity to cultural practices and beliefs can enhance client satisfaction and build a trusting professional relationship. Cultural diversity encompasses a wide range of reference points, which may include social and emotional development, age, race, religion, sexual orientation, ethnic heritage, country of origin, geographic location, and cultural beliefs and mores. Becoming culturally competent involves a certain level of interest, inquiry, and awareness of cultural differences.

Cultural differences may be considered cross-cultural, meaning the midwife and the client come from different ethnic or racial backgrounds, or they may be intercultural, where the midwife and the client come from similar ethnic or social backgrounds but have developed disparate views and beliefs, especially with regard to health care. An example of this is the home birth midwife whose client reveals that she wants access to pharmacological pain relief for labor, or a hospital-based midwife whose client calls following a surreptitiously planned home birth.

Cultural competence requires that the midwife remains open-minded, an active listener, and evaluates each woman's needs in light of the practice setting. Access to culturally competent interpreters to translate language, social customs, and mores related to women's health care can be extremely helpful. A minimum standard requires that language interpreters be available. Literal translation, however, may not always provide correct or accurate information about women's needs. Individualizing care involves taking into account the woman's chronological age, developmental stage, emotional development, sexual orientation and preferences, culture, and other social factors.

Developmental Considerations

Attention to developmental changes throughout a woman's life is essential to address the concerns that are most pressing to her. The needs of adolescent women are very different from those of women of childbearing age, as are those of the woman who is past menopause—even when they each present for the same type of visit. Midwives who frequently care for the medically underserved should remember that the effects of poverty, abuse, or marginal nutrition may impact a woman's developmental growth.

Adolescents Young women in their teens may present at various developmental stages based on age, emotional development, ethnicity, and other social and cultural factors. Compliance is frequently an issue as authority is challenged and the young woman seeks to explore the boundaries and limits put upon her.

Older Women After the childbearing years have passed, women often have a change of focus from reproductive health care to concerns surrounding general health and the fear of illness, disability, and death. Women may regress into dependence as they age, or they may continue to be as independent or dependent as they were previously.

The Mentally Challenged Such women may require coordination of specialized services in order to be provided appropriate reproductive health care. Intimate exams may require sedation or anesthesia to avoid emotional trauma, especially in the mentally challenged woman with a history of sexual violence.

The Physically Challenged Physically handicapped women may or may not have developmental delays depending on the cause of the physical challenge. Individual assessment is necessary to determine the client's developmental level and provide developmentally appropriate services. Examinations may be made more challenging by physical limitations, and ample time should be scheduled to allow for this.

Immigrant and Refugee Women may have culturally mediated variations in development, which may make interpretation of developmental stages more challenging. Accessing resources to learn about cultural variations may aid in appropriate client assessment.

Socioeconomic Challenges Any of various socioeconomic challenges may impact the rate and progression of a woman's physical, emotional, and social development. Remaining nonjudgmental offers the optimum opportunity to determine how best to identify each individual's unique needs and provide or direct women to the services that might best meet those needs.

Risk Management

Risk management is a dynamic process that evaluates and improves how care is provided on a day-to-day basis. This section will attempt to identify ways to safeguard your practice while providing quality care in our litigious society. Risk management means identifying and managing the potential risk to each woman we care for, every unborn and newborn infant, ourselves as midwives, and each of the other health professionals that become involved in the care of the women and families we serve (National Association for Healthcare Quality [NAHQ], 1998).

The process of providing care can be broken into several discrete components that occur following a client or situational assessment (American Academy of Family Physicians, 2004):

- Identification of conditions that may increase client risk or potential risk (working diagnosis)
- Potential for significant adverse effects directly related to the actual or potential risk (assessment of risk related to diagnosis)
- Potential impact of the adverse effects on the client and the provider (client- and midwife-specific hazard analysis)
- Management of risk (midwifery plan of care and provider risk management strategy)

Risk to the Client

Quantification of risk to clients is nearly impossible. Even with the surge in the number of double-blind, case-controlled studies in women's health, it is not possible to reliably identify which women are in fact at risk for which problems. New data is continually being compiled about risks associated with race, ethnicity, genetics, lifestyle, behaviors, and other factors.

By keeping abreast of new data and incorporating it into the midwife's knowledge base, she can provide information to clients that helps identify health care decisions and choices that are appropriate for them. Frank discussions about the relative risk of options for care should include the potential for unexpected outcomes, the unpredictability of individual response, and the impact and importance of self-determination.

Risk to the Unborn and Newborn

If calculating risk to the client who we can see and test and talk with is difficult, quantifying risk to the unborn, and by extension to the newborn, is virtually impossible. However, pregnant women look to their midwives as skilled professionals with the ability to identify potential problems and take corrective action to safeguard their babes in the womb.

How information is presented during pregnancy and women's health care visits may influence the client's attitude about her body, the safety of birth, the ability of the health care system to meet her and her baby's needs, and her ability to parent. Risk should be addressed in a realistic fashion that is supportive of women and birth and does not undermine traditional, alternative, or mainstream medical providers. We can foster the concept that women's bodies and birth work while still addressing the fact that there are no guarantees of perfect outcomes and that access to basic and advanced medical services is an option we are fortunate to have.

Risk to the Midwife

Each midwife needs to determine what is included in her own individual scope of practice regardless of what the professional organizations may include in their stated definitions of scope of practice. Not every midwife provides every service. A scope of practice is a dynamic entity, one that changes with experience, practice location, fatigue, staffing, distance to specialty care, and so on. Each midwife must manage individual professional risk by constantly assessing the scope of her or his midwifery practice and whether it meets the midwife's needs as well as those of the community served.

Identification of a woman with risk factors may impact midwifery management of risk in a number of respects: it may result in a transfer of care, a consultation, or continued independent management of the woman's care. It depends on the midwife's expertise and self-determined scope of practice, state laws regarding midwifery practice, and the midwife's comfort level with the level of risk involved in caring for the particular risk factor in this individual, health care setting, community, and legal climate.

Standards of practice define the expected knowledge and behaviors of the midwife according to her education, certification, and licensure status. Midwives are held accountable to national, state, and local standards. Each midwife should maintain familiarity with the professional standards, state

laws, and rules that govern her midwifery practice. Professional standards are defined by the American College of Nurse-Midwifery, the Midwives Alliance of North America, and the International Confederation of Midwives. Each of them requires knowledge of the following:

- Midwifery practice standards and recommendations
- Pathophysiology of commonly encountered conditions
- Indications for and access to medical consultation

The Risk Management Plan

The term *risk management* has acquired a negative connotation in recent years, as many liability insurance companies use this term to identify risk factors that may indicate an increased likelihood for a less than optimal outcome or chance of litigation. A comprehensive and realistic midwifery practice risk management plan demonstrates to the liability insurance carrier that the midwife seeks to provide care that is consistent with best practice, is cognizant of the risk involved in her profession, and has taken reasonable steps to limit that risk. This has been shown to contribute to the willingness on the part of the insurer to continue or extend liability insurance coverage to midwives.

A risk management plan is a helpful way to organize essential information about the various components needed to identify and manage risk in midwifery practice. The midwifery risk management plan should include practice policies and procedures that address topics such as the following (Greenwald, 2004):

- Written practice description
- Philosophy of practice
- Location(s) of practice
- Practice guidelines and standards
- The role and scope of practice for each midwife
- Medical record documentation standards

- Documentation forms that reflect care provided
- Informed consent purpose and process
- Client autonomy in decision making
- Provisions for coverage
- Indications for consultation or referral
- Collaborative practice relationships
- Plan for transfer of care or client when indicated
- Requirements for continuing education
- Education required to expand scope of practice
- Peer review and outcomes-based evaluation of care
- Client or practice-related complaints or concerns
- Licensing and professional practice issues as legally defined by state or professional organization
- Malpractice claims procedures

Midwives vary tremendously in the amount of risk they are willing to live with on a day-to-day basis. Some may prefer to work in settings where there is a physician available at all times, while others may practice in isolated settings where the nearest physician is miles away. Increased midwife autonomy may be associated with increased midwife risk, as can practicing in a setting that is antagonistic to midwives, regardless of their legal status.

Summary

Defining one's personal philosophy of midwifery care and expressing it in practice is one of the joys of midwifery. What constitutes "best care" for women, mothers, and infants is best determined individually, with standards of care used as a guide along the way. Clinical judgment is the heart and soul of midwifery care. A mindful approach practice reduces client and midwife risk, improves outcomes, and fosters collaborative relationships. This provides the opportunity for the exemplary midwife to rest better at night and continue a career for decades.

References

American Academy of Family Physicians. (2004). *Risk management and medical liability.* Retrieved December, 2004, from http://www.aafp.org/x16535.xml

American College of Nurse-Midwives [ACNM]. (2002). *Joint statement with the American College of Obstetricians and Gynecologists.* Retrieved December, 2004, from http://www.midwife.org/education/cfm?id=215

ACNM. (2004). *Philosophy of the American College of Nurse-Midwives.* Retrieved December, 2004, from http://www.midwife.org/display.cfm?id=132

American Medical Association [AMA]. (2004). *Current procedural terminology* (p. 14). Chicago: Author.

Goode, C. (2000). What constitutes the "evidence" in evidence-based practice? *Applied Nursing Research, 13,* 222–225.

Greenwald, L. (Ed.). (2004). *Perspectives on clinical risk management.* Boston: Risk Management Publications, ProMutual Group.

Kennedy, H. P. (2000). A model of exemplary midwifery practice: Results of a Delphi study. *Journal of Midwifery & Women's Health, 45,* 4–19.

National Association for Healthcare Quality (NAHQ). (1998). *Guide to quality management* (pp. 44–45). Glenview, IL: Author.

Documentation of Midwifery and Women's Health Care

2

Documentation of midwifery care should reflect the essence of midwifery: woman-oriented care focused on excellence in the processes of providing care with attentiveness to outcomes.

As professionals, midwives are continually working toward the goal of educating both clients and colleagues about how midwifery is different from medicine and nursing. Midwives strive to ensure that the difference is reflected in both midwifery education programs and the clinical experiences of those learning midwifery. Midwifery encompasses the belief that birth is essentially normal, that women have the right to be listened to and heard, and that birth and well-woman care are important events in the lives of women.

As a profession that seemingly demonstrates many of the same behaviors as obstetrics and gynecology, we need to not only demonstrate but also document how midwifery differs from obstetrics and gynecology. Although the behaviors that a midwife, a physician, a nurse-practitioner, or a physician's assistant demonstrate when providing women's health care may be similar, the origins, attitudes, and perception of the care may be radically different. If midwives truly provide woman-oriented care with a focus on excellence in the processes of providing care and attentiveness to outcomes, this should clearly be reflected in each client's medical record.

This chapter explores the process of documentation from several points of view:

- Documentation as an essential communication tool; a method of recording events and findings for future reference that follows accepted standards

- Documentation using current procedural terminology (CPT) evaluation and management criteria (E/M); a method of documentation developed by the American Medical Association that reflects the complexity and level of care provided in order to meet current reimbursement criteria

- Documentation as a means of demonstrating application of risk management and collaborative practice processes

- Documentation as a reflection of the midwifery model of care; whether or how events are recorded accurately reflects the philosophy and standards of the practice of midwifery

Thoughtful documentation can demonstrate inherent differences between the midwifery and medical models of providing women's health care. This in turn supports outcomes-based research that demonstrates improved outcomes for clients cared for by midwives. The recommendations included in this chapter should be used as a general guideline when documenting midwifery care.

Standards for Documentation

Client record document standards have been developed that allow use of the client's medical record to foster communication between professionals, verify services provided for billing and reimbursement purposes, and allow scrutiny of care provided for quality and appropriateness. To objectively evaluate medical record content, standardized criteria have been developed that are relevant to specific objectives (Johnson, 2001). Each organization that utilizes the medical record has set detailed criteria for evaluation of the content, which is based on their needs.

Documentation as Communication: Skills and Techniques

Thorough documentation provides midwives and other health care professionals with a clear view of each woman's individual presentation, concerns, and preferences for care. The client record also serves as a means of following the midwife's thought processes regarding development of the working diagnosis and ongoing plans for continued client care. Clear, concise documentation is the key

to validating quality care, and it is an integral part of any risk management program.

Each note should provide essential information that could potentially guide another health care professional in the event of a transfer of care, such as might occur following problem-oriented referral, transfer to physician care for a high-risk condition, or simple cross-coverage arrangements between midwives.

In the event of legal action, the client's medical record should ideally provide a clear picture of the client presentation, concerns, and response to care or treatment. The record should identify the midwife's evaluation process, working diagnoses, anticipatory thinking, and planning for diagnosis and treatment. The plan for follow-up care and evaluation along with the parameters for initiation of collaborative practice should be noted when indicated or applicable.

Both ACNM and MANA offer *minimum data sets* (MDS) that can be used as a tool to evaluate the adequacy of standardized client record forms used in midwifery practice. These minimum data sets have been developed to provide a tool for collecting data about the care midwives provide. Midwives seeking to improve their documentation skills may also use the MDS as a self-evaluation instrument by performing retrospective chart or medical record audits to determine form or documentation weaknesses and areas for improvement.

Thorough and complete documentation can often be brief and to the point. It is rarely necessary to provide lengthy notes. Notes may be handwritten, typed, entered into a computer data collection system, or dictated and transcribed. They may be written on a form that provides a preset format, such as a *labor flow sheet*, or written on a blank sheet of paper such as a *progress note*. Notes should reflect pertinent findings and the critical thinking that occurs during the care of each client. All notes should have, at a minimum, the following information:

- Client identification: Name, date of birth, and medical record number where applicable

- Date of service: Date and time are necessary for time-sensitive situations such as labor care or during newborn resuscitation

- Reason for encounter: This is often described in the client's own words, e.g., "It burns when I pee," or as a simple statement, such as "Onset of labor."

- Client history: This includes an expansion of the reason for the encounter, commonly known as the "chief complaint" (CC) and the history of present illness (HPI). The history includes all relevant history and subjective information provided by the client or family, including, as applicable, the review of systems (ROS), past history, family, and social history.

- Objective findings: This may include the results of the physical exam, mental status evaluation, and/or lab work, ultrasound, or other testing as indicated by the history and physical.

- Clinical impression: This is also known as the "assessment" or "working diagnosis," and may include several differential diagnoses under consideration pending lab or testing results. This may be documented as "primary symptoms," or "conditions," with differential diagnoses listed to validate testing and communicate anticipatory thinking.

- Midwifery plan of care: The plan of care may be subdivided into several categories, but essentially, it should outline all diagnostic and therapeutic measures initiated at the visit, along with further actions that are anticipated based on potential results and specific needs of the client.

To be consistent with the conventions followed during clinical assessment and documentation, each guideline in the *Clinical Practice Guidelines for Midwifery & Women's Health* is structured using this standardized system of organization. Expansion of information that could potentially be obtained during client assessment and care is provided below.

Client History: Components of the History to Consider

The history is obtained through chart review and client or family interview. It is commonly divided into several history types: the comprehensive health history, the interval history, and the problem-oriented or event-specific history. The comprehensive health history can be further subdivided into the client's past medical and surgical history, social history, and family medical history. These subtypes of the history can be again subdivided to allow for focus on specific areas of concern such as the menstrual history, obstetrical history, or genetic history.

The *review of systems* (ROS) is a review of the major body systems with the client to determine the presence or absence of signs and symptoms of disease. The comprehensive review of systems includes the following categories: constitutional symptoms; eyes, ears, nose, mouth and throat; skin; respiratory; cardiac; gastrointestinal; genitourinary; musculoskeletal; endocrine; lymphatic/hematologic; immunologic/allergic; psychiatric; and neurologic systems (American Medical Association [AMA], 2004, p. 3).

Identifying which components of the history to pursue is a skill that can assist the midwife in efficiently identifying problems or concerns and developing a working list of differential diagnoses. Components of the history that are included in the client interview should be documented, including, when applicable, the client's attitude, affect, or emotional state. The skilled diagnostician is an active listener who can discern which client responses are pertinent and use directed inquiry to elicit further information.

Physical Examination: Components of the Physical Exam to Consider

Every body system has both general and specific elements that may be evaluated during the physical examination. Thorough evaluation of the area(s) of concern is an integral part of client or patient evaluation. Components that are included during the physical exam are based on the nature of the presenting problem and the midwife's scope of practice.

While many midwives primarily care for women during the childbearing year, others provide comprehensive women's health care that includes evaluation and treatment of gynecologic and/or primary care problems and conditions.

Documentation of the physical exam is most frequently organized in a head-to-toe fashion. Following a consistent format allows for systematic client evaluation, documentation of results, and review of information. Terms used should be standard medical terms that describe the presence or absence of findings in an objective manner consistent with the anatomic area under evaluation. "Normal" is not an objective finding, as the range of normal varies widely from client to client.

Standard terminology should be used whenever possible to identify areas of note, e.g., right lower quadrant (RLQ), periumbilical, substernal. Left (L) and right (R) should be clearly identified whenever applicable. Instruments and tests used during the physical exam should be identified when necessary to describe the technique used for evaluation, for example: "A speculum was inserted in the vagina to expose the cervix" or alternatively, "Speculum exam demonstrated...."

The language should be clear, descriptive, and indicate clinical findings and any unusual client response to the exam. Notes should reflect critical thinking during the exam, such as "The left breast was noted to have an irregular fixed mass in the upper outer quadrant, into the axillary tail. The mass was approximately 2 x 3 cms, with bluish discoloration over the area, which may represent increased vascularity. The mass was firm but not hard; however, it was accompanied by palpable axillary lymph nodes. The clinical picture is highly suspicious for breast cancer in spite of a negative mammogram last week."

Clinical Impression: Differential Diagnoses to Consider

The clinical impression may be more familiar as the *assessment*, or the *diagnostic impression*. This should be a brief summary of the working diagnoses or description of presenting symptoms. These may be presented in a numbered running list from most to least important.

The clinical impression is also used for coding purposes and, while useful to document the clinician's thinking, "rule-out" is not acceptable for coding purposes, although it may be used as a way of clarifying diagnostic testing recommendations to confirm a specific differential diagnosis under consideration.

The clinical impression should identify what you believe is going on with the client based on the client history, physical examination, and any testing performed on-site. The clinical impression and differential diagnosis will then direct further evaluation and testing, the follow-up plan, and need for consultation or referral. The plan should be consistent with the differential diagnoses noted. Examples of differential diagnoses includes:

1. Preventive health visit, no other symptoms (NOS)

2. Urinary burning, urgency, and frequency

3. Pregnancy, 10 weeks gestation by LMP

4. Breast mass, L

5. Pregnancy, at 12 weeks with RLQ pain. Rule out:

   a. Appendicitis

   b. Ectopic pregnancy

   c. Ovarian cyst

Diagnostic Testing: Diagnostic Tests and Procedures to Consider

Diagnostic testing includes any tests or procedures performed to elicit additional information to accurately diagnose a problem, or evaluate an ongoing treatment plan.

Testing should be documented in a brief, straightforward manner with additional explanations necessary only in unusual situations. Testing is often documented as a numbered running list, but should be clear enough that tests ordered can be clearly identified by other health care professionals. One area where this can be confusing is when *panels* are ordered, which are often not consistent from facility to facility. For example, PIH labs (pregnancy induced hypertension or pre-eclampsia panel) may include different arrays of tests at different locations. This becomes especially important when a transfer of care is necessary and test results are pending.

Test results should be clearly documented in an easy to find location, especially when they pertain to ongoing care of a problem. Test results come under the heading of *Objective Findings* when you are writing or dictating a note. Anticipatory thinking regarding potential diagnostic test results should be documented in the record to allow continuity of care should the clinician who requested testing be unavailable to provide continued care.

Providing Treatment:
Therapeutic Measures to Consider

Therapeutic measures include the administration, ordering, or prescription of medications or treatments. Documentation of medications should include the medication name, indication for use, dosage, timing, and route of administration. When off-label medication use is prescribed, it should be documented as such, and should include documentation of relevant discussions with the client regarding clinician recommendations for off-label medication use and informed consent for such use.

Other treatments, such as physical therapy or respiratory therapy treatments, should be documented as ordered, including the indication for the treatment. For example: "Incentive spirometry TID post-op to prevent pulmonary atelectasis." .

Providing Treatment:
Alternative Measures to Consider

Alternative treatment measures include complementary and alternative therapies such as acupuncture, acupressure, homeopathy, herbal remedies, massage, and so forth. When possible, cite sources for suggested measures. Include client instructions and discussion regarding alternative, traditional, and empiric treatments.

Lack of randomized controlled trials may limit use of alternative measures in some practices, while in other practices these time-honored methods of caring for women may be used on a regular and frequent basis. Ethical practice requires discussion of known risks and benefits of all therapeutic measures and thorough documentation of the same. For example: "Client inquired about use of castor oil to stimulate labor at 41 1/7 weeks. The FHR was reactive today, cervix is soft and 1 cm. We discussed her options: expectant care, herbal or homeopathic remedies to stimulate cervical change, and the parameters for use of cervical ripening medications, or induction of labor. She was advised she may use 2–4 oz of Castor oil PO. (see *JNM*, Vol. XX, pp. *xx*). She was instructed to call with the onset of labor or..."

Providing Support:
Education and Support Measures to Consider

Client education is an integral part of most midwifery practices and as such should be clearly documented. Use of standardized client education materials can make documentation simpler and less time consuming. A simple reference to a brochure will suffice in this instance, such as "Client was given the Bleeding in Early Pregnancy handout, with instructions to call if bleeding should persist or worsen."

A master file should be kept of regularly used client education materials so the midwife may refer back as needed to see what materials were used during a specific time period. Documentation should indicate whether education and support measures were provided verbally or in writing. Written instructions or recommendations allow the client to refer back to them after the visit, and refresh her memory about what happened at the visit. Many practices use duplicate forms to document client education with a copy of the form retained in the client's medical record.

Support may also include coordination of care that is recommended, such as scheduling of diagnostic testing appointments and coordination of referrals. While review of diagnostic test results and clinical planning based on those results comes under the heading of follow-up, client notification of results that includes information about test results, options for care, and a compassionate listening ear comes under support and education.

Follow-up Care:
Follow-up Measures to Consider

Follow-up includes the actual process of documentation of all care that has been provided, including anticipatory thinking and recommendations for future care. This allows other clinicians to have a clear impression of the client visit, care provided, and anticipated potential next steps in ongoing care of this individual.

Instructions for when a client should return for care, or when follow-up care is anticipated, are key elements in the clear documentation of the midwifery plan of care. Clients must know what is expected of them in order to comply with recommendations for care. Follow-up may include returning for a scheduled visit, such as a prenatal visit, or it may be that the midwife is going to contact the client following test results, such as after a mammogram performed on a client with a suspicious breast mass.

When there is any deviation from normal or expected findings, a clear plan for follow-up should be documented. In the example above of a woman with a breast mass, the documentation might include the date that results were received, discussion with the client about options for care, plan for referral to a breast specialist, the date and time of the specialist appointment, documentation of the consult including records transferred to the specialist, and a mechanism to follow-up to verify client compliance.

For midwives who provide comprehensive women's health care, a follow-up file may be necessary to track clients and their problems. In this instance, documentation in the client record that the follow-up file has been utilized can help with tracking. A follow-up file may be a calendar, a cross-referenced index card file, or a software program that automatically generates reminders, identifies no-shows, and provides a comprehensive record of problems and follow-up contacts. Tracking of clients with unresolved problems is an integral part of any midwifery practice risk management plan.

Collaborative Practice:
Consider Consultation or Referral

Every request for consultation or referral should be clearly documented. Documentation should include the name and specialty of the provider, how the contact was made (e.g., phone, letter, or directly by the client), as well as the indication for the consult or referral and the expected type of care. Written consultation or referral requests include a brief history of the problem, essential information about the client, the type of service the client is being referred for, and expectations regarding care. A copy of the request is maintained in the client medical record. Including information about scheduled consult or referral appointments is often helpful when following up on problems.

When a consult is obtained the consultant's opinion must be documented. If the consultant provides this service via telephone, the midwife must document the content of the consultation, the consultant's recommendations for care, and application of those recommendations to the midwifery plan of care. When the consultant evaluates the client in person, the consultant is responsible for documentation of care rendered.

Referrals may be made for many types of services, such as counseling, smoking cessation, nutritional evaluation, physical therapy, psychiatric care, substance abuse treatment, alternative therapies, and medical or surgical evaluation of reproductive or other health problems.

Evaluation and Management Criteria

The American Medical Association publishes the *Current Procedural Terminology* (CPT) handbook, which is used for evaluation of documentation during coding and billing. Midwives should become familiar with this book, as well as the ICD-9-Diagnosis code book, as they are essential to appropriate reimbursement for services.

The CPT system evaluates services provided by clinicians using specific criteria that must be present in the documentation of care provided. Evaluation and management (E/M) services are based on the *level* of service provided. The level of E/M services provided are determined by evaluation of the history; physical examination; medical decision making (critical thinking); counseling and coordination of care (client education and support); nature of the presenting problem, and the amount of time required to provide care.

The H & P and the complexity of critical thinking are the *key* components used to determine the level of E/M services provided. The nature of the presenting problem, along with the provision of client education and support, are considered *contributory*, while time is considered separately. Time criteria used in E/M is based on the time spent during the face-to-face client visit. However, the time required for review of diagnostic testing, follow-up, and coordination of care is factored into the time component (AMA, 2004, pp. 2–4).

The CPT book clearly outlines the required components for evaluation of care provided. A brief overview is provided here.

The E/M evaluation considers four types of history and physical exam. The *problem focused* visit is limited to a brief history of the reason for the encounter and an exam that is limited to the affected area. The *expanded problem* focused visit adds a pertinent system review and examination of additional body systems that might be affected by the presenting problem. The *detailed* visit adds pertinent history related to the reason for the encounter, and a thorough examination of the affected area and related organ systems. The *comprehensive* visit adds a complete review of systems, comprehensive review of the client history and risk assessment, as well as either a comprehensive physical exam or thorough examination of a single organ system.

The complexity of medical decision making required is based on the complexity of reaching a diagnosis and/or formulation a management plan. The greater the number of differential diagnoses and potential plans the more complex the decision making. The more medical records, tests, or other information to be reviewed, the greater the complexity. The higher the risk of complications, morbidity, mortality or comorbidity related to health problems or recommended testing, the more complex the decision making. Decision making is evaluated as being *straightforward*, or of *low, moderate*, or *high complexity* (AMA, 2004, pp. 5–7).

Documentation as Risk Management

Exemplary midwifery practice includes understanding and implementing essential components of a risk management program to enhance midwifery care and client outcomes. Thorough documentation using a standardized format allows objective evaluation of the care provided. Each note should be written from the objective, outside observer point of view. This requires that the midwife keep in mind the adage that "If it wasn't documented, it didn't happen." While poor notes are better than no notes, thorough documentation is the ideal to strive for. Use of fill-in-the-blank forms can be a useful way to quickly record essential information, especially during busy office hours or in an emergency. These notes are best supplemented with a narrative note whenever there are unusual circumstances or findings.

The *problem list* is a convenient way to highlight ongoing acute or chronic problems. It should be kept in an easily seen location enabling all clinicians caring for the client to identify at a glance potential factors that may influence the care provided. This decreases the potential for a problem to be missed or exacerbated by an unrecognized comorbidity. The *medication list* is often adjacent to the problem list. Risk may be reduced by reviewing and updating both lists at each visit.

The *follow-up file* is a useful way to track clients with problems that require future care. While not part of the client medical record per se, it makes up a significant part of the midwife's risk management plan. When notification of abnormal results is documented in the medical record, a plan must be formulated. The follow-up file allows for tracking of whether clients return for recommended care and clinician notification when clients are noncompliant. The practice risk management plan should describe the follow-up process and indicate the procedure for utilizing the follow-up system.

Documenting Culturally Competent Care

Midwives and other health professionals have a legal and moral obligation to provide culturally competent care. An excellent resource for women's health providers is Hill's *Caring for Women Cross-Culturally*. *Cultural competence* means that professionally you are able to step outside of your own culture and obtain the vision and skills necessary to provide care in a context that is appropriate for the women who come to you for care.

The attitudes and behaviors needed to do this include a sincere interest in other cultures, the ability to communicate, and a sense of honor for the customs of others. On a more practical level the ability to access interpreter services is a key behavior that is both essential and legally mandated. Each midwife is expected to obtain or have access to information regarding specific health care problems that are racially or ethnically mediated. She should become familiar with historical events and cultural practices that may also affect health in the populations served. Each of these components should be addressed in the medical record when they are applicable. It can be a simple check box, such as:

☐ Interpreter service offered

Documentation of cultural competence may include a detailed description, such as when the informed consent process is provided through an interpreter prior to surgery or a procedure. It may be culturally appropriate to exclude the father from the birth room or to ensure a family member is present as a chaperone during intimate exams. Documentation of the cultural indications for changes or variations from usual care serves to protect the midwife and to reinforce the need for respect and awareness of cultural differences.

The essential characteristic of the culturally competent midwife is an ability to embrace diversity while retaining one's sense of personal cultural identity. To do this it may be necessary to relinquish control in select client encounters. The midwife might consider deliberate introspection following intercultural exchanges as a means to foster personal growth. Feelings of discomfort, failure, fear, frustration, anger, or embarrassment may serve to indicate a need for the midwife to examine her own personal viewpoint in order to become more culturally sensitive.

Informed Consent

Informed consent is a specific process that is designed to ensure that clients receive full information in order to participate in healthcare decision making regarding a recommended treatment or procedure. The midwife is expected to recommend a course of action and share her reasoning process with the client. Client understanding of the information provided is as important as the information itself. Discussion should be carried on in layperson's terms, and client understanding should be assessed along the way.

Complete informed consent includes discussion of the following elements (Rozovsky, 2001):

- Indications for the recommended procedure, medication, or treatment

- The accepted or experimental use of the proposed procedure, medication, or treatment

- The potential or anticipated benefits, actions, or effects of the proposed course of action

- The potential risks and adverse effects of the proposed course of action

- The potential risks and adverse effects of declining the proposed course of action

- Any urgency to undergoing the proposed course of action

- The alternatives to the proposed course of action, including potential effectiveness, risk, and benefit

- Client understanding of discussion, best demonstrated by the client paraphrasing information received and documented by direct quote (e.g., "You're going to try to turn my baby so she isn't butt first.")

- Client acceptance of the recommendation. Midwife and client signatures are preferably witnessed by a third party. Many midwives who practice in the out-of-hospital setting opt to use the informed consent process to present information on birth center or home birth. This provides opportunity for questions, discussion, and documentation of client participation in decisions.

In most cases, it is clear whether or not the client is competent to make her own decisions. The mid-wife should assess the client's ability to understand the nature of the problem, to understand the risks associated with the problem and the recommended course of action, and her ability to communicate her decision based on that understanding.

Competent clients have the right to refuse treatment following the informed consent process. This right may be limited when the client is pregnant and her decision affects her unborn child. Treatment refusal may be an indicator that further discussion is necessary in order to gain insight into the client's beliefs and understanding about the nature of the problem and recommendations for care (University of Washington School of Medicine, 2005).

Components of Common Medical Records

When documenting care provided, each category should be addressed, either with appropriate details, or with *not applicable*. This serves two purposes: it maintains the expected format of the note, and it clearly indicates what clinical components the midwife included while caring for the client.

Office Visit or Progress Note

This format is typically used for problem-oriented and well-woman office visits, as well as for progress notes during labor and postpartum. Standardized prenatal care forms typically vary from this format; however, it becomes useful during evaluation of a problem or complication during pregnancy.

- Subjective: Client interview
- Objective: Physical exam and testing
- Assessment: Differential diagnosis
- Plan: Evaluation, treatment, education, and follow-up care including coordination of care, consultations, and/or referrals

Procedure Note

The procedure note is used to provide detailed information about a procedure such as endometrial biopsy, IUD insertion, colposcopy, external version, or circumcision. This format is appropriate to use to document a procedure regardless of location, and includes the following:

- Procedure performed.

- Indication for procedure: Include diagnosis and any relevant history of present problem.

- Informed consent: Include any relevant discussion.

- Anesthesia: If used.

- Estimated blood loss: In milliliters (ml); *minimal* is accepted for EBL < 10 ml.

- Complications: Describe with treatment and client response to treatment.

- Technique: Describe techniques used, including instruments, anesthesia technique and amount used, sequence of events, and rationale for technique choices, when appropriate.

- Findings: Describe clinical findings, specimens collected and disposition of same, and client postprocedure status.

Medical Consultation or Referral

The purpose of the formal written consultation or referral request is to provide the consultant with adequate information about the client in advance to allow the consultant to focus on the problem or condition. Referral requests often include the following:

- Client introduction: Name, DOB, indication for consult or referral

- History of present problem or illness

- Type of consultation requested

- Brief client history: Allergies, medications, illnesses, surgeries, relevant social history

- Expectation for care: This portion should advise the consultant of any client education provided regarding the problem or illness. It is appropriate to advocate for the client's preferences when stating expectations for care.

Admission H & P

The admission history and physical is typically used when admitting a client to the hospital with an obstetrical, gynecological, or medical problem. However, it is also appropriate to use when admitting a client to midwifery care in labor, regardless of location.

- Admission diagnosis

- History of present condition or illness

- Past OB/GYN history

- Past medical history

- Past surgical history

- Current medications

- Allergies

- Social history

- Family history

- Review of systems

- Physical findings

- Diagnostic testing

- Plan of care

  ○ Anticipated course of care

  ○ Consults

  ○ Plan for reevaluation

Delivery Note

The delivery note is designed to summarize the pregnancy, labor, and birth in a brief but comprehensive overview of the pregnancy and labor, including detailed information about the birth and immediate postpartum and newborn periods. A typical delivery note includes the following:

- Brief review of prenatal course

- Admission status

- Course of labor

  ○ Length of each stage

  ○ ROM: time, color, FHR

  ○ Maternal and fetal response during labor

Table 2-1   Documentation Recommendations

STANDARD	PERFORMANCE MEASURES
1. Elements in the client's medical record are organized in a consistent manner.	• Client record is organized in a clear and systematic fashion. • Records are entered in chronological order.
2. Client medical records are maintained and stored in a manner that protects the safety of the records and the confidentiality of the information.	• All medical records are stored out of reach and out of view of unauthorized persons. See related standard Maintenance, Disclosure, and Disposal of Confidential Information.
3. Client name or identification number is on each document in the record.	• Client name or identification number is found on each document in the record.
4. Entries are legible.	• Handwritten entries are legible. • Notes use a consistent standardized format and language that allow the reader to review care without the use of separate legend/key.
5. Entries are dated.	• Each entry to the record is dated. • Entries generated by an outside source (e.g., referrals, consults) are also dated when reviewed. • Notes related to client encounters are in the record within 72 hours or three business days of occurrence.
6. Entries are initialed or signed by author.	• Entries are initialed or signed by the author. Author identification may be a handwritten signature, unique electronic identifier, or initials. This applies to practitioners and members of the office staff who contribute to the record. • When initials are used, there is a designation of signature and status maintained in the office. • Entries generated by an outside source (e.g., referrals, consults) are also initialed or signed when reviewed.
7. Personal and biographical data are included in the record.	• Includes information necessary to identify client and insurer and to submit claims. • Includes information related to client need for language or cultural interpreter or other communication mechanisms as necessary to ensure appropriate client care. • Information may be maintained in a computerized database, as long as it is retrievable and can be printed as needed to transfer the record to another practitioner or for monitoring purposes. • Name of the client's primary care provider is clearly indicated in the record.
8. A. Initial history and physical examinations for new patients are recorded within 12 months of a patient first seeking care or within three visits, whichever occurs first. B. Past medical history is documented and includes serious accidents, operations, and illnesses. C. Family history is documented.	• A. Initial history and physical examination for new clients is recorded within 12 months of the first visit or within three visits, whichever occurs first. If applicable, there is written evidence that the practitioner advised client to return for a physical examination. The record of a complete history and physical, included in the medical chart and done within the past 12 months by another practitioner is acceptable. Well-child exams meet this standard.

(continues)

Table 2-1   Documentation Recommendations (*continued*)

STANDARD	PERFORMANCE MEASURES
D. Birth history is documented for patients age 6 years and under.	• A. & B. History and physical documentation contains pertinent information such as age, height, vital signs, past medical and behavioral health history, preventive health maintenance and risk screening, physical examination, medical impression, and documentation related to the ordering of appropriate diagnostic tests, procedures, and/or medications. Self-administered client questionnaires are an acceptable way to obtain baseline past medical history and personal information. There is written documentation to explain the lack of information contained in the medical record regarding the history and physical (e.g., poor historians, patient's inability or unwillingness to provide information). • C. Patient record contains immediate family history or documentation that it is noncontributory. • D. Infant records should include gestational and birth history and should be age and diagnosis appropriate.
9. Allergies and adverse reactions are prominently listed or noted as "none" or "NKA."	• Medication allergies or history of adverse reactions to medications are displayed in a prominent and consistent location *or* noted as "none" or "NKA." (Examples of where allergies may be prominently displayed include on coversheet inside the chart, at the top of every visit page, or on a medication record in the chart.) • When applicable and known, there is documentation of the date the allergy was first discovered, related symptoms, and previous treatments required.
10. Information regarding social history is recorded.	• Practitioner must have documentation in the record regarding social history, such as sexual preferences and behaviors, use of tobacco, alcohol or illicit drugs (or lack thereof) in clients 12 years of age and older, who have been seen three or more times. • Cultural and developmental issues are clearly documented when present. • Health care habits and preferences are noted, including use of alternative therapies, herbal remedies, and dietary supplements.
11. An updated problem list is maintained.	• A problem list, which summarizes important client medical information, such as major diagnoses, past medical and/or surgical history, and recurrent complaints, is documented and maintained by all practitioners in the practice. • The problem list is clearly visible and accessible. • Continuity of care between multiple practitioners in the same practice is demonstrated by documentation and review of pertinent medical information.

Table 2-1   Documentation Recommendations (continued)

STANDARD	PERFORMANCE MEASURES
12. Client's chief complaint or purpose for visit is clearly documented.	• The client's chief complaint or the purpose of the visit is recorded as stated by the client. • Documentation supports that the client's perceived needs and/or expectations were addressed. • Documented history and physical are relevant to the client's reason for visit. • Telephone encounters relevant to medical issues are documented in the medical record and reflect practitioner review, including phone triage handled by office staff.
13. Clinical assessment and/or physical findings are recorded. Working diagnoses are consistent with findings.	• Clinical assessment and physical examination are documented and correspond to the client's chief complaint, purpose for seeking care, and/or ongoing care for chronic illnesses. • Documentation supports working diagnoses or clinical impressions that logically follow from clinical assessment and physical examination findings.
14. Plan of action/treatment plan is consistent with diagnosis(es).	• Proposed treatment plans, therapies, or other regimens are documented and logically follow previously documented diagnoses and clinical impressions. • Rationale for treatment decisions appears appropriate and is substantiated by documentation in the record. • Follow-up diagnostic testing is performed at appropriate intervals for diagnoses.
15. There is no evidence the patient is placed at inappropriate risk by a diagnostic or therapeutic procedure.	• The medical record shows clear justification for diagnostic and therapeutic measures. • Risk related to diagnostic and therapeutic measures is discussed with the client using accepted parameters for informed consent and clearly documented in the record.
16. Unresolved problems from previous visits are addressed in subsequent visits.	• Continuity of care from one visit to the next is demonstrated when a problem-oriented approach to unresolved problems from previous visits is documented in subsequent visit notes.
17. Follow-up instructions and time frame for follow-up or the next visit are recorded as appropriate.	• Return to office (RTO) in a specified amount of time is recorded at time of visit or following consultation, laboratory, or other diagnostic reports. • Follow-up is documented for clients who require periodic visits for a chronic illness and for clients who require reassessment following an episodic illness. • Client participation in the coordination of care is demonstrated through client education, follow-up, and return visits.

(continues)

Table 2-1   Documentation Recommendations (*continued*)

STANDARD	PERFORMANCE MEASURES
	• Implementation of a follow-up plan is documented for clients with critical values or acute conditions who do not return for care as described in the practice's risk management policy.
18. Current medications are documented in the record, and notes reflect that long-term medications are reviewed at least annually by the practitioner and updated as needed.	• Information regarding current medications is readily apparent from review of the record. • Changes to medication regimen are noted as they occur. When medications appear to remain unchanged, the record includes documentation of at least annual review by the practitioner. • There is documentation of consideration of medication, herbal, or dietary supplement interactions.
19. Health care education is noted in the record and periodically updated as appropriate.	• Education is age, developmental, and culturally appropriate. • Education may correspond directly to the reason for the visit, to specific diagnosis related issues, to address client concerns, or clarify recommendations. • Education provided to clients, family members, or designated caregivers is documented. • Examples of patient noncompliance are documented.
20. Screening and preventive care practices are in accordance with current recommendations, such as ACNM, ACOG, ASCCP, ACS, MANA, etc.	• Each record includes documentation that preventive services were ordered and performed, or that the practitioner discussed preventive services with the client, and the client chose to defer or refuse them. • Current immunization and screening status is documented. • Practitioners may document that a patient sought preventive services from another practitioner, e.g., family practitioner.
21. An immunization record is completed for members 18 years and under.	• The record includes documentation of immunizations administered from birth to present for clients 18 years and under. • When prior records are unavailable, practitioners may document that a child's parent or guardian affirmed that immunizations were administered by another practitioner and the approximate age or date the immunizations were given.
22. Requests for consultation are consistent with clinical assessment/physical findings.	• The clinical assessment supports the decision for a referral. • Referrals are provided in a timely manner according to the severity of the patient's condition. • Referral requests and expectations are clearly documented.
23. Laboratory and diagnostic reports reflect practitioner review.	• Results of all lab and other diagnostics are documented in the medical record. • Records demonstrate that the practitioner reviews laboratory and diagnostic reports and makes treatment decisions based on report findings. • Reports within the review period are initialed and dated by the practitioner, or another system of ensuring practitioner review is in place and clearly delineated in the practice's risk management policy.

STANDARD	PERFORMANCE MEASURES

Table 2-1 Documentation Recommendations (*continued*)

STANDARD	PERFORMANCE MEASURES
24. Client notification of laboratory and diagnostic test results and instruction regarding follow-up, when indicated, are documented.	• Clients are notified of abnormal laboratory and diagnostic results and advised of recommendations regarding follow-up or changes in treatment. • The record documents patient notification of results. A practitioner may document that the client is to call regarding results; however, the practitioner is responsible for ensuring that the client is advised of any abnormal results and recommendations for continued care.
25. There is evidence of continuity and coordination of care between primary and specialty care practitioners or other providers.	• Consultation reports reflect practitioner review. • Primary care provider records include consultation reports/summaries (within 60–90 days) that correspond to specialist referrals, or documentation that there was a clear attempt to obtain reports that were not received. Subsequent visit notes reflect results of the consultation as may be pertinent to ongoing client care. • Specialist records include a consultation report/summary addressed to the referral source. • When a client receives services at or through another provider such as a hospital, emergency care, home care agency, skilled nursing facility, or behavioral health specialist, there is evidence of coordination of care through consultation reports, discharge summaries, status reports, or home health reports. The discharge summary includes the reason for admission, the treatment provided, and the instructions given to the client on discharge.

Sources: Adapted from ACS, 2004; BCBS, 2004; COLA, 2004; DHHS, 2005; NHLBI, n.d.; NHLBI, 2004; USPSTF, n.d.

- ○ Labor events or interventions
- ○ Complications and treatment
- • Delivery information
  - ○ Time, date, location
  - ○ Route and method of birth
  - ○ Maternal and fetal position
  - ○ Techniques or interventions used with indication, such as:
    - ▪ Anesthesia, type, and dose
    - ▪ Episiotomy or laceration
    - ▪ Type of suture and technique of repair if done
    - ▪ Medications if used
    - ▪ Complications and treatment including client response
  - ○ Evaluation of placenta
  - ○ Estimated blood loss
  - ○ Maternal status postdelivery
- • Newborn information
  - ○ Gender
  - ○ Resuscitation, if indicated
  - ○ Apgar
  - ○ Weight
  - ○ Bonding
  - ○ Feeding, voiding, stooling
  - ○ Newborn status postdelivery

Discharge Summary

This is an appropriate format to use following a hospital admission, but it may be used for summarizing a birth center or home birth as well.

- Admission diagnosis
- History of present condition or illness
- Past medical history
- Past surgical history
- Current medications
- Allergies
- Social history
- Family history
- Review of systems
- Physical findings
- Diagnostic testing
- Hospital course
- Procedures
- Complications
- Discharge diagnosis
- Discharge medications
- Discharge instructions
- Condition on discharge

Summary

Documentation is an essential skill for midwifery and women's health practice that should be attended to with the same care and attention given to other components of clinical practice. Meticulous documentation accurately reflects the scope and nature of midwifery care, and enhances communication among health professionals who care for and about women.

References

American Cancer Society [ACS]. (2004). *American Cancer Society cancer detection guidelines.* Retrieved November 17, 2004, from http://www.cancer.org/docroot/PED/content/PED_2_3X_ACS_Cancer_Detection_Guidelines_36.asp?site

American Medical Association [AMA]. (2004). *Current procedural terminology.* Chicago: Author.

Blue Cross Blue Shield [BCBS]. (2004). *CareFirst Blue Cross Blue Shield medical record documentation standards.* Retrieved November 17, 2004, from http://www.carefirst.com/providers/html/MedicalRecord.html

Commission on Office Laboratory Accreditation [COLA]. (2004). *COLA—Clinical laboratory accreditation and education.* Retrieved November 17, 2004, from http://www.cola.org

National Heart, Lungs, and Blood Institute [NHLBI]. (n.d.). *Clinical practice guidelines.* Retrieved November 17, 2004, from http://www.nhlbi.nih.gov/guidelines

National Heart, Lungs, and Blood Institute [NHLBI]. (2004). *Seventh report of the joint national committee on prevention, detection, evaluation, and treatment of high blood pressure* (JNC 7). Retrieved November 17, 2004, from http://www.nhlbi.nih.gov/guidelines/hypertension/jnc7full.htm

Johnson, S. (2001). Documentation. In R. Carroll (Ed.), *Risk management handbook for health care organizations.* San Francisco, CA: Jossey-Bass.

Rozovsky, F. (2001). Informed consent as a loss control process. In R. Carroll (Ed.), *Risk management handbook for health care organizations.* San Francisco, CA: Jossey-Bass.

University of Washington School of Medicine. (1998). *What is informed consent?* Retrieved January 5, 2005 from http://eduserv.hscer.washington.edu/bioethics/topics/consent.html

U.S. Department of Health and Human Services [DHHS]. (2005). *National guidelines clearinghouse.* Retrieved November 17, 2004, from http://www.guideline.gov/index.aspx

U.S. Preventive Services Task Force [USPSTF]. (n.d.). *Topic index A–Z.* Retrieved November 17, 2004, from http://www.ahrq.gov/clinic/uspstf/uspstopics.htm

Care of the Woman During Pregnancy

3

The term prenatal *means* before birth. *Prenatal care is an opportunity to teach the woman how to care for her baby before she or he is born.*

There are basic components of prenatal care that are included in the core competencies of midwifery practice. For further information, the midwife is encouraged to compare the standards for basic midwifery practice that have been developed by the American College of Nurse-Midwives (ACNM), the Midwives Alliance of North America (MANA), and the International Confederacy of Midwives (ICM).

By comparing these three important standards (all available online by accessing the respective organizations' Web sites) one can gain an understanding of the expected standards for midwifery practice in the United States.

Each midwife must provide locally appropriate care. One of the limitations of a book such as this is that care varies from location to location and from provider to provider. Attempts to standardize care must, by nature, ignore the needs of individuals. The purpose of prenatal care is to identify that small, but significant, number of women whose pregnancy will deviate from the wide range of normal in a manner that may jeopardize maternal or fetal well-being.

Every woman has unique needs during pregnancy. It is a time of many changes and adjustments. Caring for women during this time of transition can foster individual autonomy and enhance self-care practices. This may improve her ability to care for her child, and to recognize her strengths as a woman and a mother.

Many of the women we see are unfamiliar with the expectations of the health care system and need some guidance to navigate the system or negotiate for care that is appropriate to their needs. Building a strong professional relationship allows for trust to develop. Trust fosters active maternal participation in health care decisions. A woman who trusts her midwife is more likely to accept the recommendations of the midwife when challenges or complications present.

The provision of prenatal care varies widely from practice to practice based on the type of women's health care professional(s) in the practice, the practice setting, and the anticipated location for labor and birth. Regional variations are also common. Be sure to familiarize yourself with local or regional resources and standards. These are not meant to dictate practice, but to provide guidelines for care that is appropriate for the majority of women.

Providing women care during pregnancy includes respecting each woman's individual desires in relation to the preferred type of health care provider, the amount of active participation in her care that she desires, her planned and preferred location of labor and birth, and methods to access medical services should they be needed. Each midwife is responsible for outlining to the pregnant client the scope of her practice and usual parameters for care.

The amount and types of testing performed during pregnancy should be determined by indications for testing or evaluation, current recommendations for practice, as well as discussion with the client regarding the risks, benefits, and alternatives to testing or evaluation processes.

Maternal participation in prenatal care encourages self-determination, and may foster the woman's resolve to surrender to the forces of labor and birth. The process of participation also builds trust. Discussion with the client demonstrates the multitude of potential options that are available and encourages flexibility on the part of both the mother-to-be and the midwife.

Diagnosis of Pregnancy

Key Clinical Information

Nature is highly motivated to maintain the species, and pregnancy can occur in spite of valiant attempts to prevent it. The diagnosis of pregnancy may be a welcome event or devastating news. Many women have mixed feelings about the changes that pregnancy will bring to their lives.

Client History:
Components of the History to Consider

- Reproductive history
  - G, P
  - Last menstrual period
  - Method of birth control
  - Symptoms of pregnancy
  - Previous STIs
- Signs or symptoms of complications
  - Pain or cramping
  - Bleeding
  - Drugs or medications taken since LMP
- Relevant social history
  - Client feelings about possible pregnancy
  - Support systems
- Relevant medical/surgical history
  - Allergies
  - Medications
  - Medical conditions
  - Surgeries
- Review of systems

Physical Examination:
Components of the Physical Exam to Consider

- Vital signs
- Thyroid
- Abdominal exam
  - Fetal heart tones
  - Fundal height
  - Abdominal tenderness
- Pelvic evaluation
  - Uterine sizing
  - Consistency of uterus
  - Color of cervix
  - Cervical motion tenderness
  - Vaginal or cervical discharge
  - Adnexal tenderness

Clinical Impression:
Differential Diagnoses to Consider

- Pregnancy, no other symptoms (NOS)
- Pregnancy complicated by
  - Ectopic pregnancy
  - Unplanned pregnancy
  - Molar pregnancy
  - Blighted ovum
- Secondary amenorrhea, related to
  - Thyroid dysfunction
  - Ovarian dysfunction
  - History of contraceptive hormone use

Diagnostic Testing:
Diagnostic Tests and Procedures to Consider

- Urine or serum HCG
- Quantitative B-HCG
- TSH
- Pelvic or vaginal ultrasound

Providing Treatment:
Therapeutic Measures to Consider

- Prenatal or other vitamin supplement with folic acid
- Iron supplementation
- Treatment of any underlying infection or condition as indicated

Providing Treatment:
Alternative Measures to Consider

- Natural prenatal vitamin supplement
- Whole foods diet
- High folate foods
- Red raspberry leaf tea
- For herbal remedies to prevent or avoid pregnancy see *A Difficult Decision: A Compassionate Book About Abortion* by Joy Gardner

Providing Support:
Education and Support Measures to Consider

- Pregnancy options counseling as indicated

- Diet and nutrition counseling
- Prenatal care
  - Usual care
  - Prenatal testing
  - Family involvement
- Practice
  - Providers
  - Medical affiliations
  - Billing arrangements
  - Birth options
    - Location(s)
  - Philosophy of care
  - Parent rights and responsibilities

Follow-up Care:
Follow-up Measures to Consider

- Document
  - Anticipated EDC
  - Relevant history
  - Clinical findings
  - Clinical impression
  - Discussion and client preferences
  - Midwifery plan of care
- Return for continued care
  - 6–12 weeks gestation for initial prenatal visit
  - ASAP if > 10 weeks gestation
  - Prenatal testing as indicated and desired

Collaborative Practice:
Consider Consultation or Referral

- OB/GYN service
  - Genetic counseling
  - Amniocentesis
  - Adoption services
  - Abortion services
  - Specialty care
- Social services
- Addiction treatment resources
- For diagnosis or treatment outside the midwife's scope of practice

Initial Evaluation of the Pregnant Woman

Key Clinical Information

The initial evaluation provides the basis for ongoing pregnancy care. Careful attention to client history, client response to the intimate questions asked during the initial interview, and to the physical exam can alert the midwife to unspoken issues. Gentle touch, coupled with an organized, systematic, yet unhurried manner is ideal during the first visit. Careful documentation of all information is essential to allow for clear communication with other health care providers, and to serve as a comprehensive background of information for the busy midwife.

Client History: Components of the History to Consider

- Cultural and demographic information
- OB/GYN history
  - Present pregnancy history
    - LMP, interval and flow
    - Signs and symptoms
  - G, P, pregnancy information and complications
  - GYN disorders or problems
  - Sexual history
  - Contraceptive history
- Health risk evaluation
- Past medical/surgical history
- Family history
- Social history
- Review of systems (ROS)

Physical Examination: Components of the Physical Exam to Consider

- Vital Signs
- Observation of general status
- HEENT
- Skin
  - Striae

- Scars, tracks, or bruises
- Cardiorespiratory system
- Breasts
- Abdomen
  - Fundal height
  - FHT
  - Fetal lie
- GI system
- Genitourinary system
  - Speculum exam
    - Vagina
    - Cervix
    - Collection of lab specimens
  - Bimanual exam
    - Uterine size, contour
    - Tenderness
    - Pelvimetry
  - Rectal exam prn
- Musculoskeletal system

Clinical Impression: Differential Diagnoses to Consider

- Pregnancy
  - Viable
  - Nonviable
  - Ectopic
- Other diagnosis related to
  - History
  - Physical exam
  - Diagnostic testing

Diagnostic Testing: Diagnostic Tests and Procedures to Consider

- Pregnancy testing
- Urine or serum HCG
- Quantitative β-HCG
- STI testing
- Chlamydia and gonorrhea testing
- VDRL or RPR
- HIV testing
- Hepatitis B surface antigen

- Pap smear
- Wet prep for BV
- Hematology and titers
- Hemoglobin and hematocrit or CBC
- Blood type, Rh factor, and antibody screen
- Sickle cell prep
- Rubella titer
- Varicella antibody screen
- TSH
- Fetal and genetic testing
- α fetal protein testing
- Cystic fibrosis testing
- Amniocentesis
- Ultrasound, vaginal or pelvic
- Tuberculosis testing
  - PPD
  - History of + PPD or BCG vaccine consider chest X-ray
- Urinalysis, with culture as indicated by history
- Group B strep culture

Providing Treatment:
Therapeutic Measures to Consider

- Prenatal vitamins with folic acid
- Iron supplementation
- Treatment of existing conditions as indicated

Providing Treatment:
Alternative Measures to Consider

- Whole foods diet
- Dietary sources of
  - Folate
  - Iron
  - Calcium
  - Fiber

Providing Support:
Education and Support Measures to Consider

- Discussion regarding
  - Diet and activity recommendations

- Danger signs and when to call
- How to access care providers
- Usual return visit schedule
- Recommended prenatal visits
- Recommended prenatal testing
  - Usual tests
  - HIV counseling
  - Amnio counseling, as indicated
- Birth options
  - Location of birth
  - Water birth
  - VBAC counseling prn
- Collaborative medical providers

Follow-up Care:
Follow-up Measures to Consider

- Document
  - Risk factors with plan for care
  - Informed consent as applicable
- Schedule return prenatal visits
  - Q 4–6 weeks through 32 weeks
  - Q 2–3 weeks 32–36 weeks
  - Weekly from 36 weeks to onset of labor
  - More frequent visits for women with risk factors
- VBAC
  - Obtain and review operative notes
  - Surgical consultation

Collaborative Practice:
Consider Consultation or Referral

- OB/GYN or perinatologist
  - Genetic or other counseling
  - Prenatal amniocentesis or CVS
  - VBAC or planned repeat Cesarean
  - History or presence of significant risk factors
- For diagnosis or treatment outside the midwife's scope of practice

Evaluation of Health Risks in the Pregnant Woman

Key Clinical Information

Prenatal care is primarily concerned with the identification of health risks that may be modified or diminished by prompt diagnosis and treatment. Health risks may have the potential to affect the health of the mother, her unborn baby, or newly born infant. Health risks may be related to diet, social habits, genetic heritage, and cultural or ethnic background and practices. Prenatal identification of health risks may offer the opportunity to diagnose or treat actual or potential conditions or provide parents with information and support to help cope with unexpected outcomes.

Client History: Components of the History to Consider

- Maternal demographic information
  - Age
  - Partner status
  - Education
- Review of personal medical history
  - Diseases or health disorders
  - Medication use, OTC or Rx
  - Surgeries
  - Alternative therapies
    - Herbs
    - Homeopathy
    - Acupuncture
- OB/GYN history
  - Prior pregnancy conditions or complications
    - Prior pregnancy losses
    - Birth defects
    - Infertility
  - STIs
  - Hx GYN procedures
    - LEEP
    - Myomectomy
    - Hysterosalpingogram
- Review of family medical history
  - Ethnic heritage
  - Hereditary or genetic health conditions
  - Cultural health habits or conditions
- Pregnancy-related risks
  - Review of health habits
  - Smoking, alcohol, and/or drug use
  - Signs or symptoms of concern
- Nutritional status
  - Usual diet
  - Caffeine use
  - Pica
- Physical activity
- Review of social situation and support
  - Presence of caring partner or support
  - Number and relationship of people in the home
  - Anticipated cultural practices during pregnancy
  - Economic situation and resources
  - Risk factors or signs of abuse
- Review of systems

Physical Examination: Components of the Physical Exam to Consider

- Physical assessment, including
  - Vital signs
  - Weight
    - Weight/height ratio (BMI)
- Evaluate for evidence of
  - Illness
  - Malnutrition
  - Exhaustion
  - Abuse
- Skin exam for signs of
  - Needle tracks
  - Bruising
  - Burns
  - Petechia
  - Lesions
- Smell for signs of
  - Tobacco or alcohol use
  - Ketosis
  - General hygiene

Clinical Impression:
Differential Diagnoses to Consider

- Pregnancy NOS
- Pregnancy at risk for adverse outcome secondary to
  - Health habits, specify
  - Genetic disorders
  - Maternal age
  - Health conditions, specify
  - Prior uterine or cervical surgery
  - GYN disorder or infection
  - Abuse
    - Physical
    - Sexual
    - Emotional
  - Substance abuse
  - Poor social support
  - Occupational hazards
- Noncompliance secondary to
  - Communication
  - Transportation
  - Limited resources
- Other diagnoses as noted

Diagnostic Testing:
Diagnostic Tests and Procedures to Consider

- Drug screening
- Cotenine testing for smokers
- HIV testing
- Hepatitis testing
- Sickle cell prep
- Hemoglobin A1c
- Alpha fetal protein, triple or quadruple screen
- Group B strep testing
- STI testing
- Level I or Level II ultrasound
- Amniocentesis
- Chorionic villus sampling

Providing Treatment:
Therapeutic Measures to Consider

- Prenatal or multivitamin with folic acid

- Smoking cessation medications
- Other medications or treatments based on diagnosis

Providing Treatment:
Alternative Measures to Consider

- Nutritional support
- Hypnosis to change health habits
- Other treatments based on diagnosis

Providing Support:
Education and Support Measures to Consider

- Allow private time to encourage disclosure
- Provide information about risks and benefits of
  - Current health behaviors
  - Prenatal tests
  - Testing options
  - Treatment options
- Genetic counseling
- Drug screening policy
- Social support services
- Cultural support services
- Diagnosis-related support groups

Follow-up Care:
Follow-up Measures to Consider

- Document
- Return visits
  - Frequency determined by
    - Client condition
    - Gestational age
  - Allow time to
    - Develop cooperative relationship
    - Observe for risk-related behaviors
  - Serial drug, cotenine, or STI testing

Collaborative Practice:
Consider Consultation or Referral

- OB/GYN service
  - Genetic screening
  - Amniocentesis or chorionic villus sampling

- ○ Termination of abnormal pregnancy
- Medical service
  - ○ As indicated for medical or specialty care
- Social service
  - ○ As indicated by lifestyle and social indicators
  - ○ Detox/drug rehabilitation
  - ○ Counseling or therapy
  - ○ Women's shelter
- For diagnosis or treatment outside the midwife's scope of practice

Ongoing Care of the Pregnant Woman

Key Clinical Information

The routine prenatal visit is anything but routine for the pregnant woman. It is each woman's brief opportunity to have her needs met and her concerns addressed, while at the same time being evaluated for the well-being of herself and her child. It provides an opportunity to look for subtle signs or symptoms that may indicate a deviation from normal. Group prenatal care provides a unique opportunity to bring together women from diverse backgrounds to meet on the common ground of childbearing.

Client History:
Components of the History to Consider

- Interval history since last visit
  - ○ Gestational age
  - ○ Maternal well-being
    - ▪ Nutrition
    - ▪ Sleep
    - ▪ Activity
    - ▪ Bowel and bladder function
    - ▪ Signs or symptoms of
      - Preterm labor
      - Pregnancy-induced hypertension (PIH)
      - Urinary tract infection
      - Vaginal bleeding or discharge
      - Exposure to infectious disease
  - ○ Fetal well-being
- Concerns

- ○ Questions
- ○ Plans related to pregnancy, labor and birth

Physical Examination:
Components of the Physical Exam to Consider

- Vital signs, including BP and weight
- Assessment of general well-being
- Abdominal exam
  - ○ Fundal height
  - ○ Fetal heart tones
  - ○ Estimated fetal weight
  - ○ Fetal lie, presentation, position, and variety
- CVA tenderness
- Examination of extremities for
  - ○ Edema
  - ○ Varicosities, phlebitis
  - ○ Reflexes
- Additional components as indicated by history

Clinical Impression:
Differential Diagnoses to Consider

- Pregnancy
  - ○ Low risk
  - ○ At risk, specify
- Additional diagnoses based on
  - ○ History
  - ○ Physical exam
  - ○ Diagnostic testing

Diagnostic Testing:
Diagnostic Tests and Procedures to Consider

- Dip urinalysis, culture prn
- Urine culture for
  - ○ History of asymptomatic bacteriuria
  - ○ History of pylonephritis
  - ○ Urinary symptoms
  - ○ Positive dip U/A
- Glucose challenge
  - ○ First trimester
    - ▪ Previous gestational diabetic
    - ▪ High risk for gestational diabetes

- 25–28 weeks gestation
  - Routine screen
  - Repeat testing in high-risk women
- Blood type and antibody screen
  - Initial prenatal labs
  - 25–58 weeks for Rh negative mothers
- Hematocrit and hemoglobin
  - Initial prenatal labs
  - 25–28 weeks
  - Q 4–6 weeks to evaluate iron replacement therapy
- Repeat STI testing as indicated
- Repeat wet mount as indicated
- Offer group B strep testing
  - 34–37 weeks gestation
  - Signs or symptoms of preterm labor
- Ultrasound evaluation
  - Pregnancy dating
  - Genetic evaluation/amniocentesis
  - Fetal growth and development
  - Placental location
  - Biophysical profile
  - Amniotic fluid index
- Additional testing as indicated
  - Sickle cell
  - TIBC, indices
  - Thyroid
  - Fasting or random glucose
  - Hgb A1C

Providing Treatment:
Therapeutic Measures to Consider

- Prenatal vitamins with folic acid
- Iron supplementation prn, such as
  - Ferro-sequels 1–2 PO daily
  - Niferex 150 1–2 PO daily
  - Ferrous gluconate 1–2 PO daily
- Calcium supplements prn, such as
  - Citracal: 200–400 mg bid
  - Tums: 500 mg 1–2 tabs daily
  - Os-cal: 1 tab 2–3 x daily
  - Other supplement of choice

- Influenza vaccine in the fall for women who (CDC, 2004)
  - Currently have a chronic respiratory disorder (e.g., asthma, chronic bronchitis)
  - Will be in the third trimester of pregnancy in December–April
  - Will be early postpartum in December–April
- Immunization update if at significant risk

Providing Treatment:
Alternative Measures to Consider

- Dietary sources of
  - Iron (see Iron Foods List)
  - Folate
    - Deep green leafy vegetables
    - Root vegetables
    - Orange juice
    - Whole grains
    - Nutritional yeast
    - Organ meats, lean beef
  - Calcium (see Calcium Foods List)
- Third trimester herbal support (Weed, 1985)
  - Red raspberry leaf
  - Dandelion leaf
  - Nettle
  - Spirulina

Providing Support:
Education and Support Measures to Consider

- Pregnancy discussion
  - Planned schedule of prenatal visits
  - Expectations related to care
    - Client/family expectations
    - Midwife/practice expectations
  - Anticipated testing
  - Fee and payment information
- Health education
  - Midwife call system
    - When and how to call
  - Importance of
    - Fetal movement
    - Nutrition and exercise

- ○ Bowel and bladder function
- ○ Feelings about pregnancy, birth, family
  - ▪ Relationship changes
  - ▪ Sexual relations in pregnancy
- Social services available
- Labor discussion
  - ○ Planned location of birth
  - ○ Preparation for labor
  - ○ Signs and symptoms of labor
  - ○ Anticipated labor care and birth options
    - ▪ Labor support
    - ▪ Pain relief
      - • Hydrotherapy
      - • Massage
      - • Positioning
      - • Acupressure
      - • Medication options
    - ▪ Perineal support
    - ▪ Episiotomy indicators
    - ▪ Transport/consult indicators
  - ○ Emergency physician coverage
  - ○ Anticipated infant care
    - ▪ Vitamin K options
    - ▪ Ophthalmic prophylaxis
    - ▪ Planned method of infant feeding
    - ▪ Transport indicators
    - ▪ Circumcision options
    - ▪ Newborn evaluation at home
  - ○ Anticipated postpartum care
    - ▪ Based on location of birth
    - ▪ 🌐 Cultural practices after birth
    - ▪ Planned help at home, resources
    - ▪ Postpartum method of birth control
  - ○ Anticipated visits for follow-up care
    - ▪ Home visits
    - ▪ Mother postpartum visits
    - ▪ Infant evaluation

Follow-up Care:
Follow-up Measures to Consider

- Document
  - ○ Findings and update problem list

- ○ Client education and expressed needs
- ○ Discussions with client/family
- ○ Client preferences for labor and birth
- ○ Plan for continued care
- ○ Informed consents
- Midwifery plan of care
  - ○ Identify
    - ▪ Alternate providers and/or location for birth
    - ▪ Client risk factors and anticipated management
    - ▪ Preferred newborn care provider(s)
  - ○ Anticipated return visit schedule
    - ▪ Q 4–6 weeks until 32 weeks gestation
    - ▪ Q 2–3 weeks from 32–36 weeks gestation
    - ▪ Weekly from 36 weeks until birth occurs
    - ▪ More frequent visits prn, specify indication
  - ○ Informed consent or consultation, as indicated, for
    - ▪ Planned out-of-hospital birth
    - ▪ VBAC
    - ▪ Cesarean birth
    - ▪ Postpartum tubal ligation

Collaborative Practice:
Consider Consultation or Referral

- Health education
  - ○ Pregnancy and/or childbirth education classes
  - ○ Diabetes education for the gestational diabetic
  - ○ Pregnancy yoga or exercise program
- Social service
- OB/GYN service
  - ○ Complications or problems during pregnancy
  - ○ Surgical consultation
- Anesthesia service
  - ○ Pre-op evaluation
- For diagnosis or treatment outside the midwife's scope of practice

Care of the Pregnant Woman with Backache

Key Clinical Information

Backache during pregnancy is a common occurrence. Client posture, body mechanics, and muscle tone may affect the strain on the back from the growing belly. Other causes of backache during pregnancy should not be dismissed without consideration, as this general symptom may be the only indication of preterm labor, pylonephritis, or renal calculi.

Client History: Components of the History to Consider

- LMP, EDC, gestational age
- Duration, severity, and location of backache
- History of complaint
  - Precipitating event, if any
  - Timing of symptoms
  - Activities that exacerbate backache
  - Medications or self-help measures used and relief obtained
- Presence of other associated symptoms
  - Presence or absence of contractions
  - Urinary symptoms
    - Frequency
    - Flank pain
  - Presence of neurologic signs or symptoms
- Past medical history
  - Back injury or disease
  - Kidney stones or pylonephritis
- Potential contributing factors
  - Body mechanics
  - Lifting at work or home
  - Physical abuse

Physical Examination: Components of the Physical Exam to Consider

- VS, including weight
- Abdominal exam
  - Abdominal muscle tone
  - Uterine size
- Back exam
  - Mobility
  - Point tenderness
  - Posture, presence of lordosis or scoliosis
  - CVA tenderness
  - Presence of muscle spasm
- Pelvic evaluation for
  - Backache accompanied by contractions
  - History suggestive of preterm labor
  - Evaluation of cervical status
- Evaluation of neurologic status
  - Muscle tone
  - Strength
  - Coordination
  - Reflexes
- Signs of physical abuse
  - Bruising
  - Burns
  - Partner presence for entire visit

Clinical Impression: Differential Diagnoses to Consider

- Backache of pregnancy
- Muscle strain or spasm, secondary to
  - Pregnancy
  - Injury
- Pregnancy complicated by
  - Pylonephritis
  - Renal calculi
  - Herniated disc

Diagnostic Testing: Diagnostic Tests and Procedures to Consider

- Urinalysis
- Urine culture in the patient with a history of UTIs
- Fetal/uterine monitoring
- Ultrasound if renal calculi are suspected

Providing Treatment:
Therapeutic Measures to Consider

- Pain relief (Murphy, 2004)
  - Acetaminophen/aspirin
    - Alternate q 4 hr
    - Use for no more than 24–48 hr
  - Naproxen/naproxen sodium
    - 200–375 mg q 8–12 hs
    - Pregnancy Cat. B
    - Avoid in late pregnancy
  - Ketoprofen (Orudis)
    - 75 mg tid
    - Pregnancy Cat. B
    - Avoid in late pregnancy
- Muscle spasm (Murphy, 2004)
  - Flexeril
    - 10 mg tid
    - Pregnancy Cat. B
- As appropriate for other confirmed diagnosis

Providing Treatment:
Alternative Measures to Consider

- Ice to affected area followed by warm packs (moist heat, castor oil, vinegar)
- Massage with liniment rubs (Foster, 1996)
  - Saint-John's-wort
    - Infused oil for massage
  - Calendula salve
  - Capsaicin salve or ointment
- Adequate calcium and magnesium intake
  - Calcium (see Calcium Foods List)
  - Magnesium (see Magnesium Foods List)
- Herbals
  - Calendula tea or tincture tid
  - Chamomile tea

Providing Support:
Education and Support Measures to Consider

- Use of good body mechanics (Varney et al., 2004)
  - Low-heeled shoes
  - Posture to minimize lordosis
  - Bend knees to lift using leg muscles
  - Avoid lifting with back
  - Avoid bending or turning from waist
- Planned back care program
  - Pelvic tilt
  - Stretching
  - Swimming
  - Yoga
- Supportive sleep environment
  - Firm mattress
  - Pillows between knees
- Mechanical support measures
  - Well-fitting, supportive bra
  - Prenatal abdominal cradle
  - Lumbar support in chair/car
  - Footstool to raise knees above hips

Follow-up Care:
Follow-up Measures to Consider

- Document
- Notify adult protective services as needed for evidence of abuse
- Return for care
  - As scheduled for gestation
  - With worsening symptoms
    - Pain
    - Numbness or tingling
  - Signs of preterm labor
  - Urinary symptoms

Collaborative Practice:
Consider Consultation or Referral

- Osteopathic manipulation
- Chiropractic manipulation
- Physical therapy
  - For posture and lifting evaluation
  - For symptom management
  - For exercise training
- OB/GYN service
  - Persistent backache
  - Persistent backache with contractions
  - Development of fever and chills
  - Positive testing for kidney involvement

○ Presence of neurologic symptoms
- For diagnosis or treatment outside the midwife's scope of practice

Care of the Pregnant Woman with Constipation

Key Clinical Information

Constipation frequently occurs in pregnant women because of the decreased motility of the intestine, as well as pressure from the enlarged uterus. Prevention of constipation requires adequate intake of both fluid and fiber accompanied by physical activity to stimulate the bowels. Determining acceptable dietary sources of fiber for each client is essential. Candid discussion regarding frequency and consistency of bowel movements is an integral part of evaluation for this common malady.

Client History:
Components of the History to Consider

- LMP, EDC, gestational age
- Onset of problem
- Bowel habits
  ○ Frequency and consistency of bowel movements
  ○ Straining
  ○ Passage of flatus
  ○ Remedies used and efficacy
- Other associated symptoms
  ○ Abdominal cramping w/ BM
    ▪ Nature of abdominal discomfort
    ▪ Location, severity
    ▪ Backache
    ▪ Contractions
  ○ Presence of blood in the stool
- Potential contributing factors
  ○ Iron therapy
  ○ Inactivity
  ○ Inadequate fluid intake
  ○ Inadequate fiber intake
  ○ Narcotic use

- Past medical history
  ○ Abdominal surgeries or PID (adhesions)
  ○ Bowel disorders
  ○ Status of appendix

Physical Examination:
Components of the Physical Exam to Consider

- Vital signs, including temp
- Abdominal exam
  ○ Auscultate bowel sounds x 4
  ○ Palpate for presence of abdominal pain
    ▪ Location
    ▪ Rebound
    ▪ Guarding
- Pelvic exam
  ○ Palpate for hard stool in rectum
  ○ Cervical evaluation if cramping present

Clinical Impression:
Differential Diagnoses to Consider

- Constipation
- Appendicitis
- Ectopic pregnancy
- Irritable bowel syndrome
- Fecal impaction
- Intestinal obstruction
- Diverticulitis

Diagnostic Testing:
Diagnostic Tests and Procedures to Consider

- Urine for specific gravity
- CBC, with differential
- Pelvic ultrasound
- Quantitative b-HCG

Providing Treatment:
Therapeutic Measures to Consider

Acute abdomen must be ruled out before treating constipation.
- Fiber therapy, such as (Murphy, 2004)
  ○ Citrucel: 1 tbs in 8 oz fluid 1–3 x daily

- ○ Metamucil: 1 tsp in 8 oz fluid 1–3 x daily
- ○ Fibercon: 1 tab with 8 oz fluids 1–4 x daily
- Stool softeners, such as (Murphy, 2004)
  - ○ Docusate sodium: 50–100 mg 1 PO QD or BID
  - ○ Docusate calcium: 240 mg 1 PO QD
- Laxatives, such as (Murphy, 2004)
  - ○ Senokot: 1 tab at hs
  - ○ Milk of magnesia
- Rectal treatments
  - ○ Glycerin suppositories
  - ○ Soapsuds enema
  - ○ Fleet enema if stool impacted
- Irritable bowel with constipation (Murphy, 2004)
  - ○ Zelnorm (pregnancy category B)

Providing Treatment:
Alternative Measures to Consider

- Increase fiber in diet
  - ○ Dried fruits, prune juice
  - ○ Whole grains, bran cereals, muffins
  - ○ Uncooked vegetables, well chewed
  - ○ Herbals
    - ▪ Psyllium seed 1 tsp TID (Foster, 1996)
    - ▪ Yellow dock root (Soule, 1996)
    - ▪ Slippery elm (Drug digest, nd)
- Increase fluid intake
  - ○ 8 cups per day
  - ○ Hot liquid in morning
    - ▪ Herb tea
    - ▪ Decaffeinated coffee
    - ▪ Hot prune juice
- Increase physical activity
  - ○ Brisk walk after hot drink
  - ○ Follow by toileting
- Bowel retraining
  - ○ Allow regular time for toileting
  - ○ Follow natural urges

Providing Support:
Education and Support Measures to Consider

- Prevention is key

- Walking helps stimulate natural peristalsis
- Fiber
  - ○ Maintain adequate fiber intake
  - ○ Helps to keep stool soft
  - ○ Must be used with adequate fluid intake
- Stool softeners
  - ○ Bring fluid to the stool to soften
  - ○ Coat stool with surfactant to help move
- Laxatives
  - ○ Stimulate peristalsis
  - ○ Should be used with caution during pregnancy
  - ○ May cause cramping
- Suppositories
  - ○ Stimulate evacuation of lower bowel
  - ○ May cause cramping
- Enemas
  - ○ Flush the lower bowel
  - ○ May cause cramping
- Lifestyle recommendations
  - ○ Need for increased fiber and fluid
  - ○ Need for activity to stimulate bowels
  - ○ Hot drink in AM may stimulate bowels
  - ○ Need for time for toileting
- Warning signs of
  - ○ Preterm labor
  - ○ Acute abdomen

Follow-up Care:
Follow-up Measures to Consider

- Document
- Return for care
  - ○ As scheduled for gestation
  - ○ Return sooner if symptoms worsen
- For emergency care
  - ○ Symptoms of acute abdomen
  - ○ Obstipation
  - ○ Symptoms of preterm labor

Collaborative Practice:
Consider Consultation or Referral

- OB/GYN service
  - ○ Threatened preterm labor

- ○ Positive occult blood in stool
- ○ Severe or persistent abdominal pain accompanied by
  - ▪ Fever
  - ▪ Abdominal rigidity or guarding
  - ▪ Obstipation
- For diagnosis or treatment outside the midwife's scope of practice

Care of the Pregnant Woman with Dyspnea

Key Clinical Information

Physiologic shortness of breath occurs in early pregnancy as the body adjusts to increase oxygen saturation to meet the baby's needs. It again becomes common in the later stages of pregnancy as the uterus pushes against the diaphragm reducing the functional residual volume of the lungs (Varney et al., 2004). Anemia, cardiac arrhythmias, and poor physical conditioning may also contribute to dyspnea during pregnancy. Evaluation of shortness of breath during pregnancy is necessary to determine whether it is physiologic or pathologic.

Client History:
Components of the History to Consider

- LMP, EDC, gestational age
- Timing of onset, duration, and severity of symptoms
  - ○ With activity vs. at rest
  - ○ Supine vs. upright
- Self-help measures or medications used
- Other associated symptoms
  - ○ Fever, chills
  - ○ Cough
  - ○ Syncope
  - ○ Peripheral edema
  - ○ Anxiety or panic symptoms
- Cardiopulmonary history
  - ○ Asthma
  - ○ Smoking tobacco or other substances

- ○ Environmental exposure to allergens, smoke, fumes
- ○ Cardiac disorders and/or symptoms
- Review of systems

Physical Examination:
Components of the Physical Exam to Consider

- Vital signs, including temperature
- Color
- Auscultation and percussion of the chest
  - ○ Respiratory rate, depth, and volume
  - ○ Cardiac rate and rhythm
  - ○ Lung fields
  - ○ Presence of abnormal breath sounds
- Observe for
  - ○ Respiratory effort
  - ○ Presence of cough
  - ○ Signs of respiratory distress
  - ○ Edema of the extremities

Clinical Impression:
Differential Diagnoses to Consider

- Physiologic SOB of pregnancy
- Dyspnea related to
  - ○ Upper respiratory infection
  - ○ Asthma
  - ○ Anemia
  - ○ Valvular heart disease
  - ○ Coronary artery disease
  - ○ Anxiety or panic disorder
  - ○ Other respiratory or cardiac disorder

Diagnostic Testing:
Diagnostic Tests and Procedures to Consider

- CBC with differential
- Sputum cultures
- TB testing
- Chest X-ray
- Pulmonary function testing

Providing Treatment:
Therapeutic Measures to Consider

- SOB of pregnancy
  - Encourage slow breathing
- Otherwise as indicated by diagnosis (see Respiratory Disorders)

Providing Treatment:
Alternative Measures to Consider

- Stretch periodically
- Maintain good posture
- Maintain slow-paced physical activity
  - Walking
  - Yoga
  - Swimming
- Use pillows as needed for comfort while at rest

Providing Support:

Education and Support Measures to Consider
- Reassurance
- Review
  - Physiologic basis of shortness of breath
  - Deliberate intercostal breathing
- Comfort measures
  - Loose-fitting clothes
  - Rest periods
  - Avoid laying flat on back
- Warning signs
  - Flulike symptoms
  - Productive cough
  - Chest pain, SOB, diaphoresis
  - Anxiety

Follow-up Care:
Follow-up Measures to Consider

- Document
- Return for care
  - As scheduled for gestation
  - Sooner for
    - Presence of warning signs
    - Persistence or worsening of symptoms
    - As needed for support

Collaborative Practice:
Consider Consultation or Referral

- Medical service
  - Evidence of decompensation
  - History or symptoms of asthma
  - Evidence respiratory infection or disorder
- Mental health service
  - Anxiety or panic attacks
- For diagnosis or treatment outside the midwife's scope of practice

Care of the Pregnant Woman with Edema

Key Clinical Information

Physiologic edema of pregnancy occurs secondary to fluid retention as the body works to increase and maintain adequate circulating fluid volume. Pressure of the pregnant uterus may cause venous stasis and force fluid out of the circulatory system and into the soft tissue. Physiologic edema and the edema associated with pregnancy-induced hypertension (PIH) may be indistinguishable. Careful evaluation for additional signs and symptoms of PIH is necessary.

Client History:
Components of the History to Consider

- LMP, EDC, gestational age
- Onset, location, duration, and severity of edema
  - Precipitating factors
  - Usual intake and urination patterns
  - Self-help measures used and their effects
  - Other associated symptoms
- Symptoms of preeclampsia
- History of
  - Preeclampsia
  - Edema with pregnancy
  - Varicose veins
- Review of systems

Physical Examination:
Components of the Physical Exam to Consider

- Vital signs
- Compare BP and WT to baseline
- Note presence or absence of facial edema
- Examination of extremities
  - Deep tendon reflexes
  - Presence of pitting edema
  - Measurement of leg circumference
  - Varicosities
  - Signs of phlebitis

Clinical Impression:
Differential Diagnoses to Consider

- Physiologic edema of pregnancy
- Edema related to
  - Excessive sodium intake
  - Preeclampsia
  - Thrombophlebitis

Diagnostic Testing:
Diagnostic Tests and Procedures to Consider

- Office urinalysis
  - Proteinuria
  - Specific gravity
  - Appearance
- Preeclampsia labs (see Preeclampsia)

Providing Treatment:
Therapeutic Measures to Consider

- Prescription support hose
  - Apply with legs elevated to maximize compression

Providing Treatment:
Alternative Measures to Consider

- Hydrotherapy TID (DiPasquale, 2003)
- Gentle massage toward heart
- Herbal support for fluid balance
  - Oat straw (Weed, 1985)
  - Red raspberry (Soule, 1996)
  - Dandelion leaf
  - Stinging nettle (Foster, 1996)

Providing Support:
Education and Support Measures to Consider

- Provide information
  - Physiologic basis of edema in pregnancy
  - Warning signs
    - Preeclampsia
    - Phlebitis
- Self-help measures
  - Continue gentle physical activity
  - Rest, elevate extremities, pillow under right hip
  - Increase fluids
  - Add salt to diet to taste if low salt intake
  - Decrease salt intake if high salt diet
- Avoid
  - Constrictive clothing
  - Diuretic medications, foods, or herbs

Follow-up Care:
Follow-up Measures to Consider

- Document
- Return for care
  - As scheduled for gestation
  - For increasing edema
  - Symptoms of preeclampsia or phlebitis

Collaborative Practice:
Consider Consultation or Referral

- OB/GYN service
  - Symptoms of preeclampsia
  - Severe progressive edema
  - Severe varicosities
  - Symptoms of phlebitis or thrombophlebitis
- For diagnosis or treatment outside the midwife's scope of practice

Care of the Pregnant Woman with Epistaxis

Key Clinical Information

Nosebleeds may occur with regularity in some pregnant women. While they are rarely of a serious nature, most women are anxious about the blood loss and may require treatment if the bleeding does not stop promptly. Epistaxis may be the presenting symptom of labile hypertension. Inhaled drug use may elevate blood pressure and lead to placental abruption or other hypertension-related complications of pregnancy.

Client History: Components of the History to Consider

- Onset, frequency, duration, and severity of bleeding
  - Precipitating factors or events
    - Allergies or URI
    - Use of inhaled drugs (e.g., cocaine, glue)
    - Use of anticoagulant medications
    - Trauma
  - Self-help measures used and efficacy
  - Associated signs and symptoms
- Past medical history
  - Epistaxis
  - Bleeding disorder
- Family history
  - Bleeding disorder

Physical Examination: Components of the Physical Exam to Consider

- Vital signs, ⏱ compare BP and P to baseline
- Examination of nares for
  - Polyps
  - Trauma
  - Erosion
  - Inflammation
- Observation for bruising

Clinical Impression: Differential Diagnoses to Consider

- Simple epistaxis of pregnancy
- Epistaxis secondary to
  - Hypertension
  - Nasal polyps
  - Inhalation drug use
  - Trauma
  - Bleeding disorder

Diagnostic Testing: Diagnostic Tests and Procedures to Consider

- Hematocrit and hemoglobin
  - Persistent, recurrent copious flow
  - Signs or symptoms of anemia
- Serial BPs
- Drug screen

Providing Treatment: Therapeutic Measures to Consider

- Normal saline nasal spray
- Nasal packing

Providing Treatment: Alternative Measures to Consider

- Herbal and dietary support:
  - Foods rich in vitamins A, C, and E
    - Deep green leafy vegetables
    - Raw garlic and onion
    - Parsley
    - Infusion of oat straw and nettle
- Treatment
  - Cold compresses of comfrey, yarrow, and/or mullein (Weed, 1985)
  - Plantain and yarrow ointment
  - Yellow dock ointment

Providing Support: Education and Support Measures to Consider

- Provide information on
  - Physiologic basis for epistaxis

○ Self-help measures
  ▪ Avoid vigorous blowing of nose
  ▪ Use humidifier or vaporizer
  ▪ Ice to bridge of nose to stop bleeding
  ▪ Pinch bridge of nose to stop bleeding

Follow-up Care:
Follow-up Measures to Consider

- Document
- Return for care
  ○ As scheduled for gestation
  ○ For bleeding unresponsive to self-help measures

Collaborative Practice:
Consider Consultation or Referral

- ENT service
  ○ Electrocautery of bleeding vessel
  ○ Nasal polyps
- Medical service
  ○ Suspected bleeding disorder
- For diagnosis or treatment outside the midwife's scope of practice

Care of the Pregnant Woman with Heartburn
Key Clinical Information

The pregnancy hormone relaxin may increase the incidence of heartburn or reflux in pregnant women beginning in early pregnancy. As pregnancy progresses, simple mechanical pressure also increases the incidence of heartburn. Women with a history of gastroesophageal reflux disease may require treatment during pregnancy. Small meals and a bland diet are often helpful.

Client History:
Components of the History to Consider

- LMP, EDC, gestational age
- Onset, frequency, timing, duration, and severity of symptoms

○ Common symptoms
  ▪ Burning epigastric pain
  ▪ Reflux
  ▪ Belching, bloating
○ Precipitating factors or events
  ▪ Foods
  ▪ Anxiety
  ▪ Positioning
○ Presence of symptoms prior to pregnancy
○ Usual diet
○ Self-help measures and efficacy

Physical Examination:
Components of the Physical Exam to Consider

- Vital signs including weight
- Fundal height

Clinical Impression:
Differential Diagnoses to Consider

- Physiologic heartburn of pregnancy
- Gastroesophageal reflux disease
- Hiatal hernia

Diagnostic Testing:
Diagnostic Tests and Procedures to Consider

- *H. pylori* testing

Providing Treatment:
Therapeutic Measures to Consider

- Antacid preparations such as
  ○ Tums
  ○ Gelusil
  ○ Amphojel
  ○ Maalox, *not recommended*
  ○ Milk of magnesia, *not recommended*
- Proton pump inhibitors (Preg. Cat B) such as (Murphy, 2004)
  ○ Aciphex 20 mg QD
  ○ Nexium 20 mg QD
  ○ Prevacid 30 mg BID
- H2 blockers (Preg. Cat B)

- ○ Axid 150 mg PO BID
- ○ Pepcid 20 mg PO BID
- ○ Tagamet 300 mg PO QID
- ○ Zantac 150 mg PO BID

Providing Treatment:
Alternative Measures to Consider

- Herbal remedies
  - ○ Chamomile tea
  - ○ Oat straw tea
  - ○ Red raspberry leaf tea
  - ○ Papaya chewable tablets (Griffith, 1999)
  - ○ Slippery elm tea or lozenges

Providing Support:
Education and Support Measures to Consider

- Information related to
  - ○ Physiologic basis of heartburn
  - ○ Warning signs
  - ○ Comfort measures
    - ■ Small frequent meals
    - ■ Maintain good posture
    - ■ Decrease intake of fatty or spicy foods
    - ■ Take food and fluids separately
    - ■ Elevate head of bed 10–30°

Follow-up Care:
Follow-up Measures to Consider

- Document
- Return for care
  - ○ As scheduled for gestation
  - ○ Persistent reflux or abdominal pain
  - ○ Indications for referral
    - ■ Persistent severe reflux
    - ■ Abdominal pain
    - ■ Signs or symptoms of ulcer or perforation

Collaborative Practice:
Consider Consultation or Referral

- Medical or gastroenterology service
  - ○ Severe symptoms unrelieved by treatment

- ○ For suspected or documented
  - ■ *H. pylori* infection
  - ■ Hiatal hernia
  - ■ GERD
  - ■ Gastric ulcer or perforation
- For diagnosis or treatment outside the midwife's scope of practice

Care of the Pregnant Woman with Hemorrhoids

Key Clinical Information

Hemorrhoids are varicosities of the anal region. They may be within the rectum, or outside the anal sphincter. The pressure of the pregnant uterus on pelvic vessels and constipation both aggravate hemorrhoids, causing bleeding, itching, and burning. Thrombosed hemorrhoids are extremely painful and frequently require treatment with incision and drainage.

Client History:
Components of the History to Consider

- LMP, EDC, gestational age
- Prior history of hemorrhoids
- Onset, duration, severity of symptoms
  - ○ Presence of bleeding, pain, itching
  - ○ Self-help measures used and efficacy
- Contributing factors
  - ○ Toileting habits
  - ○ Low-fiber diet
  - ○ Constipation or diarrhea
  - ○ Medications
    - ■ Iron supplements
    - ■ Stool softeners
    - ■ Enemas

Physical Examination:
Components of the Physical Exam to Consider

- Examination for presence of
  - ○ Hemorrhoids
    - ■ External

- ▪ Internal
- ▪ Strangulated
- ▪ Thrombosed
- Anal lesions

Clinical Impression:
Differential Diagnoses to Consider

- Hemorrhoids
- Anal fissures
- Anal trauma
- Anal herpes
- Anal fistula
- Rectal polyp
- Rectal malignancy

Diagnostic Testing:
Diagnostic Tests and Procedures to Consider

- Stool for occult blood
- Herpes culture
- STI screen
- Anoscopy

Providing Treatment:
Therapeutic Measures to Consider

- Anamantle HC: topical anesthetic and steroid (Murphy, 2004)
  - ○ Pregnancy Category B
  - ○ Apply BIX x 7 D
- Manual reduction of hemorrhoids

Providing Treatment:
Alternative Measures to Consider

- Herbal remedies (Weed, 1985)
  - ○ Bilberry tablets or capsules tid
  - ○ Comfrey compresses
  - ○ Nettle tea
- Herbal or warm water sitz baths
- Topical applications
  - ○ Witch hazel compresses
  - ○ Epsom salt compresses
  - ○ Plantain and yarrow ointment
  - ○ Yellow dock root ointment
- Knee chest position to promote drainage
- Homeopathic remedies
  - ○ Hamamelis 30x
  - ○ Arnica 30x

Providing Support:
Education and Support Measures to Consider

- Avoid
  - ○ Straining at stool
  - ○ Prolonged sitting on toilet
  - ○ Constipation or diarrhea
- Ensure adequate fiber in diet
- Topical medication use
- Signs and symptoms necessitating return for care

Follow-up Care:
Follow-up Measures to Consider

- Document
- Return for care
  - ○ As scheduled for gestation
  - ○ ASAP for thrombosed hemorrhoids

Collaborative Practice:
Consider Consultation or Referral

- OB/GYN or surgical service
  - ○ Evaluation of severe, strangulated, or bleeding hemorrhoids
  - ○ Blood in stool with no evidence of hemorrhoids or rectal fissure
  - ○ For incision and drainage of thrombosed hemorrhoids
- For diagnosis or treatment outside the midwife's scope of practice

Care of the Pregnant Woman with Insomnia

Key Clinical Information

Insomnia affects many pregnant women as they approach term. It may help to suggest it as nature's way of preparing for 2 AM feedings. However, the woman with significant sleep deprivation may have significant impairment of her ability to function on a daily basis. Starting labor with severe sleep deprivation may result in early maternal exhaustion and dysfunctional labor patterns. Mood changes may be a primary cause, or a result, of sleep deprivation.

Client History:
Components of the History to Consider

- LMP, EDC, gestational age
- Onset, duration, and severity of symptoms
  - Difficulty falling asleep
  - Wakefulness
  - Fitful sleep
  - Interruptions
    - Nocturia
    - Pain
    - Caretaking responsibilities
- Sleep habits
  - Sleep/wake patterns
    - Bedtime
    - Naps
  - Total hours sleep/24 hrs
- Social issues
  - Emotional response to sleep deprivation
  - Caffeine intake and timing
  - Meal patterns and content
  - Work hours
  - Anxieties and concerns
  - Help and support
- Other related symptoms

Physical Examination:
Components of the Physical Exam to Consider

- Assess for
  - Nutrition and hydration status
  - Evidence of sleep deprivation
  - Physical causes of sleep deprivation

Clinical Impression:
Differential Diagnoses to Consider

- Insomnia
- Insomnia secondary to
  - Pain
  - Anxiety
  - Depression
  - Substance abuse
  - Social concerns related to pregnancy
- Sleep disorder

Diagnostic Testing:
Diagnostic Tests and Procedures to Consider

- Insomnia: None indicated
- Other diagnosis: As indicated by diagnosis

Providing Treatment:
Therapeutic Measures to Consider

- 🕑 Use only when necessary
- For sleep (Murphy, 2004)
  - Ambien (pregnancy category B)
    - 5–10 mg hs
  - Benadryl (pregnancy category B)
    - 25–50 mg hs
- For therapeutic sleep (see Prolonged First Stage Labor)
  - Morphine sulfate
    - 10–15 mg IM
    - May combine with
- Vistaril 25–50 mg, or
- Phenergan 25–50 mg
    - Allows rest for 4–6 hrs
    - May be reversed with Narcan prn
  - Seconal or Nembutal
    - 100 mg PO or IM

Providing Treatment:
Alternative Measures to Consider

- Increase vitamin B intake
- Herbal remedies
  - Chamomile tea

- ○ Hops tea or tincture (after 20 weeks gestation)
- ○ Lemon balm tea
- ○ Skullcap tincture
- ○ Passion flower tea, tincture, or fluid extract tid
- Hydrotherapy
- Hypnotherapy
- Aromatherapy
- Massage

Providing Support:
Education and Support Measures to Consider

- Information related to
  - ○ Physiologic basis of insomnia
  - ○ Other factors that may interfere with sleep
    - ■ Work hours
    - ■ Caretaking requirements
    - ■ Small children
    - ■ Elderly or ill parents/family
    - ■ Sleeping arrangements
    - ■ Nighttime hunger
- Encourage a positive approach to this difficult problem
- Self-help measures
  - ○ Nap during day to maintain rest
  - ○ Warm bath before sleep
  - ○ Warm milk or comfort foods
  - ○ Massage
  - ○ Extra pillows for support
  - ○ Regular daily physical activity
  - ○ Adequate nutrition
  - ○ Limit fluids 2 hrs before bedtime

Follow-up Care:
Follow-up Measures to Consider

- Document
- Return for care
  - ○ As scheduled for gestation
  - ○ Increased visits prn for
    - ■ Evaluation and monitoring of medication use
    - ■ Emotional support

Collaborative Practice:
Criteria to Consider for Consultation or Referral

- OB/GYN service
  - ○ Maternal exhaustion
- Mental health service
  - ○ Depression
  - ○ Anxiety
- Social service
- For diagnosis or treatment outside the midwife's scope of practice

Care of the Pregnant Woman with Leg Cramps

Key Clinical Information

Leg cramps are a common occurrence during pregnancy and may interfere with a woman's ability to sleep. They are more common during the nighttime hours. Cramping may be related to an imbalance of calcium in the muscle cells, causing muscle spasms.

Client History:
Components of the History to Consider

- LMP, EDC, gestational age
- Onset, frequency, duration, and severity of cramps
  - ○ Precipitating factors
  - ○ Self-help measures used and efficacy
  - ○ Calcium and magnesium intake
  - ○ Physical activity level
- Other associated symptoms

Physical Examination:
Components of the Physical Exam to Consider

- Vital signs
- Evaluate extremities for
  - ○ Clonus
  - ○ Muscle spasm
  - ○ Varicosities
  - ○ Homan's sign

Clinical Impression:
Differential Diagnoses to Consider

- Physiologic leg cramps
- Varicose veins
- Restless leg syndrome
- Phlebitis
- Thrombophlebitis
- Deep vein thrombosis

Diagnostic Testing:
Diagnostic Tests and Procedures to Consider

- Serial calf measurements
- Venous ultrasound
- Clotting studies

Providing Treatment:
Therapeutic Measures to Consider

- Calcium supplement
- Magnesium supplement

Providing Treatment:
Alternative Measures to Consider

- Dietary sources of calcium and magnesium (see Calcium and Magnesium Foods lists)
- Acupressure
  - Pressure to posterior midcalf
  - Flex foot
- Homeopathic remedies
  - Calcarea Phos. 30x tid or with acute symptoms
  - Calcarea Carb. 30x tid or with acute symptoms
- Herbal remedies (Weed, 1985)
  - Raspberry leaf
  - Nettle
  - Dandelion

Providing Support:
Education and Support Measures to Consider

- Physiologic nature of leg cramps in pregnancy
- Self-help measures
  - Increase calcium and magnesium intake
  - Regular daily activity

- Walking
- Yoga
- Swimming
  - Keep legs warm
  - When cramp occurs
    - Flex foot
    - Massage calf toward pelvis
    - Stretch heel away from body
    - Use homeopathic remedy q 15 min x 2–4 doses
- Warning signs
  - Increasing muscle spasms
  - Swelling, pain, or redness in leg

Follow-up Care:
Follow-up Measures to Consider

- Document
- Return for care
  - As scheduled for gestation
  - For persistent leg pain or warning signs

Collaborative Practice:
Consider Consultation or Referral

- Medical service
  - For nonpregnancy related cause of leg pain
  - Phlebitis
  - Thrombophlebitis
  - Deep vein thrombosis
- For diagnosis or treatment outside the midwife's scope of practice

Care of the Pregnant Woman with Nausea and Vomiting

Key Clinical Information

While nausea and vomiting are considered a classic early pregnancy occurrence, they may cause significant dehydration and contribute to poor nutrition. In a few women the nausea and vomiting of pregnancy continue throughout the pregnancy. Hyperemesis of pregnancy most often occurs in the presence of a large amount of circulating pregnancy hormones.

Prompt treatment is required to restore fluid and electrolyte balance.

Client History:
Components of the History to Consider

- LMP, EDC, gestational age
- Onset, duration and severity of symptoms
  - Presence and frequency of vomiting
  - Symptoms of dehydration
  - Other associated symptoms
  - Self-help measures used and results
- Assess
  - Nutritional intake
  - Activity level
  - Bowel and bladder pattern
- Past medical history
  - Thyroid disorders
  - Eating disorders
- Review of systems

Physical Examination:
Components of the Physical Exam to Consider

- Vital signs, including WT and BP
- Usual prenatal evaluation, including examination for
  - Overall appearance
    - Weight loss
    - Skin turgor
    - Self-care and hygiene
  - Abdominal exam
    - Fundal height for gestational age
    - Bowel sounds

Clinical Impression:
Differential Diagnoses to Consider

- Physiologic nausea of pregnancy
- Pregnancy complicated by
  - Hyperemesis gravidarum
  - Hydatidiform mole
  - Ectopic implantation
- Mental health conditions

  - Bulimia
  - Anxiety
  - Depression
- Other medical conditions, such as
  - Cholecystitis
  - Pylonephritis
  - Gastroenteritis

Diagnostic Testing:
Diagnostic Tests and Procedures to Consider

- Urine dip for ketones and glucose
- Urinalysis
- BUN and electrolytes
- Serum albumin
- TSH
- Liver function testing
- CBC or WBC
- Pelvic ultrasound

Providing Treatment:
Therapeutic Measures to Consider

Use caution with any medications used for treatment of N & V in early pregnancy. No medications have been demonstrated to be completely safe for the developing fetus.

- IV hydration when indicated (Sinclair, 2004)
  - Hydration alone may resolve symptoms
  - Use balanced electrolyte solution
  - 500 ml bolus to start
  - Titrate to maintain urinary specific gravity in normal range
- Vitamin B_6 (pyridoxine) (Higdon, 2002)
  - 10–30 mg TID –
  - Pregnancy category A
- Meclizine Hcl (Murphy, 2004)
  - 12.5 mg bid
  - Pregnancy category B
- Meclopramide (Reglan) (Murphy, 2004)
  - 5–10 mg PO 30 min. AC
  - Pregnancy category B
- Promethazine (Phenergan) (Murphy, 2004)
  - 25 mg PO q 8–12 h

○ Pregnancy category C
- Prochlorperazine (Compazine) (Murphy, 2004)
  ○ 5–10 mg PO/IM/slow IV q 3–6 h
  ○ 15 mg spansule PO daily in AM
  ○ 10 mg spansule PO q 12 hr
  ○ Rectal 25 mg BID
  ○ Pregnancy category C
  ○ Max daily dose 40 mg/day
- Ondansetron (Zofran) (Murphy, 2004)
  ○ 4–16 mg PO q 8 hrs, prn
  ○ Pregnancy category B

Providing Treatment:
Alternative Measures to Consider

- Nutritional support
  ○ Ginger as tea, soda, cookies, etc. (Oates-Whitehead, 2004)
  ○ B vitamin foods (Weed, 1985)
    ■ Wheat germ
    ■ Molasses
    ■ Brewer's yeast
- Acupressure wristbands (Seabands) (Oates-Whitehead, 2004)

Providing Support:
Education and Support Measures to Consider

- Encourage
  ○ Small bland meals, primarily carbohydrates
  ○ Keep something in stomach, e.g., saltines, cheerios
  ○ Adequate fluids
  ○ Small bites or sips only
  ○ Use salt substitute (adds potassium)
  ○ Limit fat and increase protein
- Advise family of need for support
- Review when to call
  ○ For persistent vomiting
  ○ Symptoms of dehydration
  ○ Abdominal pain
  ○ Weakness, lethargy, confusion

Follow-up Care:
Follow-up Measures to Consider

- Document
- Return for care
  ○ As scheduled for gestation
  ○ prn for worsening symptoms
  ○ Consider hospital care for dehydration

Collaborative Practice:
Consider Consultation or Referral

- OB/GYN service
  ○ Hyperemesis
  ○ Dehydration
  ○ Molar pregnancy
- For diagnosis or treatment outside the midwife's scope of practice

Care of the Pregnant Woman with Pica
Key Clinical Information

Pica is frequently a sign of iron deficiency anemia, but may indicate other deficits in the diet. Cultural factors may influence the nonfood items women crave or eat. The most common substances consumed with pica are ice, clay, and laundry starch (Callahan, 2003).

Client History:
Components of the History to Consider

- LMP, EDC, gestational age
- Identify
  ○ Nonfood substances craved or consumed
  ○ 🌐 Cultural or ethnic expressions of pica
  ○ Social issues that may contribute to pica
    ■ Need for attention
    ■ Inadequate diet
    ■ 🌐 Cultural expectations
- Evaluate
  ○ Client's diet and nutritional resources
  ○ Use of vitamin and mineral supplements
  ○ Previous H & H
  ○ Prior history of anemia

Physical Examination:
Components of the Physical Exam to Consider

- VS, including pulse
- Assess nutritional status
- Evaluate for symptoms of anemia
  - Color of mucous membranes
  - Capillary refill
  - Orthostatic hypotension
  - Elevated heart rate

Clinical Impression:
Differential Diagnoses to Consider

- Pica of pregnancy, secondary to
  - Anemia
  - Nutrient deficiency
  - Social or cultural issues

Diagnostic Testing:
Diagnostic Tests and Procedures to Consider

- H & H
- Lead screening
- Anemia work-up prn (see Anemia)

Providing Treatment:
Therapeutic Measures to Consider

- Iron replacement therapy if anemia present (see Anemia)
- Multivitamin and mineral supplement

Providing Treatment:
Alternative Measures to Consider

- Iron rich foods (see Iron foods list)
- Sea vegetables (high in iron and trace minerals)
- Red raspberry leaf tea

Providing Support:
Education and Support Measures to Consider

- Explore concerns about pica with client
  - Stress pica may interfere with good nutrition
  - Provide or arrange for nutritional education
  - Encourage client to avoid nonfood items
    - Try offering substitute items
- Laundry starch, ice > frozen fruit pops
- Clay > food grade seaweed
- Other acceptable nutritional items

Follow-up Care:
Follow-up Measures to Consider

- Document
- Return for care
  - As scheduled for gestation
  - Follow-up labs as indicated

Collaborative Practice:
Consider Consultation or Referral

- Social services
  - WIC
  - Food stamps
  - Food bank
- OB/GYN or Medical service
  - For severe pica accompanied by anemia
  - For elevated lead levels
- For diagnosis or treatment outside the midwife's scope of practice

Care of the Pregnant Woman with Round Ligament Pain

Key Clinical Information

Round ligament pain may be a frequent occurrence between 16–20 weeks gestation. It may mimic, or mask, more serious conditions such as appendicitis or ovarian torsion. Round ligament pain may cause significant distress, especially in the athletic woman who continues to jog, or those who have highly physical jobs such as waitresses or nurse's aides. An objective pain scale is recommended to assess and document client pain

Client History:
Components of the History to Consider

- LMP, EDC, gestational age
- Evaluation of the pain
  - Onset, location, severity, duration
  - Quality of the pain
    - Intermittent vs. constant
    - Sharp or dull
    - Exacerbating factors
  - Associated symptoms
    - Cramping
    - Backache
    - Nausea and vomiting
    - Change in bowel or bladder function
- Relief measures used and efficacy

Physical Examination:
Components of the Physical Exam to Consider

- Vital signs, including temp
- Verify location of pain
- Note posture and overall appearance
- Abdominal exam
  - Palpate for tenderness
    - Note guarding
    - Rebound pain
    - Referred pain
  - Uterine exam
    - Fundal height
    - FHR
    - Presence of contractions
    - Consistency and position of uterus
- Pelvic exam
  - Cervical or vaginal discharge
  - Dilation and/or effacement
- Evaluate for CVA tenderness

Clinical Impression:
Differential Diagnoses to Consider

- Round ligament pain, NOS
- Pregnancy complicated by
  - Ectopic pregnancy
  - Preterm labor
  - Placental abruption

- Acute abdomen secondary to
  - Ovarian torsion
  - Renal calculi
  - Pylonephritis
  - PID
  - Appendicitis
  - Gallbladder disease

Diagnostic Testing:
Diagnostic Tests and Procedures to Consider

- Urinalysis
- Chlamydia and gonorrhea testing
- CBC, with diff
- Ultrasound evaluation
  - Pelvis
    - Uterus, ovaries, and tubes
    - Appendix
- Abdomen
  - Kidneys, ureters, and bladder (KUB)
  - Gallbladder

Providing Treatment:
Therapeutic Measures to Consider

- Maternity abdominal support or girdle
- Osteopathic manipulation

Providing Treatment:
Alternative Measures to Consider

- Muscle strengthening and stretching
  - Yoga
  - Swimming
  - Prenatal exercise class
- Reflexology to waist and pelvic points
- Herbal remedies
  - Red raspberry leaf tea
  - Massage with Saint-John's-wort extract
    - Soak dried flowers in olive oil

Providing Support:
Education and Support Measures to Consider

- Physiologic cause of round ligament pain
- Provide reassurance

- Self-help measures
  - Pelvic tilt
  - Warm baths
  - Applying gentle heat to area
  - Positioning
    - Knees to abdomen
    - Bending toward pain to ease ligament
    - Side-lying with pillow under abdomen
  - Limit lifting and twisting
  - Ask for help prn
- *Warning signs*
  - Onset of contractions
  - Persistent abdominal pain
  - Fever
  - Onset of nausea and vomiting
  - Vaginal bleeding or discharge
  - Pain with intercourse or BM

Follow-up Care:
Follow-up Measures to Consider

- Document
- Return for care
  - As scheduled for gestation
  - As indicated by test results
  - With onset of *warning signs*

Collaborative Practice:
Consider Consultation or Referral

- OB/GYN service
  - Abdominal pain inconsistent with round ligament pain
  - Abnormal test results
- For diagnosis or treatment outside the midwife's scope of practice

Care of the Pregnant Woman with Varicose Veins

Key Clinical Information

Varicose veins are frequently troublesome during pregnancy, and they generally worsen as the pregnancy progresses and with each subsequent pregnancy. Care must be taken to avoid trauma to the vessels, which may result in hematoma formation, superficial phlebitis, or thrombophlebitis. Good-quality support hose are helpful in easing the discomfort of significant lower limb varicosities. For women with vulvar varicosities, snug-fitting panties or even a girdle may be needed to provide needed counterpressure.

Client History:
Components of the History to Consider

- LMP, EDC, gestational age
- Onset and location of varicose veins
  - Changes with pregnancy
  - Associated symptoms
    - Pain
    - Edema
    - Redness
    - Other associated symptoms
  - Current relief measures and their effects
  - Use of medications
    - Aspirin (ASA)
    - NSAIDS
- Past medical history
  - Varicose veins
  - Superficial phlebitis
  - Thrombophlebitis

Physical Examination:
Components of the Physical Exam to Consider

- Examination of varicosities
  - Location(s)
  - Number
  - Size
  - Severity
- Serial calf measurements
- Evaluate for symptoms of
  - Superficial phlebitis
    - Heat
    - Redness
    - Tenderness
  - Deep vein thrombosis
    - Pain
    - Positive Homan's sign
    - Leg edema

Clinical Impression:
Differential Diagnoses to Consider

- Varicose veins, NOS
- Superficial phlebitis
- Deep vein thrombosis

Diagnostic Testing:
Diagnostic Tests and Procedures to Consider

- Ultrasound as indicated to R/O deep vein thrombosis (DVT)

Providing Treatment:
Therapeutic Measures to Consider

- Support garments
  - Hosiery
    - Apply after elevating legs 10 minutes
    - Prescription hose may be needed
    - Wear daily
  - Foam pad to support vulvar varicosities
    - Use with close-fitting undergarment
  - Maternity abdominal support to relieve pressure on pelvic veins
- Low dose aspirin 80 mg
  - 1 PO daily x 7 days (ACOG, 2003)
  - For symptoms of early superficial phlebitis

Providing Treatment:
Alternative Measures to Consider

- Herbal remedies
  - Bilberry tablets or capsules tid
    - Strengthens capillaries
    - Reduces platelet aggregation (Foster, 1996)
  - Nettle tea or tincture
    - Improves elasticity of vessels (Weed, 1985)
  - Oat straw tea or infusion
    - Strengthens capillaries (Weed, 1985)
- Positioning
  - Leg elevation above heart
  - Leg inversion (right-angle position)
  - Inverted yoga postures (shoulder stand against support)

Providing Support:
Education and Support Measures to Consider

- Encourage
  - Use and application of support hose
  - Rest with legs elevated
  - Regular mild exercise, especially walking or swimming
- Avoidance of
  - Constrictive clothing
  - Long periods of standing or sitting
- Medication instructions
- *Warning signs*
  - Persistent or worsening pain
  - Unilateral edema of extremity
  - Localized redness, heat, tenderness
  - Fever

Follow-up Care:
Follow-up Measures to Consider

- Document
- Return for care
  - As scheduled for gestation
  - Onset of warning signs
  - 4–7 days for suspected early superficial phlebitis
  - Evaluate closely in early postpartum period

Collaborative Practice:
Consider Consultation or Referral

- OB/GYN service
  - Severe vulvar varicosities
  - Suspected or confirmed
    - Phlebitis
    - Thrombophlebitis
- For diagnosis or treatment outside the midwife's scope of practice

References

American College of Obstetricians and Gynecologists [ACOG]. (2003). Low dose aspirin during pregnancy may lower risk of preeclampsia. (News release). Retrieved August 25, 2005, from http://www.acog.org/from_home/publications/press _releases/nr05-31-03-2.cfm

Callahan, G.N. (2003, August). Eating dirt. *Emerging infectious diseases*. Retrieved December 16, 2004, from: http://www.cdc.gov/ncidod/EID/vol9no8/03-0033.htm

Centers for Disease Control and Prevention [CDC]. (2004). *Questions & answers: Flu vaccination in the 2004-05 season*. Retrieved January 28, 2005, from http://www.cdc.gov/flu/about/qa/0405vaccination.htm

Davis, E. (1997). *Hearts and hands: A midwife's guide to pregnancy & birth* (3rd ed.). Berkeley, CA: Celestial Arts.

DiPasquale, L. R., & Lynett, K. (2003). The use of water immersion for treatment of massive labial edema during pregnancy. *American Journal of Maternal Child Nursing, 28*, 242–245.

Drug Digest. (n.d.) *Slippery elm*. Retrieved October 28, 2004, from http://www.drugdigest.org/DD/DVH/ HerbsWho/0,3923,4100%7CSlippery+elm,00.html

E-medicine. (2004). Pregnancy, *Hyperemesis gravidarum*. Retrieved December 1, 2004, from http://www. emedicine.com/emerg/topic479.htm

Foster, S. (1996). *Herbs for your health*. Loveland, CO: Interweave Press.

Frye, A. (1997). *Understanding diagnostic tests in the childbearing year.* (6th ed.). Portland, OR: Labrys Press.

Frye, A. (1998). *Holistic midwifery*. Portland, OR: Labrys Press.

Gordon, J. D., Rydfors, J. T., & Druzin, M. L. (1995). *Obstetrics, gynecology & infertility* (4th ed.). Glen Cove, NY: Scrub Hill Press.

Griffith, K.W., (1999) *Healing herbs: The essential guide.* Tucson, AZ: Fisher Books.

Higdon, J. (2002). Vitamin B_6. Retrieved July 1, 2005 from http://lpi.oregonstate.edu/infocenter/vitamins/ vitaminB6/

Morgan, G., & Hamilton, C. (2003). *Practice guidelines for obstetrics and gynecology.* Philadelphia: Lippincott-Raven.

Murphy, J. L. (Ed.). (2004). *Nurse practitioner's prescribing reference.* New York: Prescribing Reference.

Oates-Whitehead, R. (2004). Nausea and vomiting in early pregnancy. In F. Godlee (Ed.), *Clinical evidence concise* (pp. 392–394). London: BMJ Publishing Group.

Scott, J. R., Diasaia, P. J., Hammond, C. B., Gordon J. D., & Spellacy W. N. (1996). *Danforth's handbook of obstetrics and gynecology.* Philadelphia: Lippincott-Raven.

Sinclair, C. (2004). *A midwife's handbook.* St. Louis, MO: Saunders.

Soule, D. (1996). *The roots of healing.* Secaucus, NJ: Citadel Press.

Varney, H., Kriebs, J. M., & Gegor, C. L. (2004). *Varney's midwifery* (4th ed.). Sudbury, MA: Jones and Bartlett.

Weed, S. (1985). *Wise woman herbal for the childbearing year.* Woodstock, NY: Ashtree.

Bibliography

Barger, M. K. (Ed.). (1988). *Protocols for gynecologic and obstetric health care.* Philadelphia: W.B. Saunders.

Briggs, G. G., Freeman, R. K., & Yaffe, S. J. (1994) *Drugs in pregnancy and lactation* (4th ed.). Philadelphia: Williams & Wilkins.

Enkin, M., Keirce M., Renfrew, M., & Neilson, J. (1995). *A guide to effective care in pregnancy and childbirth* (2nd ed.). New York: Oxford University Press.

Godlee, F. (Ed.). (2004). *Clinical evidence concise* (Vol. 11). London: BMJ Publishing Group.

Myles, M. F. (1985). *Textbook for midwives* (10th ed.). Edinburgh, Scotland: Churchill Livingstone.

Care of the Pregnant Woman with Prenatal Variations

4

N ot every pregnancy remains uneventful. Prompt identification and treatment of prenatal variations that may result in harm to mother or baby ensures the best possible outcome.

The ability to pick up problems in pregnancy is an essential component of skilled midwifery practice. Midwives must simultaneously retain their belief that pregnancy is a normal physiologic condition while retaining a healthy respect for problems and complications that may develop (Ulrich, 2004). During optimal evaluation of potential or developing problems the midwife actively engages the mother in decision making regarding the options for care of herself and her unborn baby.

One of the hallmarks of midwifery care is fostering client autonomy and participation in self-care. While the mother may have no control over the development of problems during her pregnancy and may feel threatened by their development, the midwife can offer her a sense of control by presenting options in the areas where client choice is possible. Respect for each woman's needs is especially important when an unexpected problem develops during what was "supposed" to be a normal, uneventful pregnancy.

Many women look to their midwife to present a balanced view of the problem, diagnostic evaluation, and treatment process. Although many women may wish to be an active participant in all health care decisions, the expectation remains that the midwife will clearly recommend a course of action. Recommendations are based on the midwife's judgment of what constitutes best care for the mother and fetus in light of the presenting problem. Occasionally, the midwife's recommendations may run contrary to either the mother's preferences or standard hospital expectations for obstetric care. A clear, focused, and confidently presented midwifery plan of care with rationale backed by evidenced-based resources can be helpful in providing guidance to the client who hesitates at indicated obstetric intervention, or in the medical setting where the midwife may be pressured to intervene without clear indication.

Midwifery care of problems in pregnancy forms a continuum from least intervention to most intervention. The skilled midwife can move along this continuum in either direction and when necessary make the occasional leap from one end to the other.

Care of the Pregnant Woman with Iron Deficiency Anemia

Key Clinical Information

Iron deficiency anemia is a common diagnosis in women of childbearing age that may worsen during pregnancy. Anemia may affect the oxygenation of both mother and fetus, and result in diminished fetal growth, maternal exhaustion, and related complications such as prematurity (Graves & Barger, 2001). Prompt diagnosis and treatment of anemia with attention to the overall nutritional status of the mother is critically important for fetal well-being and for optimizing maternal health prior to the onset of labor.

Client History: Components of the History to Consider

- LMP, EDC, gestational age
- Current H & H
- Potential causes of anemia
  - Tobacco use
  - History of closely spaced pregnancies
  - Blood loss, heavy menses
  - Chronic illness
  - Malabsorption syndromes
  - Malignancy (Payton & White, 1995)
  - 🌐 Risk for thalassemia or sickle cell
    - African descent
    - Mediterranean descent
    - Asian descent
- Presence of anemia related symptoms
  - Fatigue
  - Dizziness

- Headache
- Pica (eating nonfood items such as starch or clay)
- Dyspnea
- Palpitations or tachycardia (Engstrom & Sittler, 1994)
- Usual dietary patterns
  - General nutrition
  - Dietary iron sources
  - Prenatal vitamin use
  - Iron supplement use

Physical Examination: Components of the Physical Exam to Consider

- Vital signs, including pulse and BP
- Pallor of skin and mucous membranes
- Examination for potential causes of anemia
  - Bruising
  - Bleeding

Clinical Impression: Differential Diagnoses to Consider

- Physiologic anemia of pregnancy
- Iron deficiency anemia
- Other anemia
  - Pernicious
  - Hemolytic
  - Sickle cell
  - Thalassemia

Diagnostic Testing: Diagnostic Tests and Procedures to Consider

- CBC with indices
  - Indices in simple iron deficiency anemia
    - Microcytic
    - Hypochromic

Table 4-1 Hemoglobin and Hematocrit Levels During Pregnancy

WEEK OF GESTATION	HGB (G/DL)	HCT (%)
12	11.0	33.0
16	10.6	32.0
20–24	10.5	32.0
28	10.7	32.0
32	11.0	33.0
36	11.4	34.0
40	11.9	36.0

Source: CDC, 1998.

- ▪ Serum ferritin is decreased.
- • Stool for occult blood, ova, and parasites
- • CDC range for lower limits of normal for hematocrit and hemoglobin (H & H) during pregnancy

Providing Treatment: Therapeutic Measures to Consider

- • Iron replacement therapy (CDC, 1998)
  - ○ 60–120 µg elemental iron daily
  - ○ Iron salts such as
    - ▪ Ferrous sulfate (Feosol/Slow Fe)
      - • 50–65 µg elemental iron
      - • 1 po bid
    - ▪ Ferrous gluconate (Fergon)
      - • 27 µg elemental iron
      - • 2 po bid
    - ▪ Ferrous fumarate 200 µg (Chromagen)
      - • 66 µg elemental iron
      - • 1 po bid
    - ▪ Polysaccharide iron complex (Niferex-150)
      - • 150 µg elemental iron
      - • 1–2 caps po daily (Murphy, 2004)
  - ○ Floradix iron
  - ○ Include vitamin C and folic acid

- ○ Continue through 3 months postpartum
- • IM or IV Imferon for severe or recalcitrant anemia
  - ○ May cause anaphylactic reaction
  - ○ Use with caution and following consult

Providing Treatment: Alternative Measures to Consider

- • Floradix iron plus herbs
  - ○ 2 tsp bid
  - ○ Vegetarian liquid formula
- • High iron food sources (see Iron Foods List)
- • Additional fiber to prevent constipation
- • Heme iron most easily absorbed
  - ○ Meat
  - ○ Poultry
  - ○ Fish
- • Nonheme iron
  - ○ Egg yolk
  - ○ Grains
  - ○ Vegetables
- • Cast iron cookware
  - ○ Nonenamel surface
  - ○ Adds elemental iron

Providing Support:
Education and Support Measures to Consider

- Physiologic nature of anemia in pregnancy
- Pica decreases iron absorption
- Iron supplementation recommendations
    - Dosages
    - Separate supplement from
        - Meals
        - Calcium intake
        - Fiber supplements
        - Other supplements (e.g., prenatal vitamins)
- For best absorption
    - Take with vitamin C or water
    - Take at bedtime
    - Avoid caffeine, black teas
- Common side effects include
    - GI upset, constipation, or diarrhea
    - Nausea
    - Heartburn (Engstrom & Sittler, 1994)

Follow-up Care:
Follow-up Measures to Consider

- Document
- List parameters for consultation
- Return for care
    - Repeat H & H 4–6 weeks after initiating therapy
    - Add indices for persistent anemia

Collaborative Practice:
Consider Consultation or Referral

- For nutritional consult
- For social services
    - WIC
    - Food stamps
    - Local food pantry

- Smoking cessation programs
- Medical consult
    - For abnormal indices or elevated serum ferritin
    - For anemia resistant to conventional therapy
    - For concern regarding cause of anemia
    - For diagnosis outside the midwife's scope of practice

Care of the Pregnant Woman with Fetal Demise

Key Clinical Information

Fetal demise may occur at any stage of pregnancy. No matter when it occurs, a common response is for the mother to wonder what she did wrong. Emotional support and grief counseling may be helpful to parents.

The cause of fetal demise is frequently unable to be determined. Some fetal or placental conditions are clearly incompatible with life, while other fetal loss may be related to maternal illness, heredity or unknown factors. Genetic investigation and counseling may be useful for exploring potential causes of fetal demise, particularly for the woman with a history of recurrent losses. Fetal demise is associated with an increased likelihood of maternal disseminated intravascular coagulation (DIC) (Lindsay and Hernandez, 2004).

Client History:
Components of the History to Consider

- LMP/EGA
- Regression of signs of pregnancy
    - Absence of fetal activity
    - Absence of fetal heart tones
    - Other associated signs and symptoms
- Previous HCG results
- Precipitating event(s), if any

- Idiopathic
- Trauma/physical abuse
- Substance abuse
- Diabetes mellitus
- Medication and herb use

Physical Examination:
Components of the Physical Exam to Consider

- Maternal vital signs
- Abdominal exam
  - Fundal height
  - Uterine tenderness
  - Absence of FHTs
- Pelvic exam
  - Palpation of buckled fetal skull
  - Cervical status/Bishops score

Clinical Impression:
Differential Diagnoses to Consider

- Fetal demise
  - Idiopathic
  - Cord accident
  - Chromosomal anomalies
  - Congenital anomalies
  - Ectopic pregnancy
- Blighted ovum
- False pregnancy

Diagnostic Testing:
Diagnostic Tests and Procedures to Consider

- Maternal blood work
  - CBC
  - Kleinhauer-Betke
  - Hbg A1C
  - RPR/VDRL

- Serum/urine toxicology screen
- Weekly testing in expectant management
  - PT, PTT
  - Fibrinogen, fibrin degradation products
  - Platelets
- Ultrasound
  - Absent fetal heart beat (verified by two examiners)
  - Overlapping of fetal cranial bones: Spalding's sign
  - Presence of gas in fetal abdomen: Robert's sign
- Fetal evaluation
  - Cord blood
  - Placenta to pathology
  - Skin biopsy
  - Fetal autopsy per parents request
- Genetic testing if indicated
  - Anomalies
  - Family history
  - Recurrent fetal losses

Providing Treatment:
Therapeutic Measures to Consider

- Expectant management
  - May be emotionally difficult
  - Increased risk of DIC after 3 weeks
  - Observe for onset of
    - Fever
    - DIC
    - ROM or labor
- Surgical D & E in early pregnancy
- Induction of labor
  - Laminaria or Foley catheter
  - Prostin E2 suppositories
  - Misoprostol 50–100 µg per vagina or po
  - Oxytocin drip after 32 weeks gestation

Providing Treatment:
Alternative Measures to Consider

- Natural remedies to stimulate labor
  - May not be effective before 32 weeks
  - Blue/black cohosh infusion or tincture
  - Castor oil
- Homeopathic caulophyllum thal

Providing Support:
Education and Support Measures to Consider

- Cause of death if known
- Options for birth
  - Discussion regarding labor initiation
    - Maternal preferences
    - Parameters for consultation
    - Therapeutic measures to initiate labor
  - Location for birth
  - Anticipated course of events
- Care of the body
  - May vary with gestational age
  - Family time
  - Autopsy or testing
  - Burial, cremation, or hospital disposal
- Funeral or memorial service
- Postpartum period
  - Lochia
  - Lactation suppression
- Depression
  - Support groups and community resources

Follow-up Care:
Follow-up Measures to Consider

- Document
  - Maternal response
  - Course of labor and birth

- Anomalies if any
- Care and arrangements for the fetus
- Placental disposition
- Planned follow-up
- Follow-up care
  - Weeks 1–6
    - Phone, home, or office visit
    - Results of any testing
    - Evaluation of emotional status
  - Weeks 2–6
    - Postpartum check
    - Initiation of birth control prn
    - Support

Collaborative Practice:

Consider Consultation or Referral

- For social support
  - Grief counseling
  - Support groups
- Medical/Obstetrical care
  - For fetal demise > 12 weeks gestation
  - For evidence of DIC
  - For mother who prefers surgical D & E in early pregnancy
  - For induction of labor as indicated by
    - Midwifery scope of practice
    - Maternal preference or condition
  - For diagnosis outside the midwife's scope of practice

Care of the Pregnant Woman Exposed to Fifth's Disease

Key Clinical Information

Fifth's disease is caused by the parvovirus B19. It causes childhood erythema infectiosum. It is spread by droplet, most often in the springtime. Viremia occurs 7 days after inoculation and lasts 4 days. It is common to have women who are school teachers find that their students have Fifth's disease. Fortunately, most women contract Fifth's disease as children and are not at risk for primary infection during pregnancy (*Division of Maternal-Fetal Medicine Newsletter*, 1997). Parvovirus infection during pregnancy may result in fetal hydrops, aplastic anemia, or IUGR.

Client History:
Components of the History to Consider

- Current gestation
- Blood type and Rh
- Rubella and rubeola titers
- History of recent outbreak with close contact
  - School teachers
  - Health care workers
- Symptoms of parvovirus infection
  - Rash
  - Fever
  - Malaise
  - Myalgia, arthralgia

Physical Examination:
Components of the Physical Exam to Consider

- Vital signs, including temp
- Routine prenatal surveillance
- Evaluate for
  - Rash
    - Diffuse maculopapular rash
    - Trunk and extremities
    - Occurs 16 days postinoculation
    - 5 days postresolution of virus
  - Joint and muscle pain

Clinical Impression:
Differential Diagnoses to Consider

- Fifth's disease (parvovirus B19)
- Other viral exanthema
- Allergic rash

Diagnostic Testing:
Diagnostic Tests and Procedures to Consider

- Serologic testing for parvovirus B19
  - Indicated for
    - Postexposure
    - Positive clinical signs and symptoms
    - Fetal nonimmune hydrops
  - Parvovirus B19 IgM & IgG
    - + IgM indicates recent infection
    - + IgG indicates current immunity
- AFP—As indicated by gestation
- Level II ultrasound
  - Fetal cardiac evaluation
  - Fetal hydrops

Providing Treatment:
Therapeutic Measures to Consider

- No treatment available

Providing Treatment:
Alternative Measures to Consider

- For possible exposure consider
  - Rest
  - Immune support
    - Whole foods diet, avoiding processed foods
    - Echinacea tincture 30 gtts tid × 10–14 days followed by resting period of 7 days (Foster, 1996)

Providing Support:
Education and Support Measures to Consider

- Reassure: Most adults are immune

- Explain screening and management plan

- Warning signs to report

  ○ Rash

  ○ Decreased fetal movement

- Potential for fetal compromise with infection

  ○ May have no effect

  ○ Spontaneous abortion in 1st trimester

  ○ Fetal death 2nd trimester (3–6 weeks postmaternal infection)

  ○ Nonimmune hydrops

  ○ Severe anemia

  ○ Viral-induced cardiomyopathy

- May elevate AFP

- No association of parvovirus B19 and birth defects

Follow-up Care:
Follow-up Measures to Consider

- Document

- Testing

  ○ Positive IgG: No further testing (immune)

  ○ Negative IgG: Repeat IgG in 3–4 weeks (Varney, et al., 2004)

- Return for care

  ○ 2–3 weeks postexposure

  ○ Onset of signs or symptoms

- Mother with acute illness

  ○ Follow for hydrops

    ▪ Weekly ultrasound × 12 weeks

  ○ Provide emotional support

Collaborative Practice:
Consider Consultation or Referral

- Maternal infection with parvovirus B19

- Fetus with evidence of

  ○ Hydrops

  ○ Anemia

  ○ Cardiomyopathy

  ○ Fetal demise

- For diagnosis outside the midwife's scope of practice

Care of the Pregnant Woman with Gestational Diabetes

Key Clinical Information

Gestational diabetes occurs in 4–7% of all pregnant women in the United States (ADA, 2003). There is s significant increase in fetal malformations in pregnant women with persistently elevated glucose levels. This risk is noted to be higher for women with Hgb A1c levels that are elevated early in pregnancy compared to those pregnant women whose Hgb A1c levels are normal in spite of abnormal glucose metabolism.

It is especially important to enlist the participation of the mother when gestational diabetes presents. Daily attention to diet is imperative, with food sources providing excellent nutrition and a balance of proteins, fats, and complex carbohydrates. A food diary can be very helpful in determining what foods are preferred by the client and making recommendations for changes that are culturally and financially reasonable.

Client History:
Components of the History to Consider

- G, P, gestational age

- Identify risk factors for GDM

  ○ Maternal age > 35

  ○ BMI > 25 kg/m2

Table 4-2 Screening and Diagnostic Testing for Gestational Diabetes

DOSE/TIME	PLASMA
Fasting—Normal glucose metabolism	< 105 gm/dl
Fasting hyperglycemia	> 105 < 126 gm/dl
Diagnostic of GDM—Fasting	> 126 gm/dl
Diagnostic of GDM—Nonfasting	> 200 gm/dl
50 gm glucose challenge test (GCT) 1 hr	130–140 gm/dl
100 gm glucose tolerance test (GTT) fasting	> 95 gm/dl
100 gm glucose tolerance test (GTT) 1 hr	> 180 gm/dl
100 gm glucose tolerance test (GTT) 2 hr	> 155 gm/dl
100 gm glucose tolerance test (GTT) 3 hr	> 140 gm/dl

Source: ADA, 2003.

- Previous FBS 110–125 mg/dl
- Suspected or documented previous GDM
  - Previous infant weighing > 4100 g
- Previous unexplained fetal demise
- Polyhydramnios
- Previous birth of a child with a congenital anomaly
- Ethnic heritage
  - African
  - Alaskan native
  - Hispanic
  - Native American
  - South or East Asian
  - Pacific Islands
- Family history of diabetes
- Symptoms of GDM
  - Glycosuria
  - Preeclampsia or chronic hypertension
  - Polyhydramnios

Physical Examination: Components of the Physical Exam to Consider

- VS, including weight
- Body mass index (BMI)
- Weight gain
- Monitor fundal heights
  - IUGR
  - Fetal macrosomia
  - Polyhydramnios

Clinical Impression: Differential Diagnoses to Consider

- Gestational diabetes
- Abnormal glucose metabolism
- Diabetes mellitus
- Fetal macrosomia secondary to
  - Gestational diabetes
  - Constitutionally large fetus
- Polyhydramnios

Diagnostic Testing:
Diagnostic Tests and Procedures to Consider

- Dip U/A for glucose at each prenatal visit
- Screening women *with* risk factors
    - First visit or first trimester
    - 24–28 weeks
    - 34–36 weeks
    - Onset of
        - Glucosuria
        - Macrosomia
        - Polyhydramnios
        - Pregnancy-induced hypertension
- Screening women *without* risk factors
    - 24–28 weeks
    - Testing with indications only
- No screening option for women who meet *all* of the following criteria
    - Age < 25 years
    - Normal BMI before pregnancy
    - Member of an ethnic group with a low prevalence of GDM
    - No known diabetes in first-degree relatives
    - No history of abnormal glucose tolerance
    - No history of poor obstetric outcome
- Screening methods
    - Fasting blood sugar (FBS)
    - One-hour glucose challenge test (GCT)
- If screen is elevated
    - Obtain 3-hour glucose tolerance test (GTT)
    - Consider Hgb A1c testing
- Diagnosis
    - Elevated fasting or random glucose
    - Two or more elevated blood levels in 3-hour GTT
- Maternal assessment
    - Hgb A1C

- Normal range: 4.0–8.2%
- < 6% preferable in pregnancy
    - Self-monitored blood glucose
        - All values within target range
        - Before meal and bedtime: 60 to 95 mg/dl
        - After meal
- < 120 mg/dl 2 hours after start of meal
- < 140 mg/dl 1 hour after start of meal
- Ultrasound for fetal anomalies

Providing Treatment:
Therapeutic Measures to Consider

- Dietary control
    - Caloric intake by weight
        - Underweight—40 Kcal/Kg/day
        - Average weight—30 Kcal/Kg/day
        - Overweight—24 Kcal/Kg/day
    - 6 small meals daily
        - Carbohydrates 55–60% of diet
        - Protein 12–20% of diet
        - Fat for the remainder (ADA, 2003)
- Medications
    - Glyburide (pregnancy category B)
        - Use after organogenesis
        - Consult for use and dosage
    - Initiate insulin 2-hour postprandial glucose > 120 mg/dl (ACOG, 2001)
        - Consult for use and dosages
        - Titrate to maintain glycemic control
            - FBS > 95mg/dl
            - 1-hour postprandial values >130–140 mg/dl

Providing Treatment:
Alternative Measures to Consider

- Macrobiotic or whole food diet
- Herbs

- Bilberry (Foster, 1996)
- Chicory
- Dandelion
- Nettle
- Red raspberry tea (Weed, 1985)

Providing Support:
Education and Support Measures to Consider

- Risks and benefits of options for care
- Diabetic education
  - American Diabetes Association
    - 1-800-342-2383 or e-mail askADA@diabetes.org
    - ADA publication # 4902-04 *Gestational Diabetes:What To Expect*, 4th Edition
  - Dietary control
    - Dietary recommendations for GDM
    - Physical activity recommendations
  - Medication instruction, if used
  - Daily home glucose monitoring (International Diabetes Center, 2003)
    - Meter with memory and log book
    - 6 to 7 times/day preferred until control established
      - Before and 1 to 2 hours after start of meals
      - Bedtime
    - 4 times/week minimum
      - Fasting
      - 1 to 2 hours after start of meals .
- Warning signs and symptoms
  - Decreased fetal movement
  - S/S hypoglycemia

Follow-up Care:
Follow-up Measures to Consider

- Document
- Prenatal follow up
  - Maternal and fetal evaluation
  - Blood glucose follow up
    - Evaluate result biweekly
    - Office or lab testing for validation of
      - Home monitoring results
      - Glycemic control
    - Medication use
- Fetal assessment
  - Fetal kick counts begin at 28 weeks
  - Ultrasound
    - 28–32 weeks: Begin serial U/S for
      - Asymmetric IUGR
      - Macrosomia
  - NST weekly beginning at 34 weeks
  - Biophysical profile
- Labor plan
  - Consider induction of labor at 37–38 weeks
    - Client on insulin therapy
    - Fetal macrosomia
    - Poor or marginal control
    - Based on tests for fetal well-being
  - Plan birth at facility with newborn special care
    - Anticipate RDS
  - If the EFW > 4500 grams, C/S may decrease the likelihood of brachial plexus injury in the infant (ACOG, 2001)
  - Plan for pediatric care at birth
- Postpartum follow-up
  - FBS & 2 hr pp blood sugar × 7days (International Diabetes Center, 2003)
    - Evaluate ASAP for DM with
      - FBS > 120 mg/dl, or
      - 2 hr pp bs > 160 mg/dl
  - Fasting blood sugar at 6 weeks postpartum
  - > 126 mg/dl diagnostic of DM

Collaborative Practice:
Consider Consultation or Referral

- Nutrition education and counseling
- Social services, as indicated
- Medical, obstetric or pediatric care
  - Gestational diabetic not controlled by diet
    - Initiation of insulin or glyburide
    - Ongoing medication dosage requirements
  - Fetal macrosomia, IUGR, or anomalies
  - Newborn care at birth
- For diagnosis outside the midwife's scope of practice

Care of the Pregnant Woman with Hepatitis

Key Clinical Information

Hepatitis includes a range of viral illnesses that may be transmitted via blood or body fluids. Vertical transmission of hepatitis B, C, E, and G may occur to the fetus during pregnancy. Up to 90% of babies born to hepatitis B infected mothers will be infected without treatment shortly after birth. Infected infants may become chronic carriers, or develop significant illness. Infected women may present with acute illness, or they may be chronic carriers: asymptomatic but able to transmit infection (CDC, 2002).

Client History:
Components of the History to Consider

- LMP, EDC, gestational age
- Immunization status—Hepatitis B
- Potential exposure to hepatitis
  - Health care professional
  - IV drug use, shared needles
  - Sexual contacts
  - Presence of tattoos
  - Ingestion of raw shellfish

- Hemodialysis patients
- Blood or organ recipient prior to 1992
- Immigrants from
  - Asia
  - Africa
  - Pacific Islands
  - Haiti
- Presence, onset and duration, and severity of symptoms
  - Malaise and lethargy
  - Fever and chills
  - Right upper quadrant pain
  - Jaundice
  - Nausea and vomiting (CDC, 2002)

Physical Examination:
Components of the Physical Exam to Consider

- VS, including weight
- Examine for evidence of jaundice
  - Skin
  - Mucous membranes
  - Sclera
- Palpate and percuss for
  - Liver margins
  - Splenomegaly
  - RUQ pain

Clinical Impression:
Differential Diagnoses to Consider

- Hepatitis B
- Hepatitis A
- Hepatitis C
- Cholestasis of pregnancy
- Obstructive cholelithiasis
- Other liver disorders

Diagnostic Testing:
Diagnostic Tests and Procedures to Consider

- Hepatitis B
  - Surface antibody; immunized individuals
  - Surface antigen; nonimmunized individuals
- Hepatitis profile, multiple antigen/antibody screen
- Liver function testing (LFTs)
  - SGOT (AST), SGPT (ALT), LDH, bilirubin
  - Elevation occurs during acute phase (CDC, 2002)
- Ultrasound, RUQ
  - Gallbladder (CDC, 2002)

Providing Treatment:
Therapeutic Measures to Consider

- Illness must run its course
- Supportive therapy for mother
- Consider immunization series
  - For at-risk noninfected women
  - May be used during pregnancy
  - Hepatitis B (pregnancy category C)
  - Hepatitis A (pregnancy category C)

Providing Treatment:
Alternative Measures to Consider

- Whole foods diet with minimum toxins
- Herbs
  - Milk thistle tea (Foster, 1996)
  - Silymarin 420 µg (from milk thistle) tid × 6 weeks (Wellington and Jarvis, 2001)
- Adequate rest

Providing Support:
Education and Support Measures to Consider

- Provide information about hepatitis
  - Transmission and prevention
  - Medication recommendations for infant
  - Breastfeeding
    - Not contraindicated for immunized infant
    - Not recommended for nonimmunized infant
- Discussion regarding
  - Options for care of self and infant
  - Location for birth
  - Parameters for referral

Follow-up Care:
Follow-up Measures to Consider

- Document
- Return for care
  - Per routine for carrier
  - Weekly for acute phase of infection
    - Periodic LFTs
    - Fetal evaluation with acute illness
- Administer to infant born to hepatitis B+ mother
  - Hepatitis B immune globulin
    - 0.5 ml IM in anterior thigh within 12 hrs of birth
  - Hepatitis B vaccine
    - Engerix-B 10 mcg/0.5ml
    - Recombivax HB 5 mcg/0.5ml (Murphy, 2004)
    - IM in anterior thigh shortly after birth
    - Repeat in 1 and 6 mo (CDC, 2002)

Collaborative Practice:
Consider Consultation or Referral

- Epidemiological support
- Medical care
  - Acute hepatitis, any type
  - Hepatitis C to hepatitis specialist
- Pediatric care provider consult

○ Prior to birth

○ Collaborative plan for newborn care

• For diagnosis outside the midwife's scope of practice

Care of the Pregnant Woman with Herpes Simplex Virus

Key Clinical Information

Infection of the infant with the herpes simplex virus (HSV) varies with the incidence of primary versus secondary infection. When primary infection with HSV occurs during pregnancy the perinatal infection rate may be as high as 50%. With secondary, or recurrent, HSV infection during pregnancy the perinatal infection rate diminishes to approximately 4%. Up to 60% of infants who are infected as a result of primary maternal infection will die from severe neonatal HSV, and the mother may be asymptomatic in up to 70% of instances where the infant is infected (Emmons, Callahan, Gorman, & Snyder, 1997).

Client History: Components of the History to Consider

• LMP, EDC, gestational age

• Current sexual history

• Previous history of

○ Genital or oral herpes

○ Other STIs

• Duration and quality of present symptoms

○ Location and number of vesicular lesions

▪ Oral

▪ Genital

○ Symptoms

▪ Pain

▪ Tingling

▪ Dysuria

• Primary infection associated with

○ Fever

○ Headache and photophobia

○ Malaise

○ Aseptic meningitis (CDC, 2002)

Physical Examination: Components of the Physical Exam to Consider

• VS, including temperature

• Usual prenatal evaluation

• Physical evaluation with emphasis on

○ Oral examination

○ Inguinal lymph nodes

▪ Enlargement

▪ Tenderness

○ External genitalia, buttocks, and pelvic region

○ Characteristic lesions

▪ Vesicles

▪ Shallow ulcers

• Speculum exam, prn

○ Presence of other STD symptoms

○ Cervical discharge

○ Cervical or uterine motion tenderness

Clinical Impression: Differential Diagnoses to Consider

• Herpes simplex infection (HSV)

○ Primary

○ Recurrent

• Other STI

• Genital trauma

Diagnostic Testing: Diagnostic Tests and Procedures to Consider

• Culture lesions for HSV (Quest Diagnostics, n.d.)

• Consider serum testing for HSV antibody titer. (CDC, 2002)

○ Documents primary infection

- ○ Repeat 7–10 days
- ○ Four-fold increase = primary infection (Fife, et al., 2004)
- Other SDI testing
  - ○ With symptoms
  - ○ As indicated by history

Providing Treatment: Therapeutic Measures to Consider

- Valtrex (valacyclovir hydrochloride)
  - ○ Pregnancy category B
  - ○ Pregnancy registry 1-800-722-9292 ext. 39437
  - ○ Dose: 500 μg bid × 5 days
  - ○ Begin medication within 24 hours of first symptom
- Famvir (famciclovir)
  - ○ Pregnancy category B
  - ○ Dose: 125 μg bid × 5 days
  - ○ Begin medication within 6 hours of first symptom
- Zovirax (Acyclovir)
  - ○ Pregnancy category C
  - ○ Pregnancy registry 1-800-722-9292 ext. 58465
  - ○ Topical ointment 5%
    - Apply 3 × day × 7 days
    - Initial outbreak
  - ○ 200 μg po 5 × day × 10 days
  - ○ Recurrent outbreak
    - 200 μg po 5 × day × 7 days
    - Repeat treatment prn
  - ○ Suppression or severe recurrent outbreaks
    - 400 μg po bid × 6–12 mo. (CDC, 2002)
- Acetaminophen (Tylenol) for pain relief

Providing Treatment: Alternative Measures to Consider

- Lysine
  - ○ 1000 μg po bid × 3 months
  - ○ Combine with vitamin C 500 mg
  - ○ Begin with first sign of an outbreak
- Dietary recommendations
  - ○ *Include* foods high in lysine
    - Brewer's yeast
    - Potatoes
    - Fish (Weed, 1985)
  - ○ *Avoid* foods high in arginine
    - Chocolate, coffee, cola
    - Peanuts, cashews, pecans, almonds
    - Sunflower and sesame seeds
    - Peas and corn
    - Coconut
    - Gelatin
- Garlic
  - ○ Antiviral properties
  - ○ Combine with sea vegetable for trace minerals (Weed, 1985)
- Echinacea
  - ○ Tea, tincture, tablets, or capsules
  - ○ tid × 2 weeks
  - ○ Some sources contraindicate internal use during pregnancy.
- Sitz bath or salve made with
  - ○ Lemon balm
  - ○ Calendula
  - ○ Comfrey

Providing Support: Education and Support Measures to Consider

- Information about herpes (HSV) infection
  - ○ CDC STI Hotline 1-800-227-8922

○ American Social Health Association www.ashastd.org

○ Potential effects for

- Pregnancy

- Anticipated location for birth

- Newborn

- Labor and birth plans

- Potential for Cesarean birth

• Discussion regarding

○ Treatment options

○ Labor and birth options

○ Maternal preferences

○ Midwife recommendations

• Rest and comfort measures

○ With initial outbreak

○ To enhance immune response

Follow-up Care:
Follow-up Measures to Consider

• Document

• Return for care

○ Per routine with history of herpes

○ For culture with active lesion

○ Primary herpes

- If symptoms persist > 10 days

- Worsening symptoms

• Stiff neck

• Unremitting fever

• Inability to urinate

• Labor care

○ Vaginal birth

- No active lesion

- Active lesion remote from genital region

• Occlusive dressing applied

- Limit cervical exams

- Avoid use of scalp electrode or IUPC

○ C/S recommended for active genital lesion

- Prior to ROM

- ASAP w/ PROM

- May delay with PPROM for steroid therapy

Collaborative Practice:
Consider Consultation or Referral

• For symptoms of herpes meningitis

• For collaborative labor plan

○ Presence of active lesion

○ Potential for Cesarean birth

• For pediatric follow-up post-HSV exposure (CDC, 2002)

• For diagnosis or treatment outside the midwife's scope of practice

Care of the Pregnant Woman Who Is HIV Positive

Key Clinical Information

HIV testing is recommended for every pregnant woman whose current HIV status is unknown. Many women feel threatened by the thought of HIV testing. Many states require HIV-specific pretest counseling and documentation of informed consent prior to test specimen collection. Early testing allows for prompt evaluation and the potential for antiretroviral medication, which may decrease the incidence of perinatal transmission of the infection from 13–30% to 2–8%. Vertical transmission may be reduced in babies who reach term, are appropriate weight for gestation, and are born by Cesarean. Women who are at risk for HIV infection may require additional testing during the pregnancy (Allen, 2001).

Client History:
Components of the History to Consider

• LMP, EDC, gestational age

• GYN and sexual history

- Previous HIV testing
- Number of sexual partners
- Self and/or partner(s)
  - Sexual practices
  - STIs
  - Substance abuse
    - IV drug use
    - Other substance use
  - Blood transfusions
- Abnormal pap smears
- History of opportunistic infections
  - Presence of current symptoms
    - Malaise
    - Fever
    - Cough
    - Skin lesions

Physical Examination:
Components of the Physical Exam to Consider

- VS, including temperature
- HEENT
  - Fundoscopic exam
  - Oral exam for thrush or lesions
- Skin lesions
- Respiratory system
  - Cough
  - Adventitious breath sounds
  - SOB
  - Night sweats
- Liver margins
- Lymph nodes
  - Characteristics of enlarged nodes
  - Location(s) of enlarged nodes
- Pelvic exam
  - Internal or external lesions
  - Symptoms of STIs

Clinical Impression:
Differential Diagnoses to Consider

- HIV infection
- AIDS
- STIs

Diagnostic Testing:
Diagnostic Tests and Procedures to Consider

- Pap smear
- Wet mount
- Toxoplasmosis titer
- CMV titer
- Herpes culture
- CD4 and viral load q trimester
- Liver function tests
- PPD

Providing Treatment:
Therapeutic Measures to Consider

- New onset antiretroviral therapy
  - Delay onset until after first trimester unless needed for maternal health (Burdge, et al., 2003)
    - Diminishes drug-related teratogenicity
    - Improve adherence once early nausea has passed (U.S. Public Health Service Task Force, 2004)
  - Use current facility guidelines for medication regimen
  - Management of side effects is important to maximize adherence
- Established antiretroviral therapy
- Modified antiretroviral treatment for perinatal prophylaxis
  - Intrapartum therapy
- Initiation of other therapies based on diagnosis

Providing Treatment:
Alternative Measures to Consider

- Supportive measures
- Most immune stimulating herbs *not* recommended
- Cautious use of herbals/homeopathic remedies for
  - Appetite stimulation
  - Skin integrity
  - Emotional and spiritual balance

Providing Support:
Education and Support Measures to Consider

- Provide information, listening, and discussion regarding
  - HIV and AIDS
  - Prevention and transmission
  - Benefits of testing
  - Viral load evaluation and significance
    - Perinatal transmission
    - Potential effects on baby
  - Medication and treatment options
    - Antiretroviral medication (for self and/or baby)
      - Benefits
      - Risks
      - Side effects
      - Alternatives
- Lifestyle issues
  - Encourage
    - Abstinence, *or*
    - Consistent condom use
    - Avoid shared needles

Follow-up Care:
Follow-up Measures to Consider

- Document
- Informed consent for testing

- Laboratory results
- Maternal response to
  - Diagnosis
  - Treatment recommendations
- Discussions
  - Client preferences
  - Consultations and referrals
  - Anticipated location for birth
- Follow-up care
  - Coordinate testing with primary care provider/site
  - Pediatric consult for newborn care and follow-up
  - Register with the CDC Antiretroviral Pregnancy Registry
    - 800-258-4263
    - http://www.apregistry.com
  - Observe for side effects of medications
    - May cause hepatic toxicity
    - May mimic HELLP syndrome
- Return visits
  - As indicated by prenatal course and gestation
  - For support

Collaborative Practice:
Consider Consultation or Referral

- Social support services
  - Support groups
  - Mental health referrals
  - Victim advocacy groups
  - Clean needle programs
  - Substance abuse treatment options
- Medical services
  - For all newly diagnosed HIV-positive women
  - For coordination of antiretroviral regimen
  - For HIV-positive women with
    - Onset of infection

- Decrease in CD4 cell counts
- Significant medication side effects
- For diagnosis or treatment outside the midwife's scope of practice

Inadequate Weight Gain

Key Clinical Information

Inadequate weight gain may indicate a number of medical problems. The most common cause, however, is inadequate nutrition, which may be related to poverty, substance abuse, or mental illness. Women with a history of anorexia or bulimia may have difficulty maintaining adequate intake to support growth of a healthy baby (Peery, n.d.). Overweight women may require fewer calories during pregnancy, while still demonstrating an adequate fundal growth pattern. Evaluation of fundal growth and fetal activity provide the most reliable low-tech parameters of fetal well-being when maternal weight gain is modest.

Client History: Components of the History to Consider

- LMP, EDC, gestational age
- Accuracy of LMP
- Nutritional assessment
  - Preferred diet and portion size
  - Food sources available
  - Use of enemas and laxatives
- Physical health issues
  - Activity level and general metabolic rate
  - Presence of symptoms
    - Nausea and vomiting
    - Constipation
    - Abdominal pain
    - Pica
- Prior health history, such as
  - Presence of maternal illness or infection
  - GI disorders

- Hyperthyroid
- Hepatitis
- Emotional and spiritual health issues
  - Family and personal support for pregnancy
    - Social living conditions
    - Physical abuse
  - Stress levels and coping skills
    - Physical response to stress
    - Anorexia or bulimia
  - Other mental health issues
- Substance abuse

Physical Examination: Components of the Physical Exam to Consider

- VS, including height and weight
- BMI and weight distribution
  - Prepregnancy weight
  - Interval gain
- Abdominal exam
  - Fundal height
    - For gestation
    - Fundal height growth curve
  - Bowel sounds
  - Palpation of abdomen
- Dental/oral evaluation
  - Caries
  - Abscess
- Evaluation of other symptoms

Clinical Impression: Differential Diagnoses to Consider

- Constitutionally small mother/fetus
- Small for gestational age baby
- Intrauterine growth retardation
- Malnutrition, secondary to conditions such as
  - Homelessness

- Physical abuse
- Poverty
- Substance abuse
- Physical abuse
- Eating disorder
- Mental illness

Diagnostic Testing:
Diagnostic Tests and Procedures to Consider

- Labs
  - PIH labs
  - Toxicology if drug use suspected
  - Cotenine levels (smokers)
  - TSH
  - Serum albumin
  - Hepatitis screen
- Fetal kick counts
- Ultrasound for
  - Gestational age
  - Interval fetal growth
  - Evidence of IUGR
  - AFI

Providing Treatment:

Therapeutic Measures to Consider

- Diet and nutrition counseling
  - Minimum of 1000 cal/day up to 2400 cal/day
  - Explore suitable food choices
    - Adequate protein, fat, and carbs
    - Culturally acceptable foods
    - Use of dietary supplements
- Consider hospitalization for
  - Malnutrition
  - Anorexia or bulimia
  - Significant mental illness

Providing Treatment:
Alternative Measures to Consider

- Dietary supplements
  - Spirulina (Weed, 1985)
  - Smoothies
  - Energy bars
- Homeopathic pulsatilla
  - For persistent nausea
  - Intolerance of fatty foods (Smith, 1984)
- Herbal appetite stimulants
  - May be combined for flavor and effectiveness
  - Alfalfa 500 µg daily (avoid with lupus or allergies to pollen)
  - Dandelion root tea 1 cup bid (avoid with hx gallstones)
  - Hops tea 1–2 cups daily
  - Chamomile tea 1–2 cups daily

Providing Support:
Education and Support Measures to Consider

- Provide information about
  - Weight gain and fetal growth pattern
  - Anticipated weight gain for gestation
    - IUGR babies
    - Small for gestational age babies
    - Constitutionally small babies
- Fetal kick counts
- Warning signs, such as
  - Decreased fetal motion
  - PIH signs and symptoms
- Potential effect on
  - Planned location for birth
  - Potential need for pediatric care at birth
- Importance of
  - Fundal/fetal growth over weight gain

- ○ Maternal and fetal well-being
- ○ Dietary needs during pregnancy
  - Small frequent meals
  - Balanced selection of food choices
  - Adequate caloric intake
- Provide support
  - ○ Develop plan with client
  - ○ Address client and family concerns

Follow-up Care:
Follow-up Measures to Consider

- Document
- Reevaluate weekly or biweekly for
  - ○ Interval fetal growth
  - ○ Signs and symptoms of PIH
- Address client concerns and preferences
  - ○ Nutritional counseling
  - ○ Emotional issues
- Parameters for consultation or referral

Collaborative Practice:
Consider Consultation or Referral

- Nutritional counseling
- Social service referral
- Obstetric/pediatric service
  - ○ For persistent poor weight gain accompanied by
    - Lagging fetal growth
    - Asymmetric fetal growth
    - PIH
  - ○ For transfer of care or change planned location of birth
- Medical service
  - ○ Evidence of malnutrition
  - ○ Suspected or documented
    - Mental health issues

- Medical illness
- For diagnosis or treatment outside the midwife's scope of practice

Hypertensive Disorders in Pregnancy
Key Clinical Information

Hypertensive disorders of pregnancy encompasses a broad category of conditions that includes hypertension, severe hypertension, gestational hypertension, preeclampsia, eclampsia, and HELLP syndrome. Differential diagnosis can be challenging as pregnancy-induced hypertension (PIH) may present with an uncommon array of symptoms. Onset of clinical signs and symptoms suggesting PIH should always prompt careful evaluation in order to have the opportunity to institute early treatment. Lab testing is the most reliable way to assess a woman's potential for development of PIH. Treatment improves the likelihood of the pregnancy resulting in a healthy mother, healthy baby, and it increases the potential for a vaginal birth (NIH, 2000).

Client History:
Components of the History to Consider

- LMP, EDC, gestational age
- Presence, onset, and durations of symptoms
- Evaluate for PIH risk factors (Wagner, 2004)
  - ○ Primigravida (6–8x risk)
  - ○ Multipara with previous PIH
  - ○ Maternal age < 20 and > 35
  - ○ Multiple gestation (5x risk)
  - ○ Hydatidiform mole (10x risk)
  - ○ Fetal hydrops (10x risk)
  - ○ Preexisting medical disorders
    - Essential hypertension
    - Diabetes mellitus
    - Collagen vascular disease

Table 4-3   Evaluating Hypertension in Pregnancy

HYPERTENSIVE DISORDER	SIGNS AND SYMPTOMS	CRITERIA FOR DIAGNOSIS
Chronic hypertension May be mild, moderate, or severe	Predates 20th week of pregnancy. May have cardiac enlargement, vascular changes, renal insufficiency	BP ≥ 140/90 mild/mod BP ≥ 170/110 severe 2 or more BP elevations > 4 hrs apart
Preeclampsia PIH, mild	Gestational age of ≥ 20 weeks Onset of: Elevated BP Proteinuria Elevated reflexes Fundal heights small for dates Elevated Hgb secondary to hemoconcentration Elevated serum uric acid (normal range 1.2–4.5 mg/dl)	Hypertension after 20 weeks: 1. Systolic ≥ 140 mm/hg, *or* 2. Diastolic ≥ 90 mm/hg 3. On 2 occasions ≥ 6 hrs apart New onset proteinuria: 1. 1–2+ dip, on 2. 2 specimens, in 3. Absence of UTI, *or* 4. ≥ 300 mg in 24 hr urine
Preeclampsia PIH, severe	Signs of mild PIH, plus: 1. Clonus 2. Diminished renal function (elevated BUN, diminished urinary output, serum creatinine > 1.2 mg/dl, decreased creatine clearance) 3. Headache 4. Visual disturbances 5. Epigastric discomfort 6. IUGR by ultrasound Oligohydramnios May have onset of: 1. HELLP syndrome 2. Eclampsia 3. Pulmonary edema	Hypertension: 1. Systolic ≥ 160 mm/hg 2. Diastolic ≥ 110 mm/hg 3. 2 readings ≥ 6 hrs apart Proteinuria: 1. New onset, or 2. 3–4+ dip 3. ≥ 2 Gm in 24 hr urine
Eclampsia	Grand mal seizure(s) Fetal distress Placental abruption	Gestational hypertension with seizure that is responsive to initiation of $MgSO_4$ therapy
HELLP Syndrome	Epigastric pain General malaise Abnormal coagulation profile (low fibrinogen, prolonged prothrombin time, prolonged partial prothrombin time)	Hemolysis of RBCs Elevated liver enzymes (AST, ALT, LDH) Low platelets (< 100,000)

Sources: Varney, et al., 2004; Sinclair, 2004; Roberts, 1994; NIH, 2000.

- Renal vascular disease
  - Renal parenchymal disease
- African-American or Asian heritage
- Social factors that may contribute to PIH
  - Poor nutrition
  - Tobacco use
  - Alcohol use
  - Excessive sodium intake
  - Current vasoactive drug use
    - Nasal decongestants
    - Cocaine
- Family history of PIH

Physical Examination:
Components of the Physical Exam to Consider

- Vital signs including BP and weight
- Weight: Patterns of gain
- Blood pressure evaluation
  - Two occasions > 4 hours apart
  - Allow a "rest" period following
    - Anxiety
    - Pain
    - Smoking
    - Exercise
  - Equipment of correct size should be used
  - Use same maternal position for each BP
  - Arm should be supported at level of the heart
- Evaluate extremities for
  - Presence or absence of edema
  - Deep tendon reflexes
- Abdominal exam
  - Fundal heights for evaluation of fetal growth
  - Liver margins
  - Epigastric pain
- Ophthalmic exam
  - Papilledema
  - Vessel narrowing
- Monitor pulmonary status

Clinical Impression:
Differential Diagnoses to Consider

- Pregnancy induced hypertension (PIH)
  - Preeclampsia
  - Eclampsia
- Transient hypertension
- Essential hypertension
- PIH superimposed on chronic hypertension
- HELLP syndrome

Diagnostic Testing:
Diagnostic Tests and Procedures to Consider

- Baseline PIH labs
- Note: *normal ranges may vary by lab*
  - Urine analysis for protein by dip
  - Hematocrit (normal range 10.5–14 g/dl)
  - Platelet count (normal range 130,000–400,000/ml)
  - Liver function tests
    - AST/SGOT (normal range 0–35 IU/L)
    - ALT/SGPT (normal range 5-35 IU/L)
    - LDH (normal range 0-250 IU/L)
- Coagulation studies
  - Fibrinogen
  - PT, PTT
- Renal function tests
  - Serum uric acid (normal range 1.2–4.5 mg/dl)
  - Serum albumin (normal range 2.5–4.5 g/dl)
  - Serum creatinine (normal range < 1.0 mg/dl)
  - BUN (7–25 mg/dl)
  - 24-hour urine for protein and creatinine

- Initiate based on symptoms, *or*
- When dip U/A shows > 1+ protein

- Fetal evaluation
  - Fetal kick counts—daily
  - NST and biophysical profile (NIH, 2000)
    - At diagnosis
    - Weekly
    - Biweekly for
      - AFI ≤ (5 cm)
      - EFW < 10th percentile for GA
    - Immediately with change in maternal condition (NIH, 2000)
- Ultrasound (NIH, 2000)
  - On diagnosis
  - q 3 weeks if normal
    - Amniotic fluid index
    - Fetal growth evaluation

Providing Treatment: Therapeutic Measures to Consider

- Increase calcium intake (1200 mg daily)
- Limit activity
- Low-dose aspirin therapy (Coomarasamy, Honest, Papaioannou, Gee, & Saeed Kahn, 2003)
  - For women with
    - High risk of preeclamsia
    - Chronic hypertension
    - Diabetes mellitus
    - Renal disease
  - 50–150 mg daily q hs
- Consider hospitalization
  - Bed rest not possible at home
  - Progressive signs and symptoms
- Medications for sustained BP of
  - ≥ 160 mm/Hg systolic, *or*

- ≥ 105 mm/Hg diastolic
- Hydralizine (NIH, 2000)
  - 5 mg IV or 10 mg IM
  - Repeat at 20 min intervals until BP stable
  - Repeat prn ≈ q 3 hr
  - Change med if no response by 20–30 mg
- Labetolol
  - 🔔 Do not use in women with asthma or CHF
  - 20 mg IV bolus
  - May give 40 mg IV in 10 min, followed by
    - 80 mg IV × 2 doses
    - Max dose 220 mg
  - Pregnancy category C
- Nifedipine
  - 10 mg po
  - Repeat in 30 minutes
- MgSO$_4$ Therapy
  - 4–6 gm bolus, slow IV
  - Followed by 2 gm/hr IV, *or*
  - 5 gm 50% MgSO$_4$ IM q 4 hr
  - Titrated to renal output and reflexes
    - Monitor
      - BP
      - Reflexes
      - Intake and output
      - Serum MgSO$_4$ levels
- Delivery if no improvement or condition worsens

Providing Treatment: Alternative Measures to Consider

- Balanced nutrition
  - No salt restriction
  - Whole foods diet
  - Adequate protein intake

- Garlic, 1 clove or the equivalent daily
- Cucumber, 1 daily
- Hops tea, 1 cup night in last month of pregnancy
- Hawthorn berries (Foster, 1996)
  - Best for chronic hypertension
  - Infusion: 1 cup daily
  - Tincture: 15 drops tid

Providing Support:
Education and Support Measures to Consider

- Discussion with client and family regarding
  - PIH
  - Treatment options and recommendations
  - Smoking cessation, prn
  - Drug treatment plans, if indicated
- Attention to
  - Diet
  - Rest
  - Low-key exercise with mild PIH
- Potential need for
  - Hospitalization
  - OB/GYN consultation/referral
  - Change in planned location for birth
  - Pediatric care at birth
  - Newborn special care after birth
- Indications for immediate care
  - Epigastric pain
  - Visual disturbance
  - Severe headache

Follow-up Care:
Follow-up Measures to Consider

- Document
  - Serum $MgSO_4$ 4 hrs post-initiation of therapy

- List parameters for consultation and referral
- Update plan weekly or as indicated
- Increased frequency of return visits
  - Fetal surveillance testing
  - Maternal evaluation/labs
  - Biweekly visits
  - Consider hospitalization for
    - Noncompliant client
    - Progressive signs
- Indications for delivery include
  - Gestational age > 38 weeks
  - Persistent or severe
    - Headache
    - Abdominal pain
  - Abnormal liver function tests
  - Rising serum creatinine
  - Thrombocytopenia
  - Pulmonary edema
  - Eclampsia
  - Abruptio placenta
  - Oligohydramnios
  - Nonreassuring fetal monitoring tracings
  - IUGR noted by ultrasound
  - Abnormal biophysical profile

Collaborative Practice:
Consider Consultation or Referral

- For chronic hypertension in pregnancy
- With diagnosis or suspicion of preeclampsia or PIH
- For any indications for delivery (see above)
- For diagnosis or treatment outside the midwife's scope of practice

Pruritic Urticarial Papules and Plaques of Pregnancy (PUPPP)

Key Clinical Information

Puritic uticarial papules and plaques of pregnancy is a form of urticaria that most commonly appears in the third trimester. It generally resolves within 7 days after the birth. There are no systemic disorders associated with PUPPP; therefore, treatment is aimed at relieving symptoms.

Client History:
Components of the History to Consider

- LMP, EDC, gestational age
  - Most often primipara
  - Third trimester
- Onset, duration, and severity of symptoms
  - Puritic papules begin in striae (Burkhart, 2000)
    - May have small vesicles
    - Severe itching
  - Pattern of spread
    - Abdomen and striae
    - Periumbilical area not involved
    - Trunk and limbs
    - Face, palms, and soles spared
- Other associated signs and symptoms
- Presence of allergies
  - Medications
  - Exposure to topical irritants
- Immune titers
- Exposure to viral infections
- Self-help remedies and their effects

Physical Examination:
Components of the Physical Exam to Consider

- VS, including temperature
- FHR

- Location and appearance of lesions
  - Erythematous, edematous papules
  - Urticarial plaques
  - May form papulovesicular lesions
- Evaluate prn for signs related to other differential diagnoses

Clinical Impression:
Differential Diagnoses to Consider

- PUPPPs
- Scabies
- Allergic dermatitis
  - Drug reaction
  - Poison ivy
- Impetigo
- Viral exanthema
- Herpes gestationis
- Erythema multiforme
- Cholestasis of pregnancy

Diagnostic Testing:
Diagnostic Tests and Procedures to Consider

- Evaluation of vesicular lesions
  - Herpes
  - Impetigo
  - Scabies skin prep
- Immune titers prn
  - Rubella
  - Rubeola
  - Varicella
- Liver function tests to evaluate for cholestasis
  - Alkaline phosphatase
  - Gamma glutamyl transferase

Providing Treatment:
Therapeutic Measures to Consider

- Topical antipuritic lotions
  - Calamine or caladryl (OTC)
  - Doxepin HCL 5% cream (pregnancy category B)
- Oral antihistamines
  - Diphenhydramine HCL (Benadryl)
    - 25–50 mg q 4–6 hrs
    - Pregnancy category B in third trimester
  - Loratadine (Claritin)
    - 10 mg daily
    - Pregnancy category B in third trimester
  - Cetirizine HCL (Zyrtec)
    - 5–10 mg daily
    - Pregnancy category B in third trimester
- Topical corticosteroids
  - Pregnancy category C
  - Rule out viral cause before using
    - Alclometasone dipropionate 0.05%
    - Aclovate cream or ointment
    - Hydrocortisone 1%
    - Cortisporin cream
    - Hytone cream, lotion, or ointment
    - Triamcinolone acetonide 0.025%, 0.1%, 0.5%
    - Aristocort cream
    - Kenalog cream, lotion, or ointment
- Oral steroid therapy
  - Prednisone 0.5–1 mg/kg/day po
    - Use minimum effective dose
    - Taper off when symptoms abate
  - Pregnancy category B
  - Use with caution in women with
    - Gestational diabetes
    - Hypertension (Murphy, 2004)

Providing Treatment:
Alternative Measures to Consider

- Topical relief of itching
  - Colloidal oatmeal baths
  - Calendula cream
- Herbal support
  - Yellow dock root
  - Dandelion root
- Homeopathic support
  - Cantharis
  - Rhus tox
  - Urticaria

Providing Support:
Education and Support Measures to Consider

- PUPPP not associated with fetal jeopardy
- Call if symptoms persist or worsen
- Address client concerns
- Treatment options
- Medication instructions
  - Topical steroids
    - Apply thin film only
    - Do not cover or occlude
    - May be systemically absorbed
  - Oral steroids
    - Take as directed
    - Do not stop suddenly

Follow-up Care:
Follow-up Measures to Consider

- Document
- Return for care
  - Per routine for prenatal care
  - If symptoms worsen or additional symptoms develop

Collaborative Practice:
Consider Consultation or Referral

- No relief of symptoms with treatment
- Rash accompanied by
  ○ Fever
  ○ Malaise
  ○ Rising titers
- Elevated liver function tests
- For diagnosis or treatment outside the midwife's scope of practice

Care of the Woman Who Is Rh Negative

Key Clinical Information

Rh isoimmunization or ABO incompatibility can have devastating results on both mother and baby. Infants are at risk when there is fetomaternal bleeding that initiates the process of Rh or ABO incompatibility, or if the mother became sensitized previously following blood transfusion. This may result from an Rh-positive infant that is born to an Rh-negative mother, a baby with type A or B blood born to a mother with type O blood, a baby with type B or type AB blood born to a mother with type A blood, or a baby with type A or AB blood born to a mother with type B blood.

Often the baby who is being carried when the fetomaternal bleed occurs may not have a problem, but the mother becomes sensitized. The problem will manifest itself in a subsequent pregnancy when maternal antibodies attack the fetal blood. Isoimmunization may result in fetal hydrops, congestive heart failure, and fetal anemia (Sinclair, 2004). The use of Rh immune globulin has significantly deceased the incidence of fetal isoimmunization and its sequelae.

Client History:
Components of the History to Consider

- Previous blood transfusions

- Prior obstetrical history
  ○ Unexplained fetal losses
  ○ Stillborn
  ○ Miscarriage
- Ectopic pregnancy
- Termination of pregnancy at > 8 weeks since LMP
- Rh immune globulin indicated for unsensitized Rh-negative client with
  ○ Amniocentesis
  ○ Chorionic villus sampling
  ○ External version
  ○ Trauma, such as a car accident
  ○ Placenta previa
  ○ Abruptio placenta
  ○ Fetal death
  ○ Multiple gestation
  ○ Cesarean section
  ○ 28 weeks gestation prophylaxis if father of baby is Rh positive or his Rh status is unknown
  ○ Accidental transfusion of Rh-positive blood to an Rh-negative person

Physical Examination:
Components of the Physical Exam to Consider

- Routine prenatal surveillance

Clinical Impression:
Differential Diagnoses to Consider

- Rh-negative mother
- Rh-sensitized mother
- ABO-sensitized mother

Diagnostic Testing:
Diagnostic Tests and Procedures to Consider

- Maternal—1st prenatal and repeat at 24–28 weeks for Rh-negative mothers

  ◦ Type and Rh factor

  ◦ Antibody screen (indirect Coombs)

  ◦ Antibody ID for positive antibody screen

  ◦ Early RhIG postamnio or threatened SAB may give positive titer at 24–28 week screen

- Maternal Test Results

  ◦ Titer < 1:8 anti-D—Suggests passive immunity from RhIG

  ◦ Titer > 1:8—Suggests active immunization due to Rh incompatibility

  ◦ Rh(D) negative, or type O mother

    ▪ Plan newborn follow-up

    ▪ Maternal follow-up postpartum

Providing Treatment:
Therapeutic Measures to Consider

- Offer Rh immune globulin (Pregnancy category C)

  ◦ Threatened or spontaneous miscarriage < 12 weeks give 50 *or* 300 μg IM

  ◦ Procedures or trauma give 300 μg IM

  ◦ 28–36 week prophylaxis give 300 μg IM with negative 28 week antibody screen

  ◦ Postpartum give 300 μg IM

    ▪ Provide to unsensitized Rh-negative mother with Rh-positive infant

    ▪ Give ASAP after birth, preferably within 72 hours postpartum

    ▪ Adjust dose for large fetomaternal transfusion based on lab results

- IV administration

  ◦ 9 μg RhIG/ml whole blood or 18 μg RhIG/ml of RBCs

  ◦ 800 μg q 8 hrs until total dose delivered

- IM administration

  ◦ 12 mgRhIG/ml whole blood or 24 mg RhIG/ml of RBCs

  ◦ 1200 mg q 12 hrs until total dose delivered (Moise, 2004)

Providing Treatment:
Alternative Measures to Consider

- Maintain a healthy pregnancy and placenta

  ◦ Well-balanced diet

  ◦ Decrease or eliminate fluoride intake (may interfere with placental attachment)

  ◦ Ensure adequate trace mineral intake

- Limit invasive procedures

- Avoid traumatic placental delivery

Providing Support:
Education and Support Measures to Consider

- Provide information about

  ◦ Rh and blood type status

  ◦ Rh immune globulin

  ◦ Prophylaxis and desired result

  ◦ Potential risks with Rh immune globulin

    ▪ Transfusion-type adverse reactions

    ▪ Mercury sensitivity or reaction with RhoGAM

  ◦ Potential risks without Rh immune globulin

    ▪ Maternal sensitization

    ▪ Fetal hydrops or other complications with future pregnancy

    ▪ Difficulty cross-matching blood for woman in future, e.g., following accident or surgery

    ▪ Potential for jaundice in infant due to Rh or ABO incompatibility

Follow-up Care:
Follow-up Measures to Consider

- Document
  - Indication for RhIG
  - Negative Rh and antibody status
  - Client education, discussion, and preferences
- Observe for potential blood transfusion-type reactions
  - Warmth at injection site
  - Low-grade fever
  - Flushing
  - Chest or lumbar pain
  - Poor clotting
- If mother is Rh(D) negative, or type O
  - Newborn
    - Type and Rh
    - Direct Coombs
    - Bilirubin levels
  - Maternal testing postpartum
    - Type and Rh
    - Antibody screen (indirect Coombs)
    - Antibody ID for positive antibody screen
    - Fetal red cell screen
- Kleihauer-Betke quantitative testing
  - Determine volume of fetal blood in maternal system and dosage of Rh IG to give mother
  - Performed when high risk of fetomaternal hemorrhage exists
    - Previa
    - Abruption
    - Abdominal trauma
    - Hydrops
    - Sinusoidal fetal heart rates
    - Unexplained fetal demise

Collaborative Practice:
Consider Consultation or Referral

- For Rh-negative mother with positive antibody screen
- Evidence of large fetomaternal bleed
- Transfusion-type reactions
- For diagnosis or treatment outside the midwife's scope of practice

Size–Date Discrepancy
Key Clinical Information

Size–date discrepancy has a multitude of potential contributing factors, with the most common causes including intrauterine growth retardation and gestational diabetes. Many babies, however, may simply be constitutionally small or large. Evaluation of overall interval fetal growth as well as the symmetry of growth can help determine the correct diagnosis.

Client History:
Components of the History to Consider

- LMP, EDC
- Verify gestational age
  - Estimated date of conception
  - Size at first visit
  - Date of quickening
  - Early U/S report
- OB history
  - Review fundal growth curve
  - Hypertension
  - Gestational diabetes
  - Birth weights of prior infants
- Social history
  - Diet and weight gain pattern
  - Maternal activity patterns
  - Tobacco, alcohol, or drug use

- ○ Poverty
- ○ Psychosocial factors
  - ▪ Stress
  - ▪ Mental illness
  - ▪ Abuse
- Family history
  - ○ Personal or family history of diabetes
  - ○ Hypertension
  - ○ Other preexisting disease
  - ○ 🉐 Ethnic norm for fetal weight
- Review of systems
  - ○ SOB, palpitations
  - ○ Signs or symptoms of illness
  - ○ Fetal activity

Physical Examination:
Components of the Physical Exam to Consider

- Vital signs including BP and BMI
- Weight gain/loss and pattern
- General appearance and well-being
- Palpation of thyroid
- Cardiopulmonary evaluation
- Abdominal exam
  - ○ Fundal height
  - ○ Interval growth
  - ○ Fetal lie
  - ○ FHR
- Extremities
  - ○ Reflexes
  - ○ Edema
  - ○ Physical evidence of substance abuse
- Pelvic exam
  - ○ Station of presenting part
  - ○ Evidence of ROM

Clinical Impression:
Differential Diagnoses to Consider

- Small for dates
  - ○ Incorrect dates
  - ○ Intrauterine growth retardation (IUGR)
  - ○ Small for gestational age (SGA)
  - ○ Oligohydramnios
  - ○ Constitutionally small infant
  - ○ Congenital malformations
- Large for dates
  - ○ Incorrect dates
  - ○ Large for gestational age (LGA)
  - ○ Gestational or maternal diabetes
  - ○ Multiple pregnancy
  - ○ Polyhydramnios
  - ○ Constitutionally large infant
  - ○ Fibroid uterus
- Symmetric vs. asymmetric IUGR secondary to
  - ○ Hypertension
  - ○ Underlying maternal disease or infection
  - ○ Poor nutrition

Diagnostic Testing:
Diagnostic Tests and Procedures to Consider

- Dip U/A
- Urine toxicology
- Diabetes screen
- MSAFP (may be elevated in early pregnancy)
- Maternal antiphospholipid antibody testing
- Maternal drug screen
- Symmetric IUGR
- Fetal karyotype
- Titers for
  - ○ Toxoplasmosis
  - ○ Cytomegalovirus

- ○ Herpes virus
- Preeclampsia lab profile
- Ultrasound evaluation
  - ○ Verify singleton versus multiple pregnancy
  - ○ Confirm EDC by U/S parameters
  - ○ Fetal anomaly study
  - ○ Fetal growth—May be done serially
    - ▪ Schedule at least 3 weeks apart
    - ▪ Abdominal circumference
      - • Decreased in asymmetric IUGR
    - ▪ Umbilical arterial flow studies
  - ○ AFI for oligo- or polyhydramnios
  - ○ Placenta previa
  - ○ Chronic placental abruption
  - ○ Presence of uterine fibroids
- Fetal surveillance for IUGR
  - ○ Begin as early as IUGR suspected
    - ▪ Weekly NST
    - ▪ Consider OCT or CST if NST nonreactive
  - ○ AFI—Weekly, should be > 6

Providing Treatment:
Therapeutic Measures to Consider

- Treat underlying medical condition(s), such as
  - ○ Preeclampsia
  - ○ Gestational diabetes
  - ○ Infection
  - ○ Anemia
- Substance abuse treatment
- IUGR
  - ○ Decrease maternal activity
  - ○ Left lateral position to ⇑ placental blood flow
  - ○ Ensure adequate nutrition and oxygenation

- Consider delivery if fetal compromise evident

Providing Treatment:
Alternative Measures to Consider

- Whole foods diet
- Avoid substances that may affect placental efficiency

Providing Support:
Education and Support Measures to Consider

- Provide information about
  - ○ Implications for continued care
  - ○ Options for treatment
  - ○ Parameters for intervention
- Nutritional counseling and surveillance prn
  - ○ Evaluation of intake
  - ○ Adequate hydration
  - ○ Careful food choices for maximum nutrition
- Potential for
  - ○ Serial evaluation of fetal well-being
  - ○ Change in location or providers for birth
- Provide support
- Address client and family concerns

Follow-up Care:
Follow-up Measures to Consider

- Document
- Base midwifery plan on
  - ○ Results of diagnostic testing
  - ○ Discussions with client and family
  - ○ Note indications for consultation or referral
- Anticipated follow-up

- Serial fetal surveillance (see Fetal Surveillance)
- Update plan weekly or as indicated
- Anticipate need for birth before term with
  - Positive OCT or CST
  - Oligohydramnios
  - U/S documentation of limited cranial growth
- LGA infant, anticipate potential for
  - Shoulder dystocia
- Newborn resuscitation
  - In utero
  - Postdelivery

Collaborative Practice:
Consider Consultation or Referral

- Obstetric service
  - Prenatal consultation based on maternal and fetal condition
  - Documented IUGR
  - Potential referral to high-risk OB service
  - For induction
  - For anticipated LGA infant
  - As indicated or needed during labor and birth
- Pediatric service
  - Anticipated preterm infant
  - IUGR
  - Maternal diabetes
  - Anticipated newborn resuscitation
- Social services as indicated
  - Tobacco, drug, or ETOH use
  - Poor support systems
  - WIC, food stamps, etc.

Toxoplasmosis
Key Clinical Information

Acute primary maternal infection with toxoplasmosis puts the unborn baby at risk for congenital toxoplasmosis infection. The risk of congenital fetal infection rises during pregnancy from 15% in the first trimester, to 30% during the second trimester, and peaks at 60% during the last trimester. Complications of maternal toxoplasmosis infection may include spontaneous abortion or miscarriage, fetal demise, fetal microcephaly, chorioretinitis, cerebral calcifications, and abnormalities of the cerebral spinal fluid (CDC, 2004a).

Client History:
Components of the History to Consider

- LMP, EDC
- Query regarding possible source of exposure (CDC, 2004b)
  - Cat feces, fur, and bedding
  - Raw or rare meat
  - Soil or sand
  - Contaminated water or milk
- Onset, duration, and severity of symptoms
  - Fever
  - Exhaustion
  - Sore throat
  - Swollen lymph nodes
  - Other associated symptoms

Physical Examination:
Components of the Physical Exam to Consider

- VS, including temperature
- Evaluation for
  - Lymphadenopathy
  - Liver margins

Clinical Impression:
Differential Diagnoses to Consider

- Toxoplasmosis
- Mononucleosis
- Influenza
- Other viral illness

Diagnostic Testing:
Diagnostic Tests and Procedures to Consider

- Toxoplasmosis testing
  - Preconception prn
  - Retest q trimester prn
- Types of tests
  - ELISA
  - IFA
    - If titers exceed 1:512, recent acute infection is likely
  - Possible exposure
    - IgG and IgM negative = no infection
    - IgG positive and IgM negative = previous infection/immunity
    - IgM positive = possible acute infection
- Recheck IgM in 3 weeks
- If titers rising, acute infection likely

Providing Treatment:
Therapeutic Measures to Consider

- Maternal therapy per perinatologist or OB
  - Spiromycin
  - Pyrimethamine

Providing Treatment:
Alternative Measures to Consider

- Immune support
  - Maintain quality diet
  - Rest

- Echinacea
- Emotional support and reassurance

Providing Support:
Education and Support Measures to Consider

- Prevention measures (CDC, 2004a)
  - Avoid
    - Contact with cats, cat feces, and cat bedding
    - Travel to areas with endemic toxoplasmosis
    - Handling raw meat whenever possible
- Do
  - Careful hand washing with soap and water
  - Use gloves when
    - Gardening
    - Cleaning litter or sandbox
    - Preparing raw meat
  - Cook meat to at least 150° F
  - Clean surfaces after processing raw meat
- Information and discussion about
  - Test results and diagnosis
  - Options for care
  - Recommendations for continued care
  - Optimal location for birth
  - Pediatric care for birth
  - Breastfeeding recommended

Follow-up Care:
Follow-up Measures to Consider

- Document
- Positive maternal titer
  - Ultrasound at 20–22 weeks for fetal anomalies
  - Serial ultrasounds as indicated
  - PUBS for fetal IgM and culture

- Evaluation of the newborn for congenital infection
- Return for care
  - Per prenatal routine
  - Provide ongoing support

Collaborative Practice:
Consider Consultation or Referral

- Diagnosis of acute toxoplasmosis refer to
  - Perinatology
  - Genetic counseling
  - Counseling or support group

Urinary Tract Infection in Pregnancy
Key Clinical Information

Urinary tract infection during pregnancy may have a variety of presentations. Asymptomatic bacteriuria is common in pregnancy, and acute pylonephritis will occur in up to 30% of women with previously untreated asymptomatic bacteriuria. Simple cystitis may occur during pregnancy and is extremely painful. Renal calculi may present as flank pain, accompanied by blood or leukocytes in the urine. Urinary tract infections may lead to renal damage, severe pain, and may increase risk of preterm labor.

Client History:
Components of the History to Consider

- LMP, EDC
- Current symptoms
  - Onset, duration, and severity
  - Urinary urgency, frequency, and burning
  - Fever, chills
  - Nausea, vomiting
  - Flank pain
  - Colicky pain

- Symptoms of preterm labor
- Other associated symptoms
- Review history related to
  - UTIs
  - Renal calculi
  - Recent urinary catheterization
  - Frequent intercourse
  - Voiding and fluid intake habits
  - Fetal movement (> 20 weeks gestation)

Physical Examination:
Components of the Physical Exam to Consider

- Vital signs, including temp
- Evaluation of hygiene
- Abdominal evaluation
  - FHT
  - Presence of contractions
  - Suprapubic tenderness
  - Guarding or rebound tenderness
- Signs of renal involvement
  - Fever
  - CVA tenderness
- Pelvic exam
  - Evaluate cervical length, consistency, and dilation
  - Station of presenting part

Clinical Impression:
Differential Diagnoses to Consider

- Urinary tract
  - Asymptomatic bacteriuria
  - Cystitis
  - Pylonephritis
  - Renal calculi
- Pregnancy related

- ○ Preterm labor
- ○ Preeclampsia
- ○ Concealed abruption
- ○ Ectopic pregnancy
- Appendicitis

Diagnostic Testing:
Diagnostic Tests and Procedures to Consider

- Urinalysis
  - ○ Dip
    - ■ Positive nitrites
    - ■ Positive leukocytes
  - ○ Microscopy
    - ■ Blood (RBCs)
    - ■ Pyuria (WBCs)
    - ■ Bacteria
    - ■ Casts
- Gram stain
  - ○ Positive correlates with + culture
- Urine culture and sensitivity indicated for
  - ○ Positive urinalysis
  - ○ History of UTI
  - ○ Sickle trait
  - ○ Diabetes
  - ○ Chronic renal disease
  - ○ Hypertension
  - ○ Test of cure following treatment and q 6–12 weeks
- Urine culture findings
  - ○ < 10,000 colonies
    - ■ No infection
    - ■ Treatment not indicated
  - ○ 25,000–100,000 colonies
    - ■ Asymptomatic bacteriura
    - ■ Treatment indicated
  - ○ > 100,000 colonies

- ■ Urinary tract infection if pathogenic bacteria
- ■ Contamination if mixed bacteria
- ■ Treat when UTI present
- For complicated UTI (pylonephritis, calculi)
  - ○ CBC
  - ○ Electrolytes
  - ○ BUN, creatinine
  - ○ Renal ultrasound
  - ○ Strain all urines
- Ultrasound to evaluate for
  - ○ Maternal hydronephrosis
  - ○ Calculi
  - ○ Fetal status
- For recurrent UTI screen for
  - ○ Group B strep
  - ○ Sickle cell
  - ○ G6PD
  - ○ Diabetes
  - ○ Kidney function
    - ■ BUN
    - ■ Creatinine, 24-hour creatinine clearance
    - ■ Total protein

Providing Treatment:
Therapeutic Measures to Consider

- Macrobid
  - ○ Pregnancy category B
  - ○ Simple cystitis
    - ■ 100 mg po bid × 3 days (Sinclair, 2004)
  - ○ Simple or recurrent UTI
    - ■ 100 mg po bid × 7–10 days
  - ○ Suppressive therapy
    - ■ 50–100 mg daily
- Ampicillin 500 mg
  - ○ Pregnancy category B

- 1 po qid × 7–10 days
- Sulfa trimethoprim DS
  - Pregnancy category C
  - 1 (400/80mg) po bid × 7–10 days
  - 🔔 Do not use before 13 weeks or after 36 weeks gestation
  - 🔔 Do not use with G6PD anemia
- Keflex
  - Pregnancy category B
  - 500 mg po q 12 hr × 7–10 days, *or*
  - 250 mg po QID × 7–10 days
- Pyridium, for dysuria
  - 200 mg tid after meals
  - Maximum 6 doses
  - Pregnancy category B
- Pylonephritis
  - Hospitalization
  - IV hydration
    - 200 ml/hr
    - Balanced electrolyte solution
  - Antibiotics
    - IV Cefoxitin 1–2 g q 6 hrs, or
    - Other cephalosporins
    - Change to po when afebrile × 24 hours
- Pain control
  - PCA
  - Demerol
  - Morphine

Providing Treatment:
Alternative Measures to Consider

- May be used in combination with antibiotics
- Herbals
  - Uva-ursi infusion 1 cup q 4–6 hours
  - Cranactin tablets 1–2 tablets q 4–6 hours with fluid

- Homeopathic remedies
  - Aconitum (renal discomfort, fever, and chills)
  - Cantharis (painful urination, urgency, and frequency)

Providing Support:
Education and Support Measures to Consider

- Medication instructions
- Review warning signs of progression
  - Fever and chills
  - Flank pain
  - Urinary urgency, burning
- Review perineal hygiene
  - Void after intercourse
  - Blot after voiding
  - Wipe front to back after BM
- When to call or come in for care
  - Symptoms
  - Do not resolve within 24 hrs
  - Worsen
  - Recur
- Indications for
  - Hospitalization
  - Consult or referral
- Encourage
  - Increased frequency of voiding
  - Increased fluid intake
    - Water preferable
    - Cranberry juice/tea
    - 1 cup/hr while awake
  - Avoid
    - Caffeine
    - Excess vitamin C
    - Sugars

Follow-up Care:
Follow-up Measures to Consider

- Document
- Maternal surveillance
  - Observe for improvement
  - Change antibiotics based on sensitivities
  - Culture for test of cure
  - U/A each visit for blood, nitrites, leukocytes
  - Culture each trimester
  - Suppressive therapy after 2 positive cultures
- Fetal surveillance
  - Monitor FHR and activity
  - Observe for uterine contractions
  - Evaluate for cervical changes
- Hospital discharge after
  - 24 hours on po antibiotics
  - Afebrile
  - Calculi passed
  - No signs or symptoms of preterm labor

Collaborative Practice:
Consider Consultation or Referral

- Pylonephritis
- Renal calculi
- Pain control
- Threatened preterm labor
- Recurrent cystitis or asymptomatic bacteria
- For diagnosis or treatment outside the midwife's scope of practice

First Trimester Vaginal Bleeding

Key Clinical Information

Although vaginal bleeding in the first trimester is a relatively common occurrence, it must be considered serious until all potential abnormal causes have been effectively ruled out. The precipitating cause may not readily present itself and may take some investigation to identify. Serial evaluation of quantitative β-HCG levels may assist in evaluation, as may ultrasound. Ectopic pregnancy should always be considered.

Client History:
Components of the History to Consider

- Onset, duration, and severity of bleeding
  - Color, amount, and characteristics of discharge
  - Precipitating events if any
  - Presence of cramping or abdominal pain
  - Fever or flulike symptoms
  - Presence or regression of pregnancy symptoms
  - Other associated symptoms
- Estimated gestational age
  - LMP
  - Date of conception if known
  - U/S report if done
- OB/GYN history
  - Gravida para
  - Blood type and Rh
  - Risk factors for ectopic pregnancy
    - PID
    - IUD
    - GYN surgery
  - Previous pregnancy losses
  - History related to
    - Abnormal pap smears
    - STIs
    - Infertility
    - Cesarean birth
- Potential exposure to
  - Sexually transmitted infections

- ○ Viral infections
- ○ Physical abuse or trauma

Physical Examination:
Components of the Physical Exam to Consider

- Vital signs including temperature
- FHR as appropriate for gestation
- Bimanual evaluation for
  - ○ Uterine size for dates
  - ○ Uterine tenderness
  - ○ Presence of adnexal mass or pain
- Pelvic evaluation for
  - ○ Cervical dilation
  - ○ Presence of products of conception at os or in vaginal vault
  - ○ Presence of erosion, polyps or other cervical cause of bleeding

Clinical Impression:
Differential Diagnoses to Consider

- Implantation bleeding
- Spontaneous abortion
  - ○ Threatened spontaneous abortion
  - ○ Inevitable spontaneous abortion
  - ○ Incomplete spontaneous abortion
  - ○ Complete spontaneous abortion
  - ○ Missed spontaneous abortion
- Ectopic pregnancy
- Molar pregnancy
- Cervical bleeding
  - ○ Cervicitis
  - ○ Cervical polyps
  - ○ Cervical trauma
  - ○ Cervical cancer

Diagnostic Testing:
Diagnostic Tests and Procedures to Consider

- Quantitative β-HCG x2 48 hrs apart
- Hematocrit and/or hemoglobin
- Type and Rh status
- Coagulation studies if missed abortion suspected
  - ○ Prothrombin time
  - ○ Partial prothrombin time
  - ○ Fibrinogen level
  - ○ Platelets
- Ultrasound for
  - ○ Viability

Table 4-4 Anticipated β-HCG Levels	
WEEKS POST-LMP	**ANTICIPATED HCG LEVEL**
4 weeks	Up to 425 mIU/ml
5 weeks	18–7,350 mIU/ml
6 weeks	1,080–56,500 mIU/ml
7–8 weeks	7,650–230,000 mIU/ml
9–12 weeks	25,700–288,000 mIU/ml
13–16 weeks	13,500–253,000 mIU/ml
17–24 weeks	4,060–65,500 mIU/ml

Source: Frye, 1997.

- ◦ Dating

- ◦ Placenta previa or abruptio

- ◦ Ectopic

Providing Treatment:
Therapeutic Measures to Consider

- Pelvic rest and watchful waiting

- Methotrexate for ectopic pregnancy

- Rh immune globulin for Rh negative mother (see Rh-Negative Mother)

- Iron replacement therapy

Providing Treatment:
Alternative Measures to Consider

- Await spontaneous resolution to SAB

- Encourage expulsion of products of conception with

  - ◦ Blue or black cohosh tincture

  - ◦ Homeopathic caulophyllum

- Promote healing following SAB

  - ◦ Homeopathic arnica

  - ◦ Rescue remedy

  - ◦ Herbal combinations which may include

    - ▪ Red raspberry leaf

    - ▪ Vitex berries

    - ▪ Black haw root

- Bleeding during pregnancy with rising HCG levels (Frye, 1998)

  - ◦ Red raspberry leaf

  - ◦ False unicorn root

  - ◦ Wild yam root

  - ◦ Crampbark

  - ◦ Lemon balm

Providing Support:
Education and Support Measures to Consider

- Provide emotional support

- Discuss

  - ◦ Potential for miscarriage

  - ◦ Options for care

  - ◦ Expectant care

  - ◦ Tests available

  - ◦ Potential findings

  - ◦ RhIG for Rh-negative mother

- Threatened SAB

  - ◦ Pelvic rest

  - ◦ Avoid heavy lifting

  - ◦ Call if bleeding increases or is accompanied by pain

  - ◦ If awaiting spontaneous resolution of SAB at home, call or seek care immediately if

    - ▪ Heavy bleeding with pain × $1\frac{1}{2}$ hrs

    - ▪ Faintness or weakness

    - ▪ Adnexal pain

    - ▪ Fever

- Following SAB

  - ◦ Abstain from intercourse for 2 weeks

  - ◦ Bleeding may last 7–10 days

  - ◦ Discuss birth control if desired

- Incomplete SAB

  - ◦ Provide information on options for care

- Prior to next pregnancy

  - ◦ Use multivitamin with folic acid daily

  - ◦ Improve nutrition if indicated

  - ◦ Avoid cigarettes, drugs, and alcohol

Follow-up Care:
Follow-up Measures to Consider

- Document

- 🔔 Rule out
  - Molar pregnancy
  - Choriocarcinoma
  - Ectopic pregnancy
  - Incomplete SAB
- Follow β-HCG levels
  - 48–96 hours if threatened SAB
  - Repeat q 3–5 days until
    - Clear regression
    - Appropriate increase
  - 4–6 weeks post-SAB
- Ultrasound follow-up
  - No IUP seen on ultrasound
    - Serial HCGs
    - Continued + or ⇑ HCG
- 🔔 Suspect ectopic pregnancy
- Repeat U/S 2–7 days
  - Subchorionic bleed on ultrasound
    - Follow-up ultrasound for anomalies
    - Follow β-HCG levels
- Post spontaneous abortion
  - Exam in 2–4 weeks
  - Evaluate return to nonpregnant state
  - Assess emotional status
  - Initiate birth control if desired

Collaborative Practice: Consider Consultation or Referral

- Obstetric service
  - Ectopic pregnancy
  - No IUP seen on U/S
  - Molar pregnancy
  - Excessive bleeding
  - D & C as indicated or desired
  - Cervical lesion or suspected cervical cancer

- Genetic counseling
- Other referrals prn
  - Genetic evaluation of POC
  - Evaluation for problems that can lead to SAB
    - Maternal disease (e.g., lupus, listeria, syphilis)
    - Congenital anomalies of the genital tract
    - Previous cervical surgery
    - Hormonal imbalances
    - Fibroids
- Social services
  - Mental health
  - Grief counseling

Bibliography

Bakerman, S. (1994). *Bakerman's ABC's of interpretive laboratory data.* Myrtle Beach, SC: Interpretive Laboratory Data.

Barger, M. K. (Ed.). (1988). *Protocols for gynecologic and obstetric health care.* Philadelphia: W. B. Saunders.

Briggs, G. G., Freeman, R. K., & Yaffe, S. J. (1994). *Drugs in pregnancy and lactation* (4th ed.). Philadelphia: Williams & Wilkins.

Engstrom, J. L., & Sittler, C. P. (1994). Nurse-midwifery management of iron deficiency anemia during pregnancy. *Journal of Nurse-Midwifery, 39,* 20s–34s.

Enkin, M., Keirce M., Renfrew, M., & Neilson, J. (1995). *A guide to effective care in pregnancy and childbirth* (2nd ed.). New York: Oxford University Press.

Fennell, E. (1994). Urinary tract infections during pregnancy. *The Female Patient, 19*(11), 27–35.

Foster, S. (1996). *Herbs for your health.* Loveland, CO: Interweave Press.

Frye, A. (1997). *Understanding diagnostic tests in the childbearing year* (6th ed.). Portland, OR: Labrys Press.

Frye, A. (1998). *Holistic midwifery.* Portland, OR: Labrys Press.

Gordon, J. D., Rydfors, J. T., Druzin, M. L., & Tadir, Y. (1995). *Obstetrics, gynecology & infertility* (4th ed.). Glen Cove, NY: Scrub Hill Press.

Murphy, J. L. (Ed.). (2002). *Nurse practitioner's prescribing reference.* New York: Prescribing Reference.

Murray, M. (1998, June). Advanced fetal monitoring: Antepartal and intrapartal assessment and intervention. Program presented Milwaukee, WI.

Myles, M. F. (1985). *Textbook for midwives* (10th ed.). Edinburgh, Scotland: Churchill Livingstone.

National Heart, Lung & Blood Institute [NIH]. (2000). National High Blood Pressure Education Program Web site. *Working group on high blood pressure in pregnancy.* Retrieved January 3, 2005, from http://www.nhlbi.nih.gov/health/prof/heart/hbp/hbp_preg.pdf

Nolan, T. E. (1994). Chronic hypertension in pregnancy. *The Female Patient, 19*(12), 27–42.

Phelan, J. P. (1997, October). *Intrauterine fetal resuscitation; betamimetics & amnioinfusion.* Presented at Issues & Controversies in Perinatal Practice, Bangor, ME.

Roberts, J. (1994). Current perspectives on preeclampsia. *The Journal of Nurse-Midwifery, 39,* 70–90.

Scoggin, J., Morgan, G. (1997). *Practice guidelines for obstetrics and gynecology.* Philadelphia: Lippincott-Raven.

Scott, J. R., Diasaia, P. J., Hammond, C., & Spellacy, W. et al. *Danforth's Handbook of Obstetrics and Gynecology.* Philadelphia: Lippincott-Raven.

Smith, T. (1984). *A woman's guide to homeopathic medicine.* New York: Thorsons.

Soule, D. (1996). *The roots of healing.* Secaucus, NJ: Citadel Press.

Speroff, L., Glass, R. H., & Kase, N. G. (1994). *Clinical gynecologic endocrinology and infertility* (5th ed.). Philadelphia: Williams & Wilkins.

Varney, H. (1997). *Varney's midwifery* (3rd ed.). Sudbury, MA: Jones and Bartlett Publishers.

Weed, S. (1985). *Wise woman herbal for the childbearing year.* Woodstock, NY: Ashtree.

References

American College of Obstetricians and Gynecologists [ACOG]. (2001). Practice bulletin #30, gestational diabetes. *Obstetrics & Gynecology, 98,* 525–538.

Allen, D. (2001). CDC revised recommendations for HIV screening of pregnant women. *Morbidity and Mortality Weekly Report, 50*(RR19), 59–86.

American Diabetes Association [ADA]. (2003). ADA recommendations [Electronic version]. *Diabetes Care, 26,* S103–S105.

Burdge, D. R., Money, D. M., Forbes, J. C., Walmsley, S. L., Smaill, F. M., Boucher, M., et al. (2003). Canadian consensus guidelines for the care of HIV-positive pregnant women: Putting recommendations into practice. *Canadian Medical Association Journal, 168*(13), 1671–1674.

Burkhart, C. (2000, March 25). Dermatology clinic: Itching to have a baby. *The Clinical Advisor,* 93–94.

Centers for Disease Control and Prevention [CDC]. (1998). Recommendations to prevent and control iron deficiency in the United States. *Morbidity and Mortality Weekly Report, 47,* 1–25.

Centers for Disease Control and Prevention [CDC]. (2002). Sexually transmitted diseases treatment guidelines [Electronic version]. *Morbidity and Mortality Weekly Report, 51*(No. RR-6).

Centers for Disease Control and Prevention [CDC]. (2004a). *Parasites and health: Toxoplasmosis.* Retrieved January 13, 2005, from http://www.dpd.cdc.gov/dpdx/HTML/Toxoplasmosis.htm

Centers for Disease Control and Prevention [CDC]. (2004b). *Toxoplasmosis fact sheet.* Retrieved January 13, 2005, from http://www.cdc.gov/ncidod/dpd/parasites/toxoplasmosis/factsht_toxoplasmosis.htm

Coomarasamy, A., Honest, H., Papaioannou, S., Gee, H., & Saeed Khan, K. (2003). Aspirin for prevention of preeclampsia in women with historical risk factors: A systematic review. *Obstetrics & Gynecology, 101*(6), 1319–1332.

Emmons, L., Callahan, P., Gorman, P., & Snyder, M. (1997). Primary care management of common dermatologic disorders in women. *Journal of Nurse-Midwifery, 42,* 228–253.

Engstrom, J. L., & Sittler, C. P. (1994). Nurse-midwifery management of iron deficiency anemia during pregnancy. *Journal of Nurse-Midwifery, 39,* 20s–34s.

Fife, K. H., Bernstein, D. I., Tu, W., Zimet, G. D., Brady, R., Wu, J., et al. (2004). Predictors of herpes simplex virus type 2 antibody positivity among persons with no history of genital herpes. *Sexually Transmitted Diseases, 31,* 676–681.

Foster, S. (1996). *Herbs for your health.* Loveland, CO: Interweave Press.

Frye, A. (1997). *Understanding diagnostic tests in the childbearing year* (6th ed.). Portland, OR: Labrys Press.

Frye, A. (1998). *Holistic midwifery.* Portland, OR: Labrys Press.

Graves, B., & Barger, M. (2001). A conservative approach to iron supplementation during pregnancy. *Journal of Midwifery & Women's Health, 46,* 156–166.

I am a schoolteacher and there is Fifth's disease in the school system: What do I do? (1997, December). *Division of Maternal-Fetal Medicine Newsletter, 2,* 1–2.

International Diabetes Center. (2003). *Gestational diabetes practice guidelines*. Minneapolis, MN: Author.

Lindsay, J., & Hernandez, G. (2004). Evaluation of fetal death. *E-medicine*. Retrieved March 1, 2005, from http://www.emedicine.com/med/topic3235.htm

Moise, K. J., & Brecher, M. E. (2004) Package insert for rhesus immune globulin. *Obstetrics & Gynecology, 103*, 998–999.

Murphy, J. L. (Ed.). (2004). *Nurse practitioner's prescribing reference*. New York: Prescribing Reference.

National Institutes of Health National Heart, Lung & Blood Institute [NIH]. (2000). National High Blood Pressure Education Program Working Group on High Blood Pressure in Pregnancy. Retrieved January 3, 2005, from http://www.nhlbi.nih.gov/health/prof/heart/hbp/hbp_preg.pdf

Payton, R., & White, P. (1995) Primary care for women: Assessment of hematological disorders. *Journal of Nurse Midwifery, 40*, 120–136.

Peery, M. (n.d.) *Pregnancy and eating disorders*. Retrieved December 29, 2004, from http://www.vanderbilt.edu/AnS/psychology/health_psychology/pregnancy_and_eating_disorders.htm

Quest Diagnostics. (n.d.). *HerpeSelect*. Retrieved December 28, 2004, from http://www.questdiagnostics.com/hcp/topics/herpeselect/herpeselect.html

Roberts, J. (1994). Current perspectives on pre-eclampsia. *Journal of Nurse-Midwifery, 39*, 70–90.

Smith, T. (1984). *A woman's guide to homeopathic medicine*. New York: Thorsons.

Sinclair, C. (2004). *A midwife's handbook*. St. Louis: Saunders.

Ulrich, S. (2004). First birth stories of student midwives: Keys to professional affective socialization. *Journal of Midwifery & Women's Health, 49*, 390–379.

U.S. Public Health Service Task Force (2004). Recommendations for use of antiretroviral drugs in pregnant HIV-1-infected women for maternal health and interventions to reduce perinatal HIV-1 transmission in the United States. Washington, DC: Government Printing Office.

Varney, H., Kriebs, J. M., & Gegor, C. L. (2004). *Varney's midwifery* (4th ed.). Sudbury, MA: Jones and Bartlett Publishers.

Wagner, L. K. (2004). Diagnosis and management of pre-eclampsia. *American Family Physician, 70*, 2317–2324.

Weed, S. (1985). *Wise woman herbal for the childbearing year*. Woodstock, NY: Ashtree.

Wellington, K., & Jarvis, B. (2001). Silymarin: A review of its clinical properties in the management of hepatic disorders. *BioDrugs, 15*, 465–489.

Care of the Woman During Labor and Birthing

5

Care of women in labor is the hallmark of midwifery care and remains the essence of being with woman.

Women in labor are women at their most vulnerable. Not only do they have to expend an incredible amount of energy in the process of laboring and bringing forth their children, but they also must be vigilant in protecting their birth experience, including the possible need to navigate the complexities of the health care system. Few women have the resources to attend to all of these tasks at once.

One component of being *with woman* is to foster an environment where women may give birth and feel supported during this period of intense vulnerability. In many birth settings the conditions under which women labor and birth is less than ideal. This is true throughout the world, regardless of birth location. In the United States, women from many nations and all walks of life come to midwives for birth care. These women look to midwives for safe, compassionate, maternity care. They may hold the expectation that midwives will help them navigate the health care system during the course of their pregnancy, labor, or birth. As midwives who focus on *woman-centered* care, it is essential to learn the ways of the local health care systems in order to determine how to best meet the needs of each woman who comes to us for care.

Expectations and standards for midwifery care vary geographically in the United States, as well as by birth location. Familiarity with state, regional, and local standards for birthing care can ease the way for negotiation when adopting an innovative or uncommon practice. Use of sound scientific resources is useful in developing midwifery policy, but it should not supersede the centuries of sound midwifery care that have served women so well. Nowhere in the life of a woman is individualized care more important than during labor and birthing.

During labor and birth the midwife must pay attention to verbal and nonverbal cues to evaluate the woman's response to labor. In the setting where the midwife cares for women she or he has not met previously, where there are language or cultural barriers, or other developmental or social obstacles to communication, providing sensitive care can be difficult. Midwives should explore the options and avenues open to them for overcoming these challenges, so that they may continue to be *with woman*.

Negotiating for midwifery care in the world of obstetrics poses its own set of challenges. Diplomacy and tact are essential midwifery skills, as is a comprehensive knowledge of local and state rules and regulations that impact the midwife's ability to care for her clients autonomously. The practice of midwifery is different than that of obstetrics, and midwives who practice in technologically advanced settings are more likely to be pressured into practicing obstetrics than midwifery.

Initial Midwifery Evaluation of the Laboring Woman

Key Clinical Information

Evaluation of the woman in labor is a primary midwifery skill. Evaluation of the woman in labor encompasses not only physical evaluation of both mother and baby, but also meticulous assessment of the woman's coping skills and strengths that she brings to the task of bringing forth her child. A comprehensive and accurate labor assessment forms the foundation for development of the midwifery plan of care, and may provide critical information that influences the mother's care as labor progresses. For the woman who requires Cesarean delivery or other surgical care, the labor history and physical often becomes the preoperative H & P.

Client History: Components of the History to Consider

- Verify LMP, EDC, anticipated gestational age
- Determine
  - Onset of labor
  - Frequency, length, duration of contractions
  - Status of membranes

- Presence of meconium
  - Presence of bloody show
  - Recent nutritional intake
- Perform labor risk assessment
  - Current pregnancy course
  - Prenatal lab review
  - HIV status
  - Other risk factors
- Previous OB/GYN history
- Review past medical and surgical history
  - Allergies
  - Medication and herb use
  - Previous anesthesia
  - Surgical procedures
  - Chronic and acute illnesses
  - Injuries
- Social history
- Maternal and fetal well-being
  - Fetal motion patterns
  - Coping mechanisms for labor
    - Emotional status
    - Developmental status
    - Support people
  - Preferences for labor and birth
    - 🌀 Cultural practices
    - Support for labor
    - Birth plan
- Review of systems (ROS)
  - Genitourinary system
  - Respiratory system
  - Circulatory system
  - Gastrointestinal system
  - Nervous system
  - Musculoskeletal system

Physical Examination:
Components of the Physical Exam to Consider

- Maternal and fetal vital signs
- Abdominal exam
  - Contraction pattern: frequency, duration, strength
  - Evaluate fetus
    - Fetal lie, presentation, position, and variety
    - Fetal heart rate and rhythm
- Auscultation or EFM
- Baseline heart rate
- Beat-to-beat variability
- Periodic changes
  - Estimated fetal weight
- Pelvic exam
  - Determine presenting part
  - Dilation and effacement
  - Verify status of membranes
  - Station
  - Presence of bleeding or show
  - Assess perineum and pelvic floor
- Presence of amniotic fluid
  - Nitrazine
  - Ferning
  - Meconium staining
- Extremities
  - Reflexes
  - Edema
- Preanesthesia considerations
  - Dentition
  - Airway
  - Cardiopulmonary status
  - Spine
- Evaluate additional body systems as indicated by
  - History
  - Client presentation

- Physical exam findings
- Diagnostic test results

Clinical Impression:
Differential Diagnoses to Consider

- Uterine contractions, without cervical change
- Uterine irritability, secondary to (list cause if known)
- Onset of labor at term, NOS
  - Prodromal labor
  - Early labor
  - Active labor
- Spontaneous rupture of membranes
  - Prior to onset of labor (PROM)
  - Accompanied by onset of labor
- Onset of labor, complicated by (list)

Diagnostic Testing:
Diagnostic Tests and Procedures to Consider

- Testing is performed as indicated by
  - Client history
  - Active risk factors
  - Facility or practice standards
- Urinalysis
  - Dip for protein and sugar
  - Microscopic prn
- CBC
- Type and screen/cross
- Other screening as indicated by history and physical
  - PIH labs
  - Hepatitis profile
  - Chlamydia and gonorrhea cultures
  - GBS testing
  - HIV
  - RPR/VDRL

- ○ Rubella titers
- Ultrasound
  - ○ Fetal presentation
  - ○ Amniotic fluid index (AFI)
  - ○ Biophysical profile
  - ○ Placental location and integrity

Providing Treatment: Therapeutic Measures to Consider

- Expectant management
- As indicated by mother's history or facility protocol
  - ○ Saline lock for venous access
  - ○ IV fluids for hydration, or venous access
    - GBS antibiotic prophylaxis (see GBS)
    - PIH magnesium sulfate (see PIH)
    - GDM on insulin (see GDM)
- Medications as indicated by
  - ○ Maternal history
  - ○ Fetal status

Providing Treatment: Alternative Measures to Consider

- Watchful waiting
- Oral hydration and nutrition
- Ambulation
- Hydrotherapy
- Support people present

Providing Support: Education and Support Measures to Consider

- Provide information about
  - ○ Role of birth professionals
    - Labor evaluation process
    - Expected care during labor and birth

- ○ Hydration options
- ○ Activity options
- ○ Pain relief options
  - Nonpharmaceutical
  - Pharmaceutical
- ○ Positions for birth
- Indications for
  - ○ Artificial rupture of membranes
  - ○ Internal exams
  - ○ Medications
- Provide progress updates
- Provide encouragement and support
- Provide information for informed decision making

Follow-up Care: Follow-up Measures to Consider

- Document using admission H & P
- Reevaluate for presence of progress
  - ○ As indicated by maternal and fetal status
  - ○ At least every 4–6 hours
- Monitor client responses to
  - ○ Support people
  - ○ Unfamiliar care providers
  - ○ Labor progress and information
- Note
  - ○ Anticipated progression
  - ○ Anticipatory thinking
  - ○ Consultations or referrals

Collaborative Practice: Consider Consultation or Referral

- For diagnosis or treatment outside the midwife's scope of practice

Care of the Woman in First-Stage Labor

Key Clinical Information

Ongoing evaluation of the woman in labor provides the midwife with necessary information for determining maternal and fetal well-being during labor. The range of progress during labor that is within the range of *normal* varies widely. The midwife plays a critical role in providing maternal support and reassurance, while at the same time remaining vigilant for subtle variations in maternal or fetal condition that may indicate developing, or the potential for, problems. Early identification of actual or potential problems allows problem-solving measures and treatments to be initiated proactively, with a goal of the best outcome possible for mother and baby in the given circumstances.

Client History: Components of the History to Consider

- Chart review or verbal report
- Prior labor and birth history
  - Gravida, parity
  - LMP, EDC, gestational age
  - Prenatal course
  - Birth plan or preferences
- Interval history since admission, at least q 4–6 h
  - Frequency, length, and duration of contractions
  - Pattern of labor
  - Status of membranes
  - Recent fetal and maternal vital signs
  - Maternal coping ability
- Internal exam
  - When last assessed
  - Cervical dilation, effacement
  - Presenting part and station
  - Presence of pelvic pressure
- Deviations from anticipated labor course
- Initial midwifery plan of care

Physical Examination: Components of the Physical Exam to Consider

- Maternal and fetal vital signs
  - Maternal BP, pulse, and temp
  - Fetal heart rate and rhythm
- Evaluation of fetal response to labor
  - Methods
    - Auscultation, using
      - Fetoscope
      - Doppler
    - Evaluate for 60 seconds
    - Evaluate during and following contraction
    - Electronic fetal monitoring
      - External fetal monitoring
        - Intermittent
        - Continuous
      - Internal scalp electrode
        - Not indicated for low-risk pregnancy
        - Direct ECG
        - Evaluation of abnormal FHR patterns
    - Observation of fetal activity
  - Fetal heart tones
    - At least q 30 min
    - Immediately after ROM
    - Following pain medication
      - At medication peak
    - With change in contraction pattern
    - As indicated by
      - Course of labor
      - Stage of labor
      - Previous FHR patterns
      - Evaluation of maternal response to labor

- Methods
  - Observation
  - Palpation of uterus
  - External toco
  - Intrauterine pressure catheter
- Coping ability
  - Effectiveness of support people
  - Maternal response to labor
    - (image) Cultural responses to labor
    - Maternal attitude and approach
    - Pain relief techniques and needs
- Contraction pattern
  - Duration
  - Frequency
  - Strength
  - Maternal response
- Pelvic exam
  - Cervical dilation/effacement
  - Status of membranes
  - Presenting part
  - Station
  - Position
  - Reevaluate pelvimetry
  - Assess soft tissues for distensibility
- Urinary system
  - Bladder distention
  - Urine: protein and ketones
  - Output
- Hydration and nutrition
  - Fluid intake
  - Nutritive intake
  - Nausea and vomiting
  - Energy level
- Evaluate for changes in cervical status and/or fetal descent

- Less than 4 exams decreases risk of endometritis
- With change in maternal behavior
- Prior to administration of pain medication
- With urge to push
- prn for ongoing evaluation of labor progress
- Additional assessments as indicated

Clinical Impression: Differential Diagnoses to Consider

- Progressive labor
- False or prodromal labor
- Labor complicated by
  - Abnormal fetal heart rate patterns
  - Maternal complication, such as PIH
- Labor dystocia, secondary to
  - Cephalopelvic disproportion
  - Dysfunctional labor
    - Hypotonic
    - Hypertonic
  - Fetal position, such as
    - Persistent posterior presentation
    - Breech
    - Face presentation
- Obstructed labor

Diagnostic Testing: Diagnostic Tests and Procedures to Consider

- Dip urine for protein and ketones
- Testing as indicated by
  - Labor progression and status
  - Developing maternal or fetal risk factors, such as
    - Preeclampsia
    - Suspected breech

- Obstructed labor
- Placental abruption
  - For example
    - CBC
    - Type and screen/cross
    - Ultrasound

Providing Treatment: Therapeutic Measures to Consider

- False or prodromal labor
  - Reassurance
  - Medications
    - Morphine 10–20 mg IM, with
      - Vistaril 25 mg IM
      - Consider additional 10 mg MS if no sleep in 1–2 hours
    - Seconal 100 mg po—false labor
- Hypertonic uterine dysfunction (spontaneous)
  - Reassurance
  - Hydration, po or IV
  - Rest is essential
    - Morphine 10–20 mg IM as above
- Active management of labor
  - Augmentation of labor with oxytocin infusion
  - Amniotomy
- IV access as indicated
  - Client history
  - Facility standard
  - Consider saline lock vs. continuous IV
  - Maintain IV start kit on hand for prn use
- Sedatives, anxiolytics, and antiemetics
  - Nembutal/seconal 100 mg IM
    - Early labor sedation
    - Reduces anxiety
  - Vistaril 50 mg IM

- Early or active labor
- Causes sedation
- Reduces anxiety
- May combine with analgesic to potentiate effects
  - Phenergan 25–50 mg IM or IV
    - Use in early or active labor
    - Causes sedation
    - Reduces anxiety
    - Treats nausea and vomiting
    - May combine with analgesic to potentiate effects
- Analgesic medications (Sinclair, 2004)
  - May decrease newborn respiratory drive
  - May be reversed prn with naloxone
    - ⏲ Use with caution with suspected narcotic addiction
    - Newborn dose 0.1 mg/kg IM, SQ, IV
    - Watch for rebound effect
  - Fentanyl
    - 50–100 μg IV q 1–2 h
  - Stadol (butorphanol)
    - 1–2 mg IM q 3–4 h
    - 0.5–2.0 mg IV q 1–3 h
  - Nubain (nalbuphine)
    - 10–20 mg SQ or IM or IV
  - Demerol—active labor
    - 50–100 mg IM q3–4 h
    - Demerol 12.5–25 mg IV q 1–2 h
- Regional anesthetic
  - Requires IV hydration
  - May decrease placental perfusion secondary to hypotension
  - Epidural
    - Continuous infusion possible
    - May diminish urge to push

- Intrathecal
  - Generally one-time dose
  - Lasts 2–12 hrs based on meds used
- Hydration
  - Oral fluid intake
  - IV fluids
- Consider IV access for the following conditions
  - P5 or greater
  - Overdistended uterus (e.g., twins, polyhydramnios, etc.)
  - Oxytocin administration
  - History of postpartum hemorrhage
  - Maternal dehydration or exhaustion
  - Fetal distress with fatigued mother
  - Any condition that is potentially life threatening (e.g., preeclampsia)
- Lactated Ringers or similar balanced electrolyte solution
  - Fluid bolus of 300–1000 ml
    - Prior to regional anesthesia
    - To correct dehydration or volume depletion
  - Maintenance dose of 100–200 ml/hr
  - Titrate to urinary output
- Desultory labor
  - IV oxytocin (see Augmentation of Labor)
  - Nipple stimulation
  - Enema
  - AROM if vertex well applied and station 0 or below
- Catheterize prn for distended bladder if unable to void

Providing Treatment: Alternative Measures to Consider

- Physiologic management of labor

- Watchful waiting
- Onset of active labor at ≥ 4 cms
- Allow broad time frame for progressive labor
- Encourage
  - Gentle activity
  - Food and drink
  - Rest times
- Pain relief
  - Hydrotherapy
    - Shower
    - Tub
  - Acupressure
  - Hypnobirthing
  - Massage
    - Effleurage
    - Lower back
    - Neck and shoulders
  - Ice packs
  - Hot packs
- Frequent voiding
- Position changes
  - Birth ball
  - Rocking chair
  - Hands and knees
  - Squatting
  - Side-lying
  - Walking
- Doula or support person

Providing Support: Education and Support Measures to Consider

- Active listening to maternal concerns
- Information and discussion regarding
  - Fetal and maternal well-being
  - The progress of labor

- ○ The process of labor
- ○ Any imposed limits, or medical therapies, with rationale
- Informed consent process for anticipated procedures
- Emotional support
  - ○ Presence of support people
  - ○ Access to midwife prn
  - ○ Familiar environment or objects
  - ○ Reassurance of labor as normal physiologic process
- Encourage maternal control
  - ○ Food and fluid as desired
  - ○ Position changes as desired
  - ○ Frequent voiding
  - ○ Timing of maternal and fetal evaluation

Follow-up Care:
Follow-up Measures to Consider

- Document (see Labor Notes)
- Reevaluate q 1–4 hours in active labor
  - ○ Anticipate labor progress
  - ○ Notify additional personnel as indicated

Collaborative Practice:
Consider Consultation or Referral

- As indicated by collaborative practice agreements
- For diagnosis or treatment outside the midwife's scope of practice

Care of the Woman in Second-Stage Labor

Key Clinical Information

During the second stage the fetus must traverse the bony confines of the birth canal before he or she can emerge from the womb as a newborn. The baby's position as he or she enters the pelvis contributes to the duration and difficulty of second-stage labor. Prenatal evaluation of the internal pelvic diameters, known as *pelvimetry*, can be very useful in anticipating the course of second-stage labor, and offering suggestions for maternal positioning to facilitate fetal descent.

Client History:
Components of the History to Consider

- Documented pelvimetry
- Estimated fetal weight
- Review progress of first stage
  - ○ Labor curve
  - ○ Fetal presentation and position
  - ○ Maternal positioning
  - ○ Maternal attitude and coping
  - ○ Analgesia or anesthesia
- Review progress of second stage
  - ○ Length of second stage is variable
  - ○ Second stage > 2 hrs not an indication for delivery (ACOG, 2000c)
  - ○ Progressive second stage includes
    - Presence of effective contractions
    - Steady descent
    - Maternal and fetal well-being
- Previous OB history
  - ○ Previous infants' weights
  - ○ Second-stage length
  - ○ Shoulder dystocia
  - ○ Assisted delivery
    - Forceps
    - Vacuum extractor
    - Cesarean delivery

Physical Examination: Components of the Physical Exam to Consider

- Abdominal examination
  - Evidence of fetal descent
    - Abdominal contour changes
    - Fetal position changes
    - Descent in location of FHT
- Pelvic examination
  - Verify complete dilation
  - Assess
    - Location of sutures
    - Flexion of fetal head
    - Fetal molding
    - Effectiveness of bearing down
    - Rate of descent
    - Caput formation
  - Bulging of perineum
- Fetal well-being
  - Frequent FHTs
  - FHR may decrease in midpelvis
  - Head compression may decrease FHR
    - FHR should return to > 100 between pushes
  - FHR < 90 anticipate resuscitation
- Determine maternal well-being
  - Vital signs
  - Assess hydration
  - Evaluate her energy level
  - Determine her coping ability
  - Assess for bladder distention
    - May cause second-stage obstruction
  - Perineal tissue elasticity
- Evaluate for signs or symptoms of
  - Lack of descent
  - Slow descent
  - Caput formation
  - Fetal distress
  - Maternal exhaustion
  - Perineal edema

Clinical Impression: Differential Diagnoses to Consider

- Progressive second stage
- Spontaneous vaginal birth
- Perineal integrity
  - No lacerations
  - First- or second-degree lacerations
  - Episiotomy
  - Third- or fourth-degree laceration
- Second stage, complicated by
  - Fetal distress
  - Precipitous birth
  - Meconium-stained fluid
  - Nuchal cord, state number of loops
  - True knot in cord
- Slowly progressive second stage, complicated by
  - Asynclitic presentation
  - Persistent posterior presentation
  - Shoulder dystocia
- Failure of descent during second stage
  - Obstructed labor
  - Cephalopelvic disproportion

Diagnostic Testing: Diagnostic Tests and Procedures to Consider

- None

Providing Treatment: Therapeutic Measures to Consider

- Active management of second stage (Frigoletto et al., 1995; Peaceman & Socol, 1996)

- Pushing with onset of full dilation
- Prolonged, controlled pushing
- Augmentation with oxytocin
- Episiotomy
- Assisted extension of fetal head
- Manual rotation of shoulders
- Traction for birth of baby
- Local or other anesthesia for
  - Episiotomy
  - Laceration repair prn
- Catheterization if bladder distended and unable to void
- Assisted birth
  - Manual assistance (see Shoulder Dystocia)
  - Vacuum extraction (see Vacuum Extraction)
- Clamping and cutting of the umbilical cord
  - Before birth of the shoulders for nuchal cord
  - When cord has stopped pulsing
  - Immediately following birth
  - Following birth of placenta
  - Family member may wish to cut cord
- Collect cord blood sample
  - For Rh-negative mother
  - Per facility or practice standard
  - As indicated by history

Providing Treatment: Alternative Measures to Consider

- Physiologic management of second stage (Roberts, 2002)
  - Onset of pushing with maternal urge
  - No prolonged pushing
  - No arbitrary time limits if mother and baby in good condition
  - Baby is born by mother's spontaneous expulsive efforts

- Head is allowed to restitute spontaneously
- Shoulders and body emerge spontaneously
- Assistance may be provided at any point, prn
- Positioning for second stage and birth
  - Semisitting
  - Left lateral
  - Squatting
  - Hand and knees
  - Birthing stool
  - Birthing tub
- Lithotomy position with feet braced
  - Flattens sacral spine
  - Opens midpelvis
  - Rotates symphysis anteriorly
  - Assists with
    - Persistent posterior
    - Slow descent
- Water birth
- Perineal management
  - Hot packs to perineum
  - Perineal massage
  - Perineal support
- Family participation in birth

Providing Support: Education and Support Measures to Consider

- Pushing
  - Allow for natural expulsive efforts
  - Direct pushing efforts when needed
  - Remind about pelvic pressure
  - Instruct when not to push
- Immediate care after birth
  - Discuss plan for newborn handling
    - Newborn to mother
    - Newborn to warming unit

- Initial evaluation process for baby
- Cord cutting
  ○ Remind about third stage

Follow-up Care:
Follow-up Measures to Consider

- Document (see Labor and Birth Summary)
- Provide newborn resuscitation as indicated
- Evaluate perineal integrity
  ○ Note episiotomy or lacerations
    - Extent and location(s)
    - Repair, if necessary
      • Dermabond
      • Suture
      • Medications
  ○ Provide local anesthesia, prn
  ○ Provide analgesia, prn
- IV fluids
- Observe maternal and newborn following birth
  ○ Bonding
  ○ Breastfeeding
  ○ Determine maternal stability
  ○ Signs of third stage
- Provide for ongoing care postpartum

Collaborative Practice:
Consider Consultation or Referral

- For conditions in which OB/GYN attendance may be beneficial, such as
  ○ Arrest of descent
  ○ Anticipated shoulder dystocia
  ○ Fetal distress
  ○ Repair of 3rd or 4th degree lacerations
- For conditions in which pediatric attendance may be beneficial, such as
  ○ Fetal distress

  ○ Newborn resuscitation
  ○ Shoulder dystocia
- For diagnosis or treatment outside the midwife's scope of practice

Care of the Woman in Third-Stage Labor

Key Clinical Information

Birth of the placenta signals the end of labor, and the beginning of the postpartum period. Significant blood loss may occur prior to, or following the birth of, the placenta. Active management of the third stage of labor may result in decreased maternal blood loss, and is promoted in many areas (Prendiville, Elbourne, & McDonald, 2004; Nothnagle & Taylor, 2003). It does, however, require early clamping of the umbilical cord, which may affect newborn well-being (World Health Organization, 1998; Mercer & Skovgaard, 2002). Physiologic management of third-stage labor remains a reasonable option provided the midwife is willing to act promptly in the face of any undue bleeding (World Health Organization [WHO], 1996). Hemorrhage remains the leading cause of maternal morbidity worldwide.

Complete evaluation of the placenta should include manual palpation of the maternal surface as well as visual inspection of both sides of the placenta for areas of fragmentation, divots, or torn blood vessels that may indicate retained placental parts.

Client History:
Components of the History to Consider

- Previous obstetrical history
- Risk factors for postpartum hemorrhage
  ○ Overdistended uterus
  ○ Large infant
  ○ Precipitous labor and birth

- ○ Prolonged first or second stage
- ○ Cervical manipulation
- ○ Anemia
- • Course of labor and birth

Physical Examination:
Components of the Physical Exam to Consider

- • Vital signs
- • Evaluate for tears or lacerations
  - ○ Vagina
  - ○ Periurethral area
  - ○ Rectum
  - ○ Cervix
- • Expectant management
  - ○ Observe for placental separation
    - ▪ Lengthening cord
    - ▪ Globular fundus
    - ▪ Gush of blood
- • Verify that placenta is intact (Varney et al., 2004)
  - ○ Visual exam of maternal and fetal surfaces
  - ○ Tactile exam of maternal surface
  - ○ Cord insertion and vessel pattern
  - ○ Look for gross pathological changes
  - ○ Examine for number of cord vessels (2 arteries, 1 vein)

Clinical Impression:
Differential Diagnoses to Consider

- • Third-stage labor
  - ○ Intact placenta, normal appearance
  - ○ Intact placenta with unusual cord insertion
    - ▪ Marginal cord insertion
    - ▪ Velamentous insertion of the cord
- • Third-stage labor complicated by
  - ○ Postpartum hemorrhage due to

- ▪ Vaginal lacerations
- ▪ Cervical lacerations
- ▪ Uterine atony
- ▪ Retained placental fragments
- ○ Retained placenta
  - ▪ Accreta
  - ▪ Percreta
  - ▪ Increta

Diagnostic Testing:
Diagnostic Tests and Procedures to Consider

- • Placenta to pathology for evaluation (Hargitaib, B., Marton, T., & Cox, P. M., 2004; Langston et al., 1997)
  - ○ Maternal indications
    - ▪ Retained placenta
    - ▪ Abnormal gross placental exam
    - ▪ Placental abruption
    - ▪ Diabetes
    - ▪ Chronic hypertension or PIH
    - ▪ Preterm delivery (< 35 weeks)
    - ▪ Postterm delivery (> 42 weeks)
    - ▪ Unexplained fever
    - ▪ Previous poor OB history
    - ▪ No or minimal prenatal care
    - ▪ Substance abuse
    - ▪ Unexplained elevation of α-fetal protein
  - ○ Fetal indications
    - ▪ Stillbirth
    - ▪ Neonatal death
    - ▪ Multiple gestation
    - ▪ Intrauterine growth retardation
    - ▪ Congenital anomalies
    - ▪ Hydrops fetalis
    - ▪ Admission to neonatal intensive care
    - ▪ Low 5-minute Apgar (< 6)

- Umbilical artery pH (< 7.20)
- Meconium-stained fluid
- Polyhydramnios or oligohydramnios
- Fetal cord blood testing
  - Cord blood type and Rh
  - Cord blood gasses

Providing Treatment: Therapeutic Measures to Consider

- Cord care
  - Clamp and cut cord
  - Collect cord blood sample
- Physiologic management of third stage
  - Encourage infant to nurse at breast
  - Observe for signs of placental separation
    - May take up to 30 minutes
  - Once separation has been observed
    - Place one hand on symphysis to guard uterus
    - Use gentle traction to *guide* placenta
    - Do not pull on cord
  - After delivery of placenta
    - Evaluate firmness of uterus
    - Massage to firmness prn
    - No oxytocin unless uterine atony
    - Prn give oxytocin
      - 10 units IM
      - 10–20 units in IV fluids
- Active management of third stage
  - Verify singleton infant
  - Early cord clamping not required (Miller, Lester, & Hensleigh, 2004)
  - Drain placental blood, reapply clamp
    - Reduces length of third stage (Brucker, 2001)

- Uterotonic medication
  - With birth of anterior shoulder, or
  - Following birth of entire infant
    - No prenatal ultrasound
    - Palpation of fundus to verify singleton fetus
- Assess for placental separation
- When placenta appears separated (Long, 2001)
  - Provide controlled cord traction
  - Guard uterus with one cupped hand
  - Push uterus toward maternal chest
  - Guide placenta down into vagina
- When placenta visible guide to expel
  - Twist to "rope" membranes
  - Tease membranes out as necessary
- Repair of episiotomy or lacerations
- Excessive bleeding (see Postpartum Hemorrhage)
  - Ensure IV access
  - Uterine atony
    - Fundal massage
    - Bimanual compression
    - Administer uterotonic medication
  - Lacerations
    - Locate source of bleeding
    - Clamp vessel
    - Pack PRN
    - Ensure prompt repair
  - Retained placenta or fragments
    - Perform manual exploration of uterus
    - Perform or arrange for manual removal of placenta
- Analgesic, as needed for
  - After pains
  - To facilitate laceration repair

- No signs of placental separation > 30 min.
  - No bleeding
  - Assume abnormal implantation
  - Prepare for potential surgical removal of placenta

Providing Treatment:
Alternative Measures to Consider

- Baby to breast to stimulate uterine contractions
- Allow physiologic third stage
  - Gentle birth under maternal forces
  - Avoid clamping cord until pulsations stop
  - Early breast-feeding
  - No cord traction
  - Maternal efforts for expulsion
- Allow 30–60 minutes for third stage if
  - No bleeding
  - No signs of separation
  - No maternal pain
- Herbal formulas to stimulate uterine contractions
  - Blue or black cohosh tincture
  - Shepherd's purse tincture (Weed, 1985)
- Leave cord intact until placenta births
- Allow placenta to come naturally
- Ice to perineum after birth

Providing Support:
Education and Support Measures to Consider

- Encourage mother–baby contact
- Encourage breast-feeding of baby
- Be gentle
- Provide information about
  - Third stage
  - Need for repair, if any

- Interventions, if indicated
- Show placenta at client request
- Show client firm fundus
- Advise to notify midwife or support staff if
  - Fundus boggy
  - Flow excessive
  - Concerns about baby

Follow-up Care:
Follow-up Measures to Consider

- Document (see Labor and Birth Summary)
- Postpartum evaluation
  - 1–2 hours after birth or until stable
    - Vital signs
    - Fundal/flow checks
  - Evaluate maternal–infant bonding
- Follow-up evaluation within 12–24 hours

Collaborative Practice:
Consider Consultation or Referral

- For excessive bleeding uncontrolled by
  - Oxytocin, methergine, or cytotec
  - Bi-manual compression
- As needed for
  - Vaginal lacerations beyond the midwife's scope of practice
  - Rectal lacerations
  - Cervical lacerations
  - For suspected retained placental parts
    - For placenta that is undelivered > 30–60 minutes after birth of infant
    - Accompanied by significant vaginal bleeding
- For diagnosis or treatment outside the midwife's scope of practice

Amnioinfusion

Key Clinical Information

During amnioinfusion sterile fluid such as Ringer's lactate or normal saline is instilled into the uterine cavity via intrauterine catheter to replace or dilute amniotic fluid. Amnioinfusion is recognized as an effective way to reduce fetal risks associated with cord compression, oligohydramnios, or moderate to thick meconium (Hofmeyr, 2004a, 2004b, 2004c). Some studies suggest that amnioinfusion may decrease the incidence of meconium noted below the level of the vocal cords, and may decrease the rate of Cesarean birth for fetal distress by decreasing the frequency and severity of variable decelerations, and improving umbilical cord pH (Paszkowski, 1994; Phelan, 1997).

Amnioinfusion is not without risk. It has been associated with overdistention of the uterus resulting in increased basal uterine tone and sudden deterioration of the fetal heart rate pattern (ACOG, 1995). In one 2000 study, amnioinfusion did not result in any decrease in the incidence of meconium aspiration syndrome or other respiratory disorders (Wiswell et al., 2000). Clinical indications and frequency of use of amnioinfusion vary from facility to facility.

Client History:
Components of the History to Consider

- LMP, EDC, gestational age
- Maternal vital signs, including temp
- Cervical status
- Fetal presentation
- Status of membranes
- Potential indications for amnioinfusion
  - Low AFI/oligohydramnios
  - Presence of variable decelerations associated with cord compression
  - Passage of moderate to thick meconium-stained fluid

- Contraindications to amnioinfusion (Weismiller, 1998)
  - Presence of amnionitis
  - Polyhydramnios
  - Uterine hypertonus
  - Multiple gestation
  - Known uterine anomaly
  - Severe fetal distress
  - Nonvertex presentation
  - Fetal scalp pH < 7.20
  - Placental abruption or placenta previa

Physical Examination:
Components of the Physical Exam to Consider

- Maternal vital signs, including temp
- Vaginal exam
  - Status of membranes
    - Amniotomy must be performed if SROM has not occurred
  - Dilation, effacement, and station
    - Delivery should not be imminent
  - Verify presenting part
  - Place intrauterine pressure catheter
  - Place fetal scalp electrode if desired
- Abdominal exam
  - Verify singleton fetus in vertex lie
  - Evaluate FHR
    - Variable decelerations presenting prior to 8–9 cms associated with oligohydramnios
  - Evaluate for signs of amnionitis

Clinical Impression:
Differential Diagnoses to Consider

- Amnioinfusion for treatment of
  - Variable decelerations, secondary to
    - Oligohydramnios

- Cord compression
  ◦ Meconium-stained amniotic fluid
- Procedure performed
  ◦ Bolus amnioinfusion
  ◦ Continuous amnioinfusion

Diagnostic Testing:
Diagnostic Tests and Procedures to Consider

- Pre-op labs
- Ultrasound
  ◦ AFI before amnioinfusion
  ◦ AFI after bolus

Providing Treatment:
Therapeutic Measures to Consider

- Insert IUPC if not already in place
  ◦ Use double lumen IUPC if available
- Internal fetal scalp lead or external Doppler
- Procedure
  ◦ Infuse sterile saline or Ringer's lactate into the intra-amniotic space
  ◦ Warmed solution not required
  ◦ Bolus infusion
    - For treatment of variable decelerations
    - 250–600 ml at rate of 10–15 ml/min
    - Usual bolus +/- 500 ml in 30 min
    - May follow with bolus of 250 ml after decel resolves
  ◦ Continuous infusion (Weismiller, 1998)
    - May begin with 250 ml bolus
    - 10 ml/min for 1 hour
    - Maintenance rate of 3 ml/min
    - May take 20–30 minutes to see effect
- Management of fetal distress
  ◦ Maternal position changes
  ◦ Oxygen therapy

- Terbutaline therapy
- Emergency C-section
- 🔔 Do not delay preparations for Cesarean birth while performing amnioinfusion
- Assess uterine resting tone and FHT continuously

Providing Treatment:
Alternative Measures to Consider

- Watchful waiting
- Oligohydramnios
  ◦ Maternal hydration
  ◦ Left-lateral positioning
- Meconium-stained fluid
  ◦ Assess for addition risk factors for fetal distress
- Variable decelerations
  ◦ Maternal positioning to optimize FHR
  ◦ Avoid stimulation of labor
  ◦ Provide gentle birth environment
- Prepare for resuscitation of baby

Providing Support:
Education and Support Measures to Consider

- Address concerns about baby
- Provide information to allow informed consent
- Address client and family concerns
- Risks, benefits, and alternatives
  ◦ For indications benefits often outweigh risks
  ◦ Safety and efficacy have been well documented
  ◦ Elevated risk of endometritis/chorioamnionitis (Tucker, 2004)
  ◦ Not indicated for prophylaxis
- Educate regarding client requirements
  ◦ Positioning for procedure

○ Confined to bed postprocedure

• Continuous fetal and maternal monitoring

Follow-up Care:
Follow-up Measures to Consider

• Document (see Procedure Notes)

• Observe for complications

  ○ Deterioration of FHR

  ○ Uterine hypertonus

  ○ Cord prolapse

  ○ Uterine scar separation

  ○ Amniotic fluid embolism

  ○ Placental abruption

  ○ Signs or symptoms of infection

• Monitor and document

  ○ Maternal and fetal response

  ○ Progress of labor

Collaborative Practice:
Consider Consultation or Referral

• OB/GYN service

  ○ With indication(s) for amnioinfusion

  ○ For potential surgical consult

  ○ For complications related to amnioinfusion

• Pediatric service

  ○ Fetal distress

  ○ Meconium aspiration syndrome

  ○ Newborn resuscitation

• For diagnosis or treatment outside the midwife's scope of practice

Assisting with Cesarean Section

Key Clinical Information

Many midwives have expanded their clinical practice to include assisting with Cesarean birth and/or gynecologic surgery (ACNM, 1998). By first assisting, the midwife may provide greater continuity of care to women and greater versatility within her clinical practice. First assisting skills enhance the midwife's ability to perform perineal repairs when needed, and lead to a greater appreciation of the complexities of the female body. Working with the surgeon provides an opportunity to develop another facet of the midwife's collaborative relationship.

Client History:
Components of the History to Consider

• Review OB history

  ○ Prenatal labs

  ○ Admission labs

  ○ Course of labor/interval history

  ○ Indication for C-section

    ▪ Maternal

    ▪ Fetal

    ▪ Urgent vs. scheduled

• Medical history

  ○ Allergies

  ○ Medication or herb use

  ○ Medical conditions

    ▪ Asthma

    ▪ Cardiac dysfunction

    ▪ Respiratory disorders

    ▪ Scoliosis

  ○ Previous surgeries

    ▪ Response to anesthesia

• General

• Regional

• Review of systems

• Social history

  ○ Support systems

  ○ Smoking

  ○ Alcohol or drug use

• Client concerns

Physical Examination:
Components of the Physical Exam to Consider

- Maternal and fetal vital signs
- Admission physical, with focus on
  - Cardiopulmonary system
  - GI system
  - Fetal presentation, EFW
- Preoperative considerations
  - Maternal body mass index
  - Mobility of
    - Jaw
    - Neck
    - Back
  - Positioning limitations

Clinical Impression:
Differential Diagnoses to Consider

- Primary Cesarean section for
  - Maternal indication
  - Fetal indication
- Repeat Cesarean section
  - Scheduled
  - In labor
  - Following VBAC attempt

Diagnostic Testing:
Diagnostic Tests and Procedures to Consider

- Pre-op labs (see Preparing for Cesarean Section)
- Additional testing as indicated
  - Ultrasound localization of placenta
  - Preeclampsia labs
  - Coagulation studies

Providing Treatment:
Therapeutic Measures to Consider

- Ensure IV access and patency
- Ensure airway patency
- Assist with induction of general or regional anesthesia prn
- Assist surgeon with (Rothrock, 1993)
  - Prep
  - Draping
  - Retraction
  - Suctioning
  - Extraction of infant and placenta
  - Hemostasis
  - Suturing
- Procedure
  - Abdomen opened in layers
    - Skin
    - Subcutaneous fat
    - Fascia
    - Muscle
    - Peritoneum
  - Bladder flap created
  - Uterine incision made
    - Follow scalpel with suction
    - Rotate bladder blade to provide exposure
    - Incision extended with scissors or bluntly
  - Rupture of membranes
  - Remove bladder blade
  - Head/ buttocks delivered
    - Manually
    - Vacuum extractor
    - Piper forceps for after-coming head with breech
  - Fundal pressure for birth of body
  - Suction mouth and nares
  - Clamp and cut cord

- Collect cord blood
- Administration of medications by anesthesia
  - Meds given after cord is clamped
  - Oxytocin
  - Antibiotics
  - Anxiolytics
  - Narcotics
  - Antiemetics
- Placenta
  - Spontaneous expulsion, associated with
    - Decreased risk infection
    - Decreased blood loss
  - Manual removal of placenta
    - Identification of attachment location
    - Opportunity to learn skill
  - Surgeon preference
- Uterus inspected and cleared of debris
- Uterus closed in layers
  - Assistant "follows" suture
  - Uterus exteriorized or left in situ
- Inspection of other organs; ovaries, tubes, appendix
- Closure of layers per surgeon preference (Ethicon, 2004)
  - Assistant "follows" or sutures
- Sterile dressing applied

Providing Treatment:
Alternative Measures to Consider

- Allow/encourage support person(s)
  - Pre-op area
  - Holding area
  - Operating room
  - Recovery room (PACU)
- Encourage mother to hold baby after initial evaluation

- Allow support person(s) to care for infant until mother able

Providing Support:
Education and Support Measures to Consider

- Provide emotional support
- Advise client of routines related to
  - Anesthesia
  - C-section procedure
  - Newborn care
  - Recovery room
  - Postoperative course
- Active listening to client and family concerns

Follow-up Care:
Follow-up Measures to Consider

- Document post-op care provided
- Ensure adequate pain control
  - Long-acting spinal or epidural medications
  - Patient-controlled analgesia (PCA)
  - IM narcotics
  - po narcotics
  - po NSAIDs
- Post-op labs: CBC or H & H
- Physical exam
  - Vital signs
  - Reproductive system
  - Cardiopulmonary system
    - Assess for signs or symptoms of
      - Anemia
      - Hypovolemia
    - Incentive spirometry
  - GI system
    - Auscultate for bowel sounds
    - Note passage of flatus
    - Passage of stool

- ○ Urinary system
  - ■ Ensure voiding post-catheter removal
  - ■ Assess for
    - • Urinary retention
    - • Postvoid residual
    - • Urinary tract infection
    - • Bladder injury
    - • Bladder spasm
- • Assess for signs and symptoms of post-op complications
  - ○ Thrombus or embolism
  - ○ Atalectasis
  - ○ Infection
  - ○ Illeus
  - ○ Emotional difficulties
- • Evaluate client's emotional response to
  - ○ Events and procedure
  - ○ Newborn
  - ○ Parenting demands
- • Evaluate for postpartum depression risk
- • Other post-op follow-up
  - ○ Advance diet as tolerated
  - ○ Ambulate when full sensation
  - ○ DC Foley when able to ambulate
  - ○ DC IV/saline lock when taking po fluid well

Collaborative Practice:
Consider Consultation or Referral

- • OB/GYN service
  - ○ Presence of intraoperative or post-op complications
  - ○ For post-op care per collaborative practice agreement
  - ○ For diagnosis or treatment outside the midwife's scope of practice

Caring for the Woman Undergoing Cesarean Birth
Key Clinical Information

In many settings the midwife may help prepare the client who will have her child born via Cesarean. This provides a wonderful opportunity to provide women with education and support. The mother who was anticipating a planned birth center or home birth may need additional assistance in coping with the disappointment of the unexpected change in birth plans and in assimilating the procedure and its outcome. Any mother who undergoes Cesarean delivery may have conflicting feelings about her labor and birth experience and can benefit from the midwife's gentle care.

Client History:
Components of the History to Consider

- • See First Assisting with Cesarean Section
- • Indication for Cesarean
- • Client response to need for Cesarean
- • Complete maternity admission history
  - ○ OB/GYN history
  - ○ Medical and surgical history
  - ○ Review of systems
  - ○ Labs
  - ○ Social history
- • Interval labor history as applicable

Physical Examination:
Components of the Physical Exam to Consider

- • Complete maternity admission physical
- • Physical examination related to indication for Cesarean

Clinical Impression:
Differential Diagnoses to Consider

- • Cesarean section

- Primary, secondary to
  - Obstetrical or fetal indication(s)
- Repeat, secondary to
  - Obstetrical or fetal indication(s)
  - Patient preference
  - Previous incision type
  - Onset of labor
  - Following VBAC attempt
- Obstetrical or fetal indication(s)
  - Fetal indications
    - Fetal distress
    - Malpresentation
    - Multiple gestation
    - Congenital anomalies
    - Preterm birth
  - Maternal indications
    - CPD
    - Dysfunctional labor
    - Preeclampsia
    - Diabetes mellitus
    - Preterm labor
    - Placenta previa
    - Placental abruption
    - Uterine rupture

Diagnostic Testing:
Diagnostic Tests and Procedures to Consider

- Preoperative labs
  - Urinalysis
  - CBC with diff
  - Type and screen or type and cross
- Other necessary labs as indicated by maternal/fetal status
  - Fetal lung maturity assessment
  - Preeclampsia labs
  - Clotting studies

- Antibody identification

Providing Treatment:
Therapeutic Measures to Consider

- NPO (6 hour minimum preferred)
- IV access and fluids
  - LR, D5LR, NS or similar balanced electrolyte solution
  - 14–20 gauge IV catheter
  - Bolus of 500–1000 ml if regional anesthesia anticipated
  - Maintenance rate 100–150 ml/hr
- Foley catheter
  - May insert in
    - L & D/admission unit
    - Holding area
    - Following regional anesthesia
- Notify appropriate personnel of pending surgery
  - OB/GYN
  - Anesthesia
  - Nursing or operating room supervisor
  - Pediatrics
- Medications per anesthesia
- Maternal and fetal monitoring as indicated

Providing Treatment:
Alternative Measures to Consider

- Failure to progress is common cause of primary C/S
- Based on indication for Cesarean consider
  - Watchful waiting
  - Pain management
  - Rest and nutrition
  - Augmentation of labor
  - VBAC

- Provide emotional support
  - Allow/encourage family or support person(s) in OR
  - Engage mother in decision making where possible

Providing Support:
Education and Support Measures to Consider

- Obtain informed consent
  - Discuss indication(s) for Cesarean birth
  - 🌐 Provide interpreter as necessary
  - Risks
    - Infection
    - Bleeding
    - Injury
      - Bowel or bladder
      - Fetus
      - Uterus
      - Blood loss
  - Benefits
    - Delivery in controlled environment
    - Expedited delivery
    - C/S *may* decrease risk to mother or baby, based on indication for Cesarean birth
      - Breech/transverse lie
      - CPD
      - Severe PIH
      - Pre-term fetus
  - Alternatives to procedure
    - Continued labor
    - Vaginal birth, based on indication(s)
- Discuss recommendations and process with family
  - Unless time is critical allow for maternal input

- Maternal participation in decision making may impact
    - Feelings about surgical delivery
    - Bonding with baby
    - Self-image as woman
- Considerations for client and family education
  - Time in OR and postanesthesia unit
  - If support person(s) can stay with mother
  - Expected care for baby following birth
  - Anticipated postoperative care
- Provide emotional support related to
  - Indication for Cesarean birth
  - Change in
    - Birth plans
    - Birth attendant
    - Birth location

Follow-up Care:
Follow-up Measures to Consider

- Document
- Assist at surgery if qualified (see Assisting with Cesarean Birth)
- Remain with client if possible during surgery
- Review experience with client postpartum
- Provide post-op care as applicable
- Obtain operative note for records

Collaborative Practice:
Consider Consultation or Referral

- OB/GYN service
  - Confirmed or suspected indication for Cesarean birth as indicated by
    - The midwife's scope of practice
    - Practice setting
    - Client preference
    - Collaborative practice agreement

○ Development of complications postoperatively

- Pediatric service
  ○ Newborn care at birth
- Anesthesia service
  ○ Pre-op evaluation
  ○ Post-op pain control, prn
- For diagnosis or treatment outside the midwife's scope of practice

Caring for the Woman with Umbilical Cord Prolapse

Key Clinical Information

Cord prolapse is a true clinical emergency. Unless compression is removed from the cord, the fetus will be deprived of oxygen and may suffer brain and organ damage. While Cesarean birth is one method of resolving cord prolapse, maternal positioning, and manual replacement of the cord may help diminish cord compression. Cord prolapse is more common in women who have polyhydramnios, a fetal presentation other than vertex, and during spontaneous, or artificial, rupture of the membranes when the head or presenting part is not engaged in the pelvis.

Client History: Components of the History to Consider

- LMP, EDC, gestational age
- Identify risk factors for cord prolapse
  ○ Polyhydramnios
  ○ Multiple pregnancy
  ○ Nonvertex presentation
  ○ Compound presentation
- Status of membranes
- Fetal heart rate
  ○ Previously documented FHR/FHT
  ○ Fetal heart rate changes

- Maternal medical or obstetric problems

Physical Examination: Components of the Physical Exam to Consider

- Diagnosis and prevention
  ○ Avoid ROM unless presenting part is engaged
  ○ Evaluate FHR following ROM
    - Severe bradycardia = likely cord prolapse
    - Severe FHR drop with resolution = potential occult cord or true knot in cord
- Abdominal exam
  ○ Evaluation of fluid volume
  ○ Determination of fetal lie and presentation
  ○ Estimation of fetal weight
- Vaginal exam
  ○ Determine presenting part(s)
  ○ Station, cervical dilation
- Risk for cord prolapse
  ○ Floating presenting part
  ○ Bulging bag of waters
  ○ Ballooning or hourglass membranes

Clinical Impression: Differential Diagnoses to Consider

- Cord prolapse
  ○ Occult
  ○ Frank
- Fetal distress due to cord compression

Diagnostic Testing: Diagnostic Tests and Procedures to Consider

- Pre-op labs STAT if not obtained previously
  ○ CBC
  ○ Type and screen/cross
  ○ Urinalysis

Providing Treatment:
Therapeutic Measures to Consider

- In presence of suspected cord prolapse
  - Discontinue any oxytocin if running
  - O_2 by mask at 6–8 L
  - Positioning
    - Knee chest position, or
    - Trendelenberg position with left lateral tilt
  - Elevation of presenting part off of cord
    - Manually
    - Insert Foley catheter
      - Instill 500 ml sterile saline into bladder to lift presenting part of cord
      - Clamp off catheter
      - Release clamp when prepped for Cesarean
  - Cord care
    - Cover cord with warm saline-soaked gauze
    - Minimize manipulation to prevent cord spasm
    - Maintain elevation of presenting part until delivery
  - Continuous evaluation of FHR
- Terbutaline
  - To decrease contractions and uterine tone
  - 0.25 mg sq., or
  - 0.125–0.25 mg IV
- If infant continues to deteriorate
  - Attempt rapid vaginal birth if fully dilated
  - Prep for urgent Cesarean
  - Attempt manual reduction of cord
    - Especially if there is delay for C/S

Providing Treatment:
Alternative Measures to Consider

- Attempt to reduce prolapse
  - Position mother left lateral Trendelenberg
  - Abdominally lift presenting part
  - Manually attempt to reinsert cord into uterus
  - Evaluate for fetal response
  - Maintain knee-chest position until
    - Presenting part is well applied to cervix or engaged
    - FHR is within normal range
    - Monitor FHR closely
- If unable to reduce cord prolapse
  - Keep cord warm and moist
  - Maintain knee chest or Trendelenberg position
  - Arrange for surgical delivery
- Rescue Remedy at pulse points

Providing Support:
Education and Support Measures to Consider

- Education
  - Include cord prolapse in informed consent
    - Breech births
    - Polyhydramnios
- During emergency
  - Briefly explain to nature of emergency
  - Keep client and family advised of what is happening
  - Provide emotional support
- Following emergency
  - Compassionate listening
  - Information about the emergency

Follow-up Care:
Follow-up Measures to Consider

- Evaluate FHR continuously following treatment
  - Auscultation
  - Electronic fetal monitoring
- Following delivery
  - Document, as soon as possible after delivery

○ Provide client with information about events as applicable

○ Encourage client to verbalize feelings, understanding

- Consider peer review

  ○ Overall case review

  ○ Learning experience

  ○ Maternal and fetal outcomes

Collaborative Practice: Consider Consultation or Referral

- OB/GYN service

  ○ Conditions that may lead to cord prolapse

  ○ Suspected or confirmed cord prolapse

  ○ Fetal distress unresponsive to therapy

- Pediatric service

  ○ Fetal distress unresponsive to therapy

  ○ Newborn resuscitation

  ○ Newborn evaluation following emergency

- Social service

  ○ Counseling

  ○ Support group

- For diagnosis or treatment outside the midwife's scope of practice

Care of the Woman with Failure to Progress in Labor

Key Clinical Information

Failure to progress is a common diagnosis that may have multiple components. Delay in progression may be related to the effectiveness of uterine contractions, the size of the mother's pelvis in relation to the size of the fetus, fetal position or anatomy, or psychosocial factors that inhibit labor progress. The challenge to the midwife is to identify and treat the specific component(s) causing the delay. "Failure to progress" is a catchall description. When labor does not progress the suspected mechanism(s) should be clearly identified in order to systematically select the appropriate treatments.

In some instances fetal size or positioning may slow the progression of labor, while the uterus works hard to literally push past the difficulty. Time and patience may be rewarded with slow but steady progress. When the uterus is not working efficiently, as in desultory labor, augmentation of labor via oxytocin may help prevent prolonged labor and avoid unnecessary Cesarean birth. Patience is essential as many women do not follow the accepted labor curve, but need to find their own pace for labor and birth.

Client History: Components of the History to Consider

- G, P, LMP, EDC, gestational age
- Review of labor

  ○ Onset of labor

  ○ Progress of labor

  ○ Fetal response to labor

  ○ Maternal response to labor

  ○ Status of membranes

    ▪ Color of fluid

    ▪ Length of rupture

  ○ Oral intake of food or fluids

  ○ Positions used and results

  ○ Estimated fetal weight

  ○ Previous clinical evaluation of fetal lie

- Previous labor and delivery history
- Inquiry into potential barriers to labor progress

  ○ 🌐 Cultural

  ○ Developmental

  ○ Emotional or social

  ○ Physical

    ▪ Positioning

    ▪ Hydration

- Nutrition
- Voiding

Physical Examination:
Components of the Physical Exam to Consider

- Maternal and fetal vital signs
- Evaluate for signs of exhaustion
  - Tachycardia
  - Ketonuria
  - Trembling
  - Lethargy
- Maternal attitude
  - Fear or anxiety
  - Tension
- Abdominal exam
  - Fetal lie, presentation, position,
  - Estimated fetal weight
  - Signs of engagement
  - Uterine contractions; frequency, duration, intensity
  - Bladder distension
- Pelvic exam
  - Cervix
    - Dilation and effacement
    - Position
    - Edema or asymmetry of cervix
  - Presenting part
    - Verification of presenting part
    - Application to the cervix
    - Station
    - Asyncliticism
    - Caput formation
    - Molding
  - Assess pelvimetry
- Fetal vital signs
  - FHR/FHT; short- and long-term variability

- Fetal activity
- Fetal response to stimulation

Clinical Impression:
Differential Diagnoses to Consider

- Slowly progressive labor
- Presence of a protraction disorder
  - Dilation
  - Descent
- Presence of an arrest disorder
  - Arrest of dilation
  - Arrest of descent
- Potential causes
  - Dysfunctional labor
  - Fetopelvic dystocia
  - Cervical entrapment
  - Cephalopelvic disproportion
  - Fetal presentation or position
  - Fetal anomalies or cord entanglement
  - Maternal fear or stress reaction

Diagnostic Testing:
Diagnostic Tests and Procedures to Consider

- Urine for ketones
- Uterine pressure catheter to evaluate uterine contractions
- Pre-op labs if consideration for potential C-section

Providing Treatment:
Therapeutic Measures to Consider

- Watchful waiting
- Assess maternal environment for stress factors
  - Fear and pain
  - Light and noise
  - Family or staff members

- Hydration
  - po clear liquids
  - IV bolus of 500 ml of solution suitable for labor
    - Maintain at 125–200 ml/hr
- Rest, if maternal and fetal status is stable
  - Consider MS 10–20 mg IM in early labor
    - Have Narcan immediately available
  - Pain relief to facilitate rest/relaxation
- Clinical repositioning techniques
  - Flex vertex with fingers
  - Release entrapped cervix
  - Hip press to open midpelvis
- Active management of labor (Institute for Clinical Systems Improvement, 2004)
  - Oxytocin (see Augmentation of Labor)
  - Amniotomy
- Empty bladder
- Antibiotic prophylaxis
  - Not indicated with negative GBS
  - ROM > 18 hours or per facility recommendations
  - Maternal fever or elevated WBC

Providing Treatment: Alternative Measures to Consider

- Watchful waiting
- Explore emotional issues that may interfere with labor
  - Fear
  - Previous trauma, such as rape, abortion
  - Family issues (e.g., gender of infant, history of abuse)
  - Deadlines related to
    - Labor management
    - Interventions

- Encourage position changes
  - Hands and knees
  - Side-lying
  - Walking
  - Rocking chair
  - Semisitting
- Empty bladder, bowels
- Hydrotherapy
  - Tub
  - Whirlpool
  - Shower
- Flat on back with knees flexed may encourage descent
  - Opens pelvic inlet
  - Flattens sacrum
  - Move upright once vertex descends
- Use upright positions once head enters pelvis
  - Squatting
  - Squatting bar
  - Birth stool
  - Standing
  - Sitting
    - Birth ball
    - Bed
    - Chair
    - Toilet
- If contractions slow secondary to fatigue
  - Mother and fetus are both stable
    - Sleep
    - Provide nutrition and hydration
    - Allow more time
    - Close monitoring of maternal and fetal well-being
- Stimulate contractions
  - Nipple stimulation

○ Herbal remedies (see Augmentation of Labor)

Providing Support:
Education and Support Measures to Consider

• Discuss findings with client, family
   ○ Options available
   ○ Address client and family concerns
   ○ Formulate plan with patient
      ▪ Potential need to transport if out-of-hospital
      ▪ Recommendations for midwifery care
• Increased potential for augmentation with
   ○ Prolonged ROM
   ○ Desultory labor
• Increased potential for Cesarean with
   ○ Protracted active labor
   ○ Failure to descend
   ○ Maternal or fetal exhaustion

Follow-up Care:
Follow-up Measures to Consider

• Reassess
   ○ At least every 1–3 hours
   ○ Following initiation of treatments
   ○ With maternal or fetal indication
• Update plan after each assessment
   ○ Maternal and fetal response
   ○ Interval change
   ○ Clinical impression
   ○ Discussions with client and family
   ○ Planned course of action

Collaborative Practice:
Criteria to Consider for Consultation or Referral

• OB/GYN service

○ For persistently nonprogressive labor
○ Suspected CPD
○ Fetal malposition
○ For fetal or maternal distress
○ For transport
○ For diagnosis or treatment outside the midwife's scope of practice
• Pediatric service
   ○ Fetal distress

Care of the Woman with Group B Strep
Key Clinical Information

On average 10–30% of women are colonized, either vaginally or rectally, with Group B streptococcus (GBS). GBS may cause maternal urinary tract infection, amnionitis, postpartum endometritis, or wound infection. As many as 50% of infants, born to colonized mothers, may become colonized with GBS. Up to 4% of colonized infants develop significant complications related to GBS infection (CDC, 2002; Jolivet, 2002).

Early onset GBS disease occurs in the presence of maternal colonization accompanied by additional risk factors associated with GBS disease. The rate of early-onset GBS disease has diminished significantly since the institution of antibiotic prophylaxis in the early 1990s. Late onset GBS disease is defined as GBS disease that occurs between 1 week and several months of age. Late onset GBS disease occurs in up to 20% of newborns with GBS sepsis. Complications of neonatal GBS infection includes meningitis, pneumonia, and sepsis. The associated newborn mortality rate for the 1990's was 4-6% (Schuchat, 1998).

Client History:
Components of the History to Consider

• G, P, EDC
• Review prenatal course
   ○ GBS cultures

- Performed at 35–37 weeks
- Rectovaginal
- Urine
- Note documented discussions
  - GBS status
  - Antibiotic prophylaxis in labor
- GBS status unknown
  - Evaluate risk factors for risk-based management
- Identify risk factors for neonatal sepsis (CDC, 2002)
  - African-American women
  - + GBS culture
  - GBS bacteriuria in pregnancy
  - Previous infant with GBS sepsis
  - Previous amnionitis
  - PPROM
  - Prolonged ROM
  - Maternal fever (> 38°C/100.4°F) in labor
  - Preterm birth/low birth weight
- Review labor course
  - Onset and progression of labor
  - Fetal and maternal vital signs
  - ROM
    - Odor and color
    - Anticipated time from ROM to birth

Physical Examination:
Components of the Physical Exam to Consider

- Vital signs
- Usual maternal and fetal labor evaluation
- Evaluate for symptoms of chorioamnionitis
  - Febrile mother
  - Significant and persistent fetal tachycardia
  - Odor to amniotic fluid
  - Uterine tenderness (late sign)

- Observe newborn immediately following birth for symptoms of sepsis
  - Pallor and poor tone
  - Respiratory distress
  - Slow, irregular pulse

Clinical Impression:
Differential Diagnoses to Consider

- Group B strep
  - Colonization
  - Infection
- Amnionitis
- GBS negative with signs or symptoms of infection
  - Consider other organisms
  - Maternal fever of unknown origin
  - Fetal distress or appearance of sepsis

Diagnostic Testing:
Diagnostic Tests and Procedures to Consider

- Obtain culture at 35–37 weeks gestation
  - Distal vagina to rectum, through anal sphincter
  - Self-collect an option
  - Use selective broth medium for GBS
  - Urine culture
- CBC with diff
- Cultures at delivery
  - No GBS results available
    - Amnion/placenta
    - Baby's axilla, groin, or ear fold

Providing Treatment:
Therapeutic Measures to Consider

- Follow current CDC recommendation (CDC, 2002)

- GBS negative—no treatment
- GBS unavailable
  - Use risk-based strategy
  - Offer antibiotics with anticipated
    - Delivery at < 37 weeks gestation
    - Intrapartum fever (> 38°C/100.4°F)
    - ROM > 18 hours
- GBS positive—offer treatment based on
  - Positive culture this pregnancy
  - Previous infant with GBS disease
  - GBS bacteriuria in current pregnancy
  - Labor onset at < 37 weeks gestation
  - Local standards for risk factors
  - Client preferences
- Intrapartum prophylaxis *not* required
  - Previous pregnancy with positive GBS culture
  - Planned Cesarean without labor or ROM
  - Negative culture this pregnancy
  - Client preferences
- Allow time for 2 doses of antibiotics prior to delivery
- Note antibiotic allergies
  - PCN allergy
    - Not at risk for anaphylaxis
      - Cefazolin
    - High risk for anaphylaxis
      - Clindamycin
      - Erythromycin
      - Vancomycin
- Penicillin G
  - 5 million U IV followed by
  - 2.5 million U q 4 hours until delivery
- Ampicillin
  - 2 g IV followed by
  - 1 g q 4 hours until delivery

- For PCN allergy
  - Clindamycin
    - 900 mg IV q 8 hours until delivery
  - Erythromycin
    - 500 mg IV q 6 hours until delivery
- Oral therapy for expectant management of PROM
  - Not included in current CDC recommendations
  - PROM < 37 weeks gestation
  - Begin at 18 hours ROM
    - Amoxicillin 500 mg po tid
    - For PCN allergy
- Clindamycin 300 mg po q 6 hr
  - Client obtains temp q 4–6 hours while awake
    - Call with temp > 37.8°C
  - Change to IV chemoprophylaxis
    - Onset of active labor
    - Temp > 38°C

Providing Treatment: Alternative Measures to Consider

- Expectant management with or without screening
- For clients on antibiotic prophylaxis
  - Replace bacteria in gut via
    - Acidophilus capsules
    - Live culture yogurt
- Immediate evaluation and treatment of symptomatic newborn

Providing Support: Education and Support Measures to Consider

- Discuss
  - Practice routine regarding GBS screening
  - Treatment options if GBS +

- Provide information to allow informed decision making
  - Current CDC recommendations
  - Risks and benefits of antibiotics
  - Individual risk for GBS disease in infant
  - Alternatives to current recommendations
- Provide information regarding neonatal sepsis
  - May occur from birth through 3 months
  - Seek care immediately if any symptoms develop
  - Symptoms
    - Lethargy
    - Pallor
    - Poor feeding
    - Fever
    - Abnormal cry (ACNM, 1997)

Follow-up Care:
Follow-up Measures to Consider

- Document all discussions
  - GBS culture results
  - Treatment plan options
  - Client preferences for care
  - Risk factors for GBS infection
- Schedule regular newborn assessment

Collaborative Practice:
Consider Consultation or Referral

- OB/GYN service
  - Women with intrapartum fever (> 38°C/100.4°F)
  - Women with + GBS and preterm labor or PROM
  - Signs or symptoms of amnionitis
  - Transfer of care or birth location due to GBS status or symptoms

- Pediatric service
  - GBS + client with abnormal FHR pattern
  - Infant whose mothers have received antibiotic
  - Newborn conditions
  - Symptomatic infants
- For diagnosis or treatment outside the midwife's scope of practice

Care of the Woman Undergoing Induction or Augmentation of Labor

Key Clinical Information

Induction or augmentation of labor may be initiated for a wide variety of indications.

Practices vary tremendously toward the approach to induction and augmentation. Maternal involvement in the decision-making process is essential, as stimulation of labor may contribute to maternal feelings of failure or success based on maternal motivation and attitude toward the induction or augmentation process.

Client History:
Components of the History to Consider

- Prenatal record review
  - LMP, EDC, gestational age
  - Estimated fetal weight
- Identify indication for induction/augmentation
  - Desultory or nonprogressive labor
  - PROM
  - Maternal fever
  - + GBS culture
  - Time limits post-SROM for delivery
  - Chorioamnionitis
  - Postterm pregnancy (≥ 42 weeks)
  - Moderate or severe PIH
  - Maternal diabetes mellitus

BISHOP'S SCORE	0	1	2	3
Dilation (cms)	0	1–2 cms	3–4 cms	5–6 cms
Effacement	0–30%	40–50%	60–70%	80+%
Station	-3	-2	-1/0	+1/+2
Consistency	Firm	Medium	Soft	N/A
Position	Posterior	Midposition	Anterior	N/A

Table 5-1   Bishop's Score

Source: Bishop, 1964.

- ○ Maternal medical problems
- ○ Fetal risk in utero
- ○ Fetal demise
- Contraindications to induction or augmentation
  - ○ Abnormal lie
  - ○ Placenta previa
  - ○ Vasa previa
  - ○ Classical uterine incision
  - ○ Active genital herpes
  - ○ Invasive cervical cancer
- Misoprostol contraindications
  - ○ VBAC
  - ○ Asthma
- Obtain labor admission history or review interval labor history

Physical Examination:
Components of the Physical Exam to Consider

- Maternal and fetal vital signs
- Assess fetal and maternal well-being
  - ○ Contraction status
  - ○ Frequency, duration, strength
    - ▪ Palpation
    - ▪ External or internal monitoring
- Pelvic exam

- ○ Bishop's score (9 or more is considered favorable)
- ○ Pelvimetry to rule out CPD
- Pelvic exam
  - ○ Cervical status
    - ▪ Effacement
    - ▪ Dilation
    - ▪ Consistency
  - ○ Status of membranes
  - ○ Descent of presenting part

Clinical Impression:
Differential Diagnoses to Consider

- Induction of labor for indications such as
  - ○ PROM
  - ○ Preeclampsia
  - ○ Postterm pregnancy (≥ 42 weeks)
  - ○ Maternal diabetes mellitus
  - ○ Maternal medical problems
  - ○ Fetal risk in utero
  - ○ Fetal demise
- Augmentation of labor for
  - ○ Dysfunctional labor
  - ○ Uterine inertia

Diagnostic Testing:
Diagnostic Tests and Procedures to Consider

- Fetal evaluation
  - NST/CST
  - Biophysical profile
  - Amniotic fluid index
  - Fetal kick counts
- Fetal surveillance
  - Intermittent auscultation of FHT
  - Continuous fetal monitoring
- Pre-op labs
  - CBC
  - Urinalysis
  - Type and screen (or red top tube to hold)
  - Other labs as indicated

Providing Treatment:
Therapeutic Measures to Consider

- Cervical-ripening agents (Summers, 1997)
  - Prostin E2
    - Prepidil
    - Cervidil
    - Hospital compounded prostin E2 gel 2-6 mg
  - Misoprostol (may result in induction)
    - Off-label use
    - 🔔 Informed consent recommended
    - 25 μg maximum recommended dose
    - po or in posterior vaginal fornix
    - Repeat doses q 3–6 hours
  - Laminaria
  - Foley catheter balloon
    - Place inside internal os
    - Fill with 30 ml fluid
    - Tape to client's thigh
- Induction/augmentation

- Amniotomy
- Oxytocin infusion
  - 10 units oxytocin/1000 ml IV solution such as LR
  - Titrate to 3 contractions q 10 minutes
  - Rates vary, examples include
    - 0.5 to 2 mU/min
    - Increase 1–2 mU/min q 15–60 min
  - Maximum dose 20–40 mU/min
- Potential complications
  - Overstimulation of the uterus
  - Fetal distress
  - Underdosing and maternal exhaustion
  - Water intoxication (oxytocin)

Providing Treatment:
Alternative Measures to Consider

- Repeated fetal surveillance and patience
- Cervical ripening/initiation of labor (Falcao, nd; Summers, 1997)
  - Nipple stimulation
  - Sexual intercourse
  - Castor oil 2–4 oz po
  - Stripping of membranes
  - Herbs
    - Evening primrose oil
      - Apply to cervix with exam
    - Blue/black cohosh (Weed, 1985)
      - Tea or tincture
      - Take in small doses
      - Titrate to 3 contraction q 10 min
  - Homeopathic remedies
    - Caulophyllum (Weed, 1985)
    - Cimicifuga
    - Pulsatilla

Providing Support:
Education and Support Measures to Consider

- Outline recommendations for care
  - Indication for induction or augmentation
  - Obtain informed consent
  - Client/family preferences
- Potential for
  - Transport if out-of-hospital
  - IV access
  - Fetal monitoring
- Potential restrictions with induction/augmentation
  - NPO
  - Clear liquids
  - IV oxytocin
  - Electronic fetal monitoring
  - Limited mobility
  - Operative assistance at birth
    - Vacuum extraction
    - Forceps
    - C-section
- Provide support

Follow-up Care:
Follow-up Measures to Consider

- Document
- Address client preferences
- Evaluate maternal/fetal status at regular intervals
  - Evaluate for progress
  - Per indication for induction/augmentation
  - Update plan after each evaluation
- Ensure access to emergency services prn
- Encourage client to express feelings and concerns

Collaborative Practice:
Consider Consultation or Referral

- OB/GYN service
  - Prior to induction or ripening per collaborative practice agreement
  - Women requiring C-section or other assisted birth
  - As needed for transport
- Pediatric service
  - For evidence or suspicion of fetal compromise
- For diagnosis or treatment outside the midwife's scope of practice

Care of the Woman with Meconium-Stained Amniotic Fluid

Key Clinical Information

Meconium-stained amniotic fluid occurs in approximately 2–18% of all pregnancies with increasing frequency as term is approached and passed (Wiswell et al., 2000; Yoder, 1994; Hernandez et al., 1993). While, it is more common in the postdates pregnancy, it can also occur before term. Meconium-aspiration syndrome (MAS) affects 5–12% of babies born through meconium-stained amniotic fluid, or 1–3% of all live infants (Hernandez et al., 1993). MAS may occur when the fetus born through meconium-stained fluid breathes meconium into the lungs, but it occurs more often as a prenatal occurrence in the already compromised fetus. Suctioning the baby's mouth and nose before the birth of the shoulders is the single most important action to decrease potential chemical irritation or mechanical blockage of the airway from meconium aspiration.

Client History:
Components of the History to Consider

- Verify EDC, gestational age

- Assess fetal well-being
  - Reassuring FHR pattern
  - Patterns of fetal activity
- Characteristics of meconium in fluid
  - Thin
  - Moderate
  - Thick
  - Particulate
- Risk factors for meconium aspiration syndrome (Hernandez et al., 1993, Wiswell et al., 2000)
  - Maternal factors
    - < 5 prenatal visits
    - Oligohydramnios
    - Term or postterm pregnancy
  - Labor risk factors
    - Consistency of meconium
    - Abnormal FHR patterns
    - Precipitous birth
    - Cesarean delivery
  - Fetal factors
    - Advancing gestational age (> 42 wks)
    - Lack of suctioning before birth of shoulders
    - Apgar of < 7 (1 or 5 minutes)

Physical Examination:
Components of the Physical Exam to Consider

- Abdominal exam
  - FHT in relation to contractions
  - Fetal mobility
  - Fluid adequacy (thick meconium may = oligohydramnios)
  - Frequency, duration, and strength of contractions
  - Fetal lie, presentation (meconium common with breech)
- Pelvic exam
  - Cervical status
  - Confirmation of presentation
  - Station of presenting part
  - Amnioscopy offers
    - Visualization of fluid through intact membranes
    - Ability to maintain intact membranes
    - Information for earlier decision making regarding
- Additional personnel for birth
- Transport in utero, as indicated

Clinical Impression:
Differential Diagnoses to Consider

- Meconium-stained amniotic fluid
  - Thin, watery
  - Moderate
  - Thick, particulate
- Term fetus, NOS
- Fetal distress
- Fetus at risk for meconium-aspiration syndrome

Diagnostic Testing:
Diagnostic Tests and Procedures to Consider

- Amnioscopy for early evaluation of fluid color
- Evaluation of fetal well-being
  - Intermittent auscultation
  - Electronic fetal monitor
    - External
    - Internal
- Ultrasound
  - Amniotic fluid index
  - Fetal presentation
- Preoperative labs
  - Persistent or worsening fetal distress
  - Arrest of dilation or descent
  - Per facility standard

Providing Treatment:
Therapeutic Measures to Consider

- Amnioinfusion (see Amnioinfusion)
  - Moderate to thick meconium
  - With nonreassuring FHR changes (Hofmeyr, 2004a)
- Birth in gravity neutral position
  - Allows time to suction on perineum
  - At birth of the head suction
    - Nares
    - Mouth
    - Pharynx
- Prepare for potential outcomes
  - Vigorous newborn receives routine care
  - Follow-up suctioning for newborns who are
    - Not vigorous
    - Initially vigorous but develop respiratory distress
    - Intubation and suction using endotracheal tube preferred (AAP/AHA, 2000)
  - Neonatal resuscitation
  - Neonatal transport

Providing Treatment:
Alternative Measures to Consider

- Expectant management
- Gentle birth
- Suctioning method determined by midwife scope of practice

Providing Support:
Education and Support Measures to Consider

- Most healthy term babies with meconium-stained fluid will not develop MAS
- Encourage maternal participation in prevention of MAS

- No pushing until mouth and nose are suctioned
- Gravity neutral positioning for birth
- No stimulation until airway is cleared
- Importance of maternal attention to newborn
- Advise client of potential risk with meconium
  - Meconium aspiration syndrome
  - Trauma potential with intubation
- Advise of potential for interventions
  - Transport if out-of-hospital birth planned
  - Amnioinfusion
  - Intubation of newborn
  - Oxygen for newborn
  - Newborn special care
  - Antibiotic therapy for infant
- No treatment for baby with MAS increases risk for
  - Severe respiratory disorders
  - Newborn death
- Provide ongoing information
  - In labor
  - At birth
  - If newborn needs special care

Follow-up Care:
Follow-up Measures to Consider

- Have all resuscitation equipment on hand and tested
- Anticipate newborn vigor at birth
  - Professional skilled in intubation present if possible
  - Additional personnel for newborn resuscitation, prn
- Document

Collaborative Practice:
Consider Consultation or Referral

- OB/GYN service

- ○ Abnormal FHR patterns
- ○ Thick or particulate meconium
- ○ Documented or suspected oligohydramnios
- ○ For change in planned location of birth
- Consider hospital birth in presence of
  - ○ Meconium-stained amniotic fluid, *and*
  - ○ Postdates pregnancy, *or*
  - ○ Abnormal FHR pattern
- Pediatric service
  - ○ Presence of meconium
  - ○ Anticipate compromised newborn
  - ○ Newborn resuscitation
  - ○ Respiratory distress in neonate
- For diagnosis or treatment outside the midwife's scope of practice

Caring for the Woman with Multiple Pregnancy

Key Clinical Information

Midwives attend women with multiple pregnancies in some settings. Early identification of the multiple pregnancy provides an opportunity to address potential complications before they arise. In the home birth setting, the midwife assumes the responsibility for advising parents of the increased risk of adverse outcomes with multiple pregnancy when birth occurs in the home (Mehl & Medrona, 1997; ACOG, 1998b). Regardless of planned birth location, the midwife must have a means to provide access to obstetrical or pediatric care should it be indicated. Incidence of multiple gestation may be as high as 3%, and is associated with increased risk for preterm labor, preterm rupture of membranes, intrauterine fetal growth retardations, twin-to-twin transfusion and perinatal death (Sinclair, 2004).

Client History: Components of the History to Consider

- LMP, EDC, gestational age

- Contributing factors for multiple gestation
  - ○ Family history of multiples
  - ○ Personal history of multiples
  - ○ Use of fertility drugs
  - ○ In vitro fertilization (ACOG, 1998b)
- History suggestive of multiple gestation
  - ○ Fundal growth pattern
  - ○ Size > dates by exam
  - ○ Fetal motion not detected by 18–20 weeks size
  - ○ Elevated AFP results
- Multiple pregnancy complications
  - ○ Increased incidence of
    - ▪ Fetal anomalies
    - ▪ Spontaneous abortion
    - ▪ Fetal demise
    - ▪ Preeclampsia
    - ▪ Preterm labor
      - • Uterine irritability
      - • Cervical changes
      - • Preterm PROM
    - ▪ Polyhydramnios
    - ▪ Placental abruption
- Other pregnancy considerations
  - ○ Rh status
  - ○ Medical conditions
- Social support
  - ○ Nutrition status
  - ○ Working or living conditions
  - ○ Response to multiple gestation

Physical Examination: Components of the Physical Exam to Consider

- Interval weight gain
- Abdominal exam
  - ○ Interval fundal growth pattern

Table 5-2   Meconium Algorithm

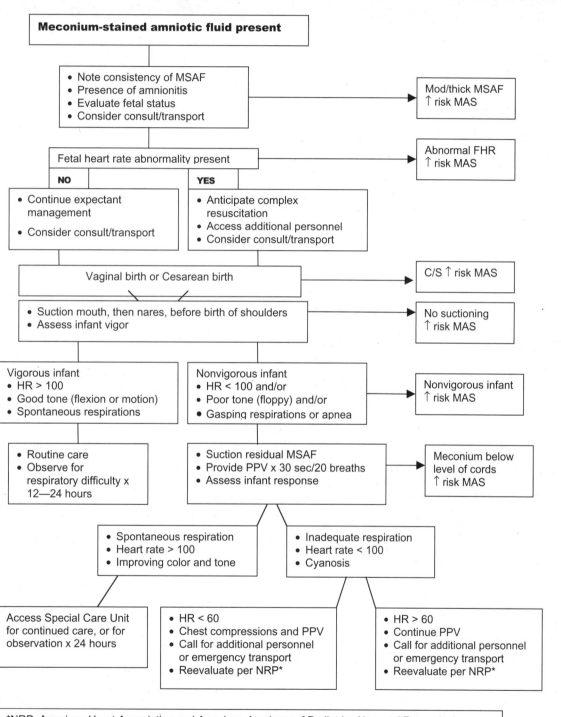

Meconium-stained amniotic fluid present

- Note consistency of MSAF
- Presence of amnionitis
- Evaluate fetal status
- Consider consult/transport

→ Mod/thick MSAF ↑ risk MAS

Fetal heart rate abnormality present

→ Abnormal FHR ↑ risk MAS

NO
- Continue expectant management
- Consider consult/transport

YES
- Anticipate complex resuscitation
- Access additional personnel
- Consider consult/transport

Vaginal birth or Cesarean birth

→ C/S ↑ risk MAS

- Suction mouth, then nares, before birth of shoulders
- Assess infant vigor

→ No suctioning ↑ risk MAS

Vigorous infant
- HR > 100
- Good tone (flexion or motion)
- Spontaneous respirations

Nonvigorous infant
- HR < 100 and/or
- Poor tone (floppy) and/or
- Gasping respirations or apnea

→ Nonvigorous infant ↑ risk MAS

- Routine care
- Observe for respiratory difficulty x 12—24 hours

- Suction residual MSAF
- Provide PPV x 30 sec/20 breaths
- Assess infant response

→ Meconium below level of cords ↑ risk MAS

- Spontaneous respiration
- Heart rate > 100
- Improving color and tone

- Inadequate respiration
- Heart rate < 100
- Cyanosis

Access Special Care Unit for continued care, or for observation x 24 hours

- HR < 60
- Chest compressions and PPV
- Call for additional personnel or emergency transport
- Reevaluate per NRP*

- HR > 60
- Continue PPV
- Call for additional personnel or emergency transport
- Reevaluate per NRP*

*NRP: American Heart Association and American Academy of Pediatrics Neonatal Resuscitation Program recommendations from the Neonatal Resuscitation Textbook (2000).

- ○ Size > dates on two or more occasions
- ○ Multiple small parts felt on palpation
- ○ Two fetal hearts heard via Doppler or fetoscope
- Pelvic exam
  - ○ Cervical length and dilation

Clinical Impression: Differential Diagnoses to Consider

- Multiple pregnancy, with increased risk for
  - ○ Structural anomalies
  - ○ Chromosomal anomalies
  - ○ Preterm labor
  - ○ Preterm rupture of membranes
  - ○ Fetal discordance

Diagnostic Testing: Diagnostic Tests and Procedures to Consider

- MSAFP
- Amniocentesis
- Ultrasound evaluation for
  - ○ Gestational age
  - ○ Presence of multiple gestation
  - ○ Presence of anomalies
  - ○ Amniocentesis
  - ○ Placenta(s) and membranes
    - ▪ Monochorionic
    - ▪ Dichorionic, diamniotic
  - ○ Fetal gender(s)
  - ○ Interval growth
  - ○ Cervical evaluation
    - ▪ Width
    - ▪ Length
    - ▪ Funneling
- Antepartum surveillance

- ○ Not indicated for uncomplicated multiple gestation (ACOG, 1998b)
- ○ For complications of multiple gestation, such as
  - ▪ IUGR
  - ▪ Abnormal AFI
  - ▪ Discordant fetal growth
  - ▪ PIH
  - ▪ Fetal anomalies
  - ▪ Monoamniotic twins
- Nonstress testing
- Biophysical profile

Providing Treatment: Therapeutic Measures to Consider

- Not recommended (ACOG, 1998b)
  - ○ Cervical cerclage
  - ○ Bed rest
- Selective fetal termination
  - ○ Common with in vitro fertilization
  - ○ May pose ethical challenges
- Treat
  - ○ Preterm labor (see Preterm Labor)
  - ○ Preterm ROM (see PROM)
  - ○ Preeclampsia (see Preeclampsia)
- Delivery should occur by 40 weeks
- Vertex—Vertex twins
  - ○ Anticipate vaginal birth
  - ○ Second twin may require time to be born
  - ○ C/S for same indications with singleton birth (ACOG, 1998b)
- Vertex—Nonvertex twins
  - ○ Consider vaginal birth for second twin over 1500 g
  - ○ Consider Cesarean birth based on
    - ▪ Fetus weight (under 1500 g)
    - ▪ Maternal preference

- Clinician skill and experience
- Nonvertex first twin
  - Cesarean delivery is usual
  - Vaginal delivery of nonvertex first twin has not been studied
  - Potential for locked twins with breech-vertex twins
- Ongoing evaluation of second fetus following first birth
  - Ultrasound
  - Electronic fetal monitoring
  - Close observation for complications
    - Cord prolapse
    - Placental abruption
    - Abnormal fetal heart rate pattern (ACOG, 1998b)
  - Stimulation or augmentation of labor prn
    - Oxytocin
    - Amniotomy
  - For deteriorating fetal status
    - Internal podalic version prn
    - Breech extraction
    - Cesarean delivery of second twin

Providing Treatment:
Alternative Measures to Consider

- Diagnosis of twins via clinical exam
- Out of hospital birth
  - Uncomplicated multiple gestation
  - Maternal preference
  - Informed choice considerations
  - Risk factors for individual
  - Midwife skill and experience
  - Distance/time to emergency care
- Multiple births hold increased risk regardless of birth location (Mehl & Medrona, 1997)

- Poor outcomes at home birth may hurt home birth
- Freedom of choice includes ready access to care as needed
- In hospital birth
  - Vaginal birth
  - Birth room
  - Minimum of people
  - Opportunity to meet staff beforehand
  - Negotiation of preferences
  - Ability to see and touch babies immediately
  - Care provided in family's presence
  - Rooming in and breastfeeding fostered
- Cesarean birth
  - Support people present
  - Ability to see and touch babies immediately, if stable
  - Care provided in family's presence
  - Rooming-in and breast-feeding fostered

Providing Support:
Education and Support Measures to Consider

- Discussion and education regarding multiple gestation
  - Anticipated care during pregnancy
  - Information on testing or surveillance
    - Procedures
    - Results
    - Implications
    - Options and recommendations
- Active listening to client
  - Individual needs
  - Preferences
  - Collaborative planning of care
  - Options for high-risk care as indicated

Follow-up Care:
Follow-up Measures to Consider

- Document
- Increased frequency of prenatal visits
  - By gestational age
  - As indicated by results of testing
  - In presence of any complicating factors
  - As term approaches (third trimester)
- Identification of risk factors
  - Problem list
  - Update plan as changes occur
- Labor, anticipate potential complications
  - Preterm labor (see Preterm Labor)
  - Preterm ROM (see PROM)
  - Uterine inertia
  - Placental abruption
  - Postpartum hemorrhage

Collaborative Practice:
Consider Consultation or Referral

- OB/GYN service
  - For all multiple pregnancies per midwife scope of practice
  - For multiple gestation with complications
    - Maternal complications
    - Fetal complications
  - Triplet or greater multiple pregnancy
  - Maternal preference
- Pediatric service
  - Presence of prenatal complications
  - Immediate newborn care at birth
- Social service
  - Mothers of twins support group
  - Grief support group for pregnancy losses
  - Other support services
- For diagnosis or treatment outside the midwife's scope of practice

Caring for the Woman with a Nonvertex Presentation

Key Clinical Information

Breech presentation is the most common nonvertex presentation, occurring in 3–4% of term singleton pregnancies. Breech and other nonvertex presentations carry an increased risk of complications over a vertex presentation. The relative safety of breech birth may be affected by the skill and experience of the birth attendant. Women's preferences for care should be taken into account during discussions of options.

ACOG recommends external version to convert breech or transverse lie to vertex presentation to decrease the risks associated with nonvertex presentations and avoid unnecessary Cesarean birth (ACOG, 2001). Current recommendations include offering planned Cesarean to women with term breech babies in an attempt to decrease perinatal morbidity and mortality (Hannah et al., 2000). Planned Cesarean for nonvertex presentation does not apply to those women who refuse surgical delivery, those in advanced labor when birth is imminent at the time of diagnosis, or those whose second twin is a nonvertex presentation.

Client History:
Components of the History to Consider

- LMP, EDC
- Previous maternity history
  - Previous breech births
  - Previous birth weights of children
  - Presence of uterine scars
- Contraindications for vaginal breech birth
  - Inexperienced birth attendant
  - Maternal preference
  - Birth attendant preference
  - Suspected CPD
  - Large baby
  - Nonreassuring FHR patterns

- Maternal or fetal complications
- Previous
  - Shoulder dystocia
  - Desultory labor
  - Protracted labor
- Current pregnancy history
  - Methods of dating pregnancy
  - Current gestation
  - Rh status
  - Placental location
  - Presence of labor
- Contributing factors to nonvertex presentation
  - Polyhydramnios
  - Lax abdominal muscle tone
  - Multiparity
  - Prematurity
  - Multiple gestation
  - Placenta previa
  - Hydrocephalus
  - Fetal or uterine anomalies (Varney et al., 2004)

Physical Examination:
Components of the Physical Exam to Consider

- Diagnosis of nonvertex presentation
  - Abdominal exam
    - Leopold's maneuvers
    - Determine fetal presentation, lie, and variety
    - Estimate fetal weight
    - Note abdominal muscle tone
    - Uterine tone
    - Fetal heart rate and location
- Pelvic exam
  - Clinical pelvimetry
  - Cervical status

Clinical Impression:
Differential Diagnoses to Consider

- Pregnancy, nonvertex presentation
  - Presentation, note lie
    - Breech
    - Transverse
    - Face
  - Gestation
    - Preterm
    - Term
    - Postterm

Diagnostic Testing:
Diagnostic Tests and Procedures to Consider

- Ultrasound
  - Confirmation of fetal position
  - Evaluation of placental position
  - Version may be performed under U/S guidance
- External cephalic version
  - Fetal evaluation
    - Preprocedure
    - During and postprocedure
    - Continuous fetal monitoring
    - NST and/or BPP
  - Maternal
    - IV access
    - Preoperative labs

Providing Treatment:
Therapeutic Measures to Consider

- External cephalic version (ACOG, 2000b)
  - Success rates of 35–86%
  - More successful in
    - Multiparous women
    - Transverse or oblique lie
  - Use of tocolytics

- For nulliparous women
- For all women
  - Rh immune globulin for Rh-negative women
  - Ready access to emergency Cesarean birth
- Method, following fetal evaluation
  - Have client empty bladder (Frye, 1998)
  - Client relaxes with knees bent and supported
  - Abdominal muscles must be relaxed
  - Attempt forward roll using gentle steady pressure
  - Lift breech from pelvis
  - Encourage head toward pelvis with gentle pressure and flexion
  - Attempt backward roll if forward roll not successful
  - Two practitioners may work together to encourage fetus to turn
  - Stop in the presence of
    - Fetal bradycardia
    - Maternal pain
    - Unsuccessful version
    - Successful version
- Vaginal breech birth
  - More successful in women with
    - Adequate pelvis
    - Previous vaginal birth
    - Skilled birth attendant
  - Higher risk of perinatal complications versus
    - Vaginal vertex birth postversion
    - Planned Cesarean birth

Providing Treatment:
Alternative Measures to Consider

- Breech tilt position
  - Use 5 minutes 3–4 times daily
  - Hips higher than head on tilt board
    - Music at maternal feet to encourage fetus to turn
- Moxibustion (Frye, 1998)
  - Burn Moxa cone 15 minutes daily
  - Outer corner of little toe nailbed
- Homeopathic pulsatilla (Frye, 1998)
  - Potency: 200C
  - One dose tid
  - Use with breech tilt

Providing Support:
Education and Support Measures to Consider

- Provide information on risks, benefits and availability of
  - Vaginal breech birth
  - External cephalic version
  - Planned Cesarean birth
- Obtain informed consent for planned birth or procedure
  - Perinatal risk with planned vaginal breech ≈ 5%
  - Perinatal risk with planned cesarean for breech ≈ 1.6% (ACOG, 2001)
  - Perinatal risk includes
    - Fetal injury or death
    - Neonatal injury or death
  - Maternal risk deemed equivalent for C/S vs. vaginal breech
- Encourage questions regarding options
- Consider maternal preferences in jointly determining plan for care

Follow-up Care:
Follow-up Measures to Consider

- Document
- Reconfirm

- Fetal position prior to birth
- Maternal preference for planned birth or procedure
- Persistent breech
  - Repeat version attempt
  - Reconsider vaginal breech or planned Cesarean
- Document
  - All discussions
  - Informed consent/informed choice
  - Maternal preferences for care
- For planned vaginal breech birth
  - Plan access to emergency care
  - Estimate fetal weight
  - Plan for birth
    - Number and type and skill of birth attendants
    - Presence of resuscitation team for newborn
    - Plan for emergency care
  - Procedure for vaginal breech birth (El Halta, 1996)
    - Evaluate fetal well-being frequently
    - Allow lull between first- and second-stage labor
      - Mother may have urge to push before full dilation
      - Avoid head entrapment by ensuring full dilation
    - Keep "hands off" baby and perineum
      - Allow baby to stretch tissues slowly
      - Avoid stimulation of baby
    - Allow baby to birth to above umbilicus
      - At this point cord compression is likely
      - *Gently* pull down a loop of cord
    - Encourage maternal pushing

- Keep baby in anterior position
- Allow baby to birth until nape of neck can be seen
- Do not pull on baby
- Arms and legs may need gentle assistance to be born
  - To birth face and head
    - Wrap baby's body in warm towel
    - Head may be guided into pelvis with gentle rotation of body
    - Assistant provides suprapubic pressure
    - Gently swing baby on to mother's abdomen
    - As face appears suction mouth and nose
    - Keep baby warm as head molds and is born
  - If birth does not occur promptly
    - Cut episiotomy
    - Use Ritgen maneuver prn
    - Do not pull on baby, severe injury may result

Collaborative Practice: Consider Consultation or Referral

- OB/GYN service
  - For nonvertex presentation
  - For Cesarean delivery
    - For failed version
    - Maternal preference
    - For nonvertex presentations
    - Contraindications to vaginal breech birth
- Pediatric service
  - For newborn care following vaginal breech birth
- For diagnosis or treatment outside the midwife's scope of practice

Caring for the Woman with Postpartum Hemorrhage

Key Clinical Information

Postpartum hemorrhage is defined as a blood loss of greater than 500 ml at delivery, or within the first 24 hours following vaginal birth (Varney et al., 2004). Postpartum hemorrhage is a leading cause of maternal mortality worldwide. Anemia may be a significant contributor to delayed postpartum healing and predispose to infection. Hemorrhage may be the primary indicator of retained placental tissue, uterine fatigue, significant lacerations, or disorders of coagulation. The primary cause of postpartum hemorrhage is uterine atony (Long, 2001).

Client History: Components of the History to Consider

- Past OB history
  - Prior history of postpartum hemorrhage
  - Grand multiparity
- Ethnic history
  - Asian
  - Hispanic
- Course of labor
  - Gestational age
  - H & H at onset of labor
  - Effectiveness of uterine contractions
  - Length of each stage
  - Oxytocin administration
  - Placental delivery and status
  - Genital tract laceration
- Risk factors for hemorrhage
  - Preterm delivery
  - Overdistension of the uterus
    - Fetal macrosomia
    - Polyhydramnios
    - Multiple gestation
  - Prolonged third stage (Brucker, 2001)
  - PIH, HELLP syndrome
    - $MGSO_4$ use
    - Low platelets
  - Operative delivery
    - Vacuum extraction
    - Forceps
    - Uterine manipulation, i.e., version
  - Placenta previa or abruption
  - Chorioamnionitis
  - Fetal demise
  - DIC
- Medical history
  - Bleeding disorders
  - Asthma (prostin)
  - Hypertension (methergine)

Physical Examination: Components of the Physical Exam to Consider

- Evaluate cause of bleeding
  - Uterine atony
  - Lacerations
  - Retained placenta or fragments
  - Coagulopathy
- Evaluate bladder, empty prn
- Evaluate for shock (EBL > 500 ml)
  - Rapid, thready pulse
  - Rapid, shallow respirations
  - Pale clammy skin and mucous membranes
  - Anxiety or lack of affect
- Placenta undelivered
  - Evaluate the uterus for placental separation
    - Uterus globular, firm
    - Fundus rises and is mobile
    - Cord lengthens

- ○ Assess for lacerations
- ○ Consider manual removal of partially separated placenta
- Placenta delivered
  - ○ Examine placenta for completeness
  - ○ Evaluate the uterus for atony
    - ■ If atony present
      - • Massage fundus
      - • Bimanual compression
      - • Consider retained placental fragments
  - ○ If no atony
    - ■ Evaluate for traumatic source of bleeding
      - • Cervical lacerations
      - • Vaginal lacerations
      - • Uterine rupture
    - ■ Reexamine placenta for absent fragments

Clinical Impression:
Differential Diagnoses to Consider

- Postpartum hemorrhage, secondary to
  - ○ Uterine inertia
  - ○ Genital tract laceration(s)
  - ○ Retained placental tissue
  - ○ Clotting dysfunction

Diagnostic Testing:
Diagnostic Tests and Procedures to Consider

- CBC
- H & H
- Platelets
- Type and cross-match
- Liver function tests
- Preeclampsia labs
- Labs to confirm suspected coagulopathy
- Ultrasound evaluation for

- ○ Retained placental tissue
- ○ Hematoma formation

Providing Treatment:
Therapeutic Measures to Consider

- Preventive measures
  - ○ Controlled birth of infant to minimize tissue trauma
  - ○ Physiologic management of third stage
    - ■ Clients with no risk factors for PPH
  - ○ Active management of third stage
    - ■ Clients with risk for PPH
    - ■ All clients
  - ○ Massage uterus until firm once placenta born
  - ○ Encourage breast-feeding and skin contact with infant
- PPH placenta in situ
  - ○ Bleeding indicates partial separation
  - ○ Manual exploration and removal may be necessary
    - ■ Do not pull on cord
    - ■ Procedure
      - • Insert sterile gloved hand into vagina
      - • Follow cord to placenta
      - • Move hand laterally to find edge
      - • Wedge fingertips under leading edge of placenta
      - • Sheer placenta off uterine wall using short strokes
      - • Remove placenta
      - • Treat for PPH with placenta delivered
      - • Potential need for follow-up D & E
- PPH with placenta delivered, assess
  - ○ Placenta for completeness
  - ○ Tissues for lacerations
  - ○ Maternal vital signs

- Perform bimanual compression
  - If uterus fails to contract well
  - Decreases blood supply to large uterine vessels
  - Will not diminish bleeding due to lacerations
  - Technique
    - One hand in vagina against lower uterine segment
      - Form into fist in anterior fornix
    - Second hand on abdomen
      - Cup posterior wall of uterus
    - Bring hands firmly together
      - Uterus will be compressed between hands
      - Maintain steady pressure until bleeding controlled
      - Order uterotonic medications (Varney et al., 2004)
- Medications
  - Oxytocin 10 U IM, or 20–40 U/1000 ml IV fluids
  - Misoprostol (Cytotec) (Lokugamage et al., 2001; Walraven, Dampha, Bittaye, Sowe, & Hofmeyr, 2004)
    - 200–800 mcg rectally
    - Thermostable uterotonic agent
    - Low incidence of side effects
    - Onset of action rapid
    - Half-life (oral) is 20–40 min (Rx Med, n.d.)
  - Methergine 0.2 mg IM (Murphy, 2004)
    - May follow with 0.2 mg po q6 hours
    - Indicated for persistent boggy uterus
    - Avoid in client w/ HTN
  - Hemabate 250 µg IM
    - Significant side effects
    - Not preferred first-line therapy
  - Prostin 15 M, 0.25 mg IM
- IV therapy
  - Large bore catheter(s)
  - D5LR, LR, Normosol or other similar solution
  - 10 units oxytocin/500 ml IV fluids
  - Run rapidly until atony subsides
  - Use second IV prn for fluid replacement
- Uterine exploration for retained placental tissue
  - May need D & E under anesthesia
- Replacement blood transfusion
  - For EBL > 1000 ml or signs of shock
  - Blood products
    - Whole blood
    - Packed RBCs
    - Other blood components as indicated
- For shock
  - Additional IV access
  - O$_2$ by mask
  - Trendelenberg or shock position
  - Foley catheter
  - Monitor I & O closely
- Extreme bleeding
  - Packing
    - Deep vaginal or cervical lacerations
    - While awaiting surgical repair
  - Aortic compression
    - Emergency measure while awaiting surgical care
  - Surgical control of bleeding
    - Repair of lacerations
    - Suture ligature of bleeding vessels
    - Dilation and evacuation of retained placenta fragments
    - Hysterectomy or uterine artery ligation in extreme cases

Providing Treatment:
Alternative Measures to Consider

- Preventives
  - Nettle or alfalfa leaf infusion (Weed, 1985)
    - Given during pregnancy
    - Immediately following birth of baby
  - Motherwort tincture
- Treatment of hemorrhage due to atony
  - Shepherd's purse tincture (Soule, 1995)
  - Tincture of
    - Blue cohosh
    - Shepherd's purse
    - Motherwort
  - Breast stimulation
  - Homeopathic
    - Caulophyllum
    - Arnica
    - Rescue remedy

Providing Support:
Education and Support Measures to Consider

- Discuss and arrange transport if out of hospital
- Following resolution of hemorrhage discuss
  - Occurrence of hemorrhage
  - If symptomatic, call for help before arising
  - Take iron replacement therapy as directed
    - Dietary sources
    - Supplements
  - Rest and adequate nutrition are essential for healing
  - Reinforce signs and symptoms of infection
    - How to recognize
    - When and how to call
- Active listening

Follow-up Care:
Follow-up Measures to Consider

- Document
- Observe for
  - Persistent bleeding
  - Signs of hypovolemia or anemia
    - Weakness
    - Dyspnea
    - Syncope
- CBC/H & H
  - First postpartum day
  - Repeat if bleeding continues
  - 4–6 week check

Collaborative Practice:
Consider Consultation or Referral

- OB/GYN service
  - Hemorrhage that does not respond
    - Immediately to treatment
    - As expected with appropriate treatment
  - Signs and symptoms of shock
  - For transport from out of hospital
  - For suspicion of
    - Retained placental fragments
    - Severe vaginal lacerations
    - Cervical lacerations
    - Uterine rupture
- For diagnosis or treatment outside the midwife's scope of practice

Postterm Pregnancy

Key Clinical Information

Postterm pregnancy is defined as pregnancy that has exceeded 42 completed weeks. Approximately 10% of women will go past term. There is no evidence that induction is beneficial for the uncomplicated postterm pregnancy. ACOG recommends beginning fetal surveillance by 42 weeks, although many practices begin surveillance prior to 42 weeks gestation (ACOG, 2004b). There are no firm guidelines on what constitutes a reasonable time frame for initiation of fetal surveillance in the postdate pregnancy. Induction may be indicated for either maternal or fetal indications, but not simply for 42 weeks gestation. Recent literature review shows a mild rise in perinatal mortality beginning at 43 weeks gestation (Hart, 2002).

Client History:
Components of the History to Consider

- Assess EDC using multiple parameters
  - LMP
  - β-HCG
  - Uterine size at first visit
  - Initial FHR
    - Fetoscope or stethoscope 18–20 wks
    - Doppler 10–14 wks
  - Quickening
  - Fundal height at umbilicus at 20 weeks
  - Early ultrasound
- Postdates risk assessment
  - Fetal macrosomia
  - Fetal postmaturity syndrome
  - Oligohydramnios
  - Meconium aspiration syndrome
- Review history for additional factors that may prolong pregnancy
  - Adrenal hyperplasia
  - Maternal psychosocial stresses
- Assess
  - Ongoing nutrition
  - Fetal activity and changes
  - Contraction patterns
  - Maternal concerns and state of mind

Physical Examination:
Components of the Physical Exam to Consider

- Weight
- Abdominal examination
  - Fetal presentation, position, lie, and variety
  - Fetal flexion and engagement
  - Estimated fetal weight
  - Palpate for
    - Fluid adequacy
    - Presence of contractions
- Pelvic examination
  - Perform Bishop's score
  - Verify presenting part
  - Reassess pelvimetry

Clinical Impression:
Differential Diagnoses to Consider

- Postterm pregnancy (≥ 42 weeks)
  - No other symptoms (NOS)
  - Decreased fetal movement
  - Abnormal BPP/NST results
  - Fetal macrosomia
- Term pregnancy (< 42 weeks)
- Pregnancy complicated by
  - Uncertain dates
  - Decreasing AFI
  - Other complications

Diagnostic Testing:
Diagnostic Tests and Procedures to Consider

- Fetal surveillance
  - Daily fetal kick counts
  - Nonstress test
    - Weekly
    - Biweekly

- Biophysical profile
  - Weekly
  - Biweekly
- AFI as separate indicator
- Contraction stress testing (ACOG, 2004b)

Providing Treatment:
Therapeutic Measures to Consider

- Watchful waiting; requires
  - Close observation of maternal and fetal well-being
  - Informed choice
  - Willingness to intervene prn
- Cervical ripening (see Induction of Labor)
  - No demonstrated benefit over expectant care for healthy mother and fetus (ACOG, 2004b)
  - As indicated by maternal or fetal status
    - Preeclampsia
    - Gestational diabetes
    - Nonreassuring fetal surveillance
  - Generally followed by induction of labor
- Induction (see Induction of Labor)
  - As indicated by maternal or fetal status

Providing Treatment:
Alternative Measures to Consider

- Watchful waiting (see previous section)
- Alternative measures for cervical ripening/induction (see Induction of Labor)

Providing Support:
Education and Support Measures to Consider

- Discuss potential risks and benefits of
  - Expectant management
  - Interventions

- Review or teach
  - Postdates is *after* 42 weeks
  - Fetal kick count
  - Process of labor
  - When to call
- Discuss labor options
  - Obtain informed consent
  - Expectant care
  - Elective intervention
  - Indicated intervention
  - Any potential change in location or anticipated care for labor and birth
- Listen to and note client and family
  - Preferences
  - Concerns

Follow-up Care:
Follow-up Measures to Consider

- Fetal surveillance
  - Schedule to evaluate fetal status q 4–7 days
  - Review results promptly
- Document ongoing plan
- Anticipate potential for complications (ACOG, 2004b)
  - Meconium-stained amniotic fluid
  - Shoulder dystocia
  - Postpartum hemorrhage
  - Elevated chance of Cesarean
  - Newborn respiratory distress

Collaborative Practice:
Consider Consultation or Referral

- OB/GYN service
  - Pregnancy post 41–43 weeks
  - Nonreassuring fetal testing

- ○ Concerns regarding reasons for postdates status
- ○ Change in location of birth due to fetal status/postdates
- Pediatric service
  - ○ Anticipatory for postdates baby
  - ○ As indicated by
    - Nonreassuring fetal surveillance
    - Meconium-stained amniotic fluid
    - Shoulder dystocia
    - Cesarean delivery
    - Newborn respiratory distress
- For diagnosis or treatment outside the midwife's scope of practice

Caring for the Woman with Pregnancy-Induced Hypertension in Labor

Key Clinical Information

Approximately 5–7% of pregnant women will develop pregnancy-induced hypertension or PIH (see Hypertensive Disorders in Pregnancy). Prompt identification of PIH offers the opportunity for early treatment, which may increase the likelihood of vaginal birth, and decrease the potential for maternal or fetal harm (Livingston et al., 2003). The woman who presents with PIH during labor may initially appear fine; therefore, systematic evaluation for PIH is warranted in all women with *any* clinical indicators suggestive of PIH (Roberts, 1994).

PIH frequently causes elevations in maternal BP, urinary protein, serum uric acid, and liver function tests. The maternal circulating blood volume is diminished resulting in hypovolemia in spite of generalized peripheral edema. Placental and renal blood flow is frequently diminished. Platelets may fall well below the normal range. HELLP syndrome is associated with a greater incidence of maternal morbidity, including a greater incidence of seizures, epigastric pain, nausea and vomiting, significant proteinuria

and stillbirth (Martin et al., 1999). Severe preeclampsia may result in maternal or perinatal death (Chandrasekhar & Datta, 2002). Seizures may be the first sign of PIH, and may occur 24–48 hours postpartum (Katz et al., 2000).

Client History: Components of the History to Consider

- Prenatal history
  - ○ EDC, LMP
  - ○ Review of preeclampsia labs if any
  - ○ Vasoactive drug use (e.g., nasal decongestants, cocaine)
- Labor history, as applicable
- Maternal BP
  - ○ During pregnancy
  - ○ During evaluation
- Presence and onset of symptoms
  - ○ Symptoms of end-organ involvement
    - Persistent headache
    - Epigastric pain
    - Visual disturbance
- Evaluate for PIH risk factors
  - ○ History of essential hypertension
  - ○ Hydatidiform mole (10x risk)
  - ○ Fetal hydrops (10x risk)
  - ○ Primigravida (6–8x risk)
  - ○ Hypertension in previous pregnancy, other than first
  - ○ Diabetes
  - ○ Collagen vascular disease
  - ○ Persistent nausea and vomiting
  - ○ Renal vascular disease
  - ○ Renal parenchymal disease
  - ○ Multiple gestation (5x risk)
  - ○ African-American and other minority women

○ Age < 20 and > 35

- Other complicating medical factors
- Family history

Physical Examination:
Components of the Physical Exam to Consider

- Blood pressure readings
  ○ Intact equipment of correct size should be used
  ○ Use same maternal position for each BP
  ○ Arm should be supported at level of the heart
- Evaluation for pitting edema
  ○ Face
  ○ Hands
  ○ Feet and lower legs
- Deep tendon reflexes
  ○ Patellar, Achilles
  ○ 3+ or clonus indicates CNS irritability
- Optic fundi for evidence of edema or hemorrhage
- Evaluate pulmonary status
- Evaluate fetal status
- Pelvic exam, as indicated
  ○ Bishop's scope prior to induction
  ○ Labor progress

Clinical Impression:
Differential Diagnoses to Consider

- Labor complicated by, or
- Induction of labor or C/S for
  ○ Gestational hypertension
  ○ PIH superimposed on chronic hypertension
  ○ Preeclampsia
  ○ Eclampsia
  ○ HELLP syndrome

○ Preexisting undiagnosed essential hypertension

Diagnostic Testing:
Diagnostic Tests and Procedures to Consider

- Baseline preeclampsia/pre-op labs
  ○ Urinalysis
  ○ CBC w/ differential
    ■ Platelet count (normal range 130,000–400,000/ml)
    ■ Elevated HCT may indicate severity of hypovolemia
  ○ Serum uric acid (normal range 1.2–4.5 mg/dl)
  ○ Type and screen or cross-match
  ○ Renal function testing
    ■ BUN
    ■ Creatinine (normal range < 1.0 mg/dl)
  ○ Liver function testing (LFTs)
  ○ Coagulation studies, in presence of
    ■ Abnormal LFTs
    ■ Abruptio placenta (Frye, 1997)
- Fetal surveillance
  ○ Biophysical profile
  ○ Amniotic fluid index
- Fetal monitoring, observe for
  ○ Decreased beat-to-beat variability
  ○ Periodic late decelerations

Providing Treatment:
Therapeutic Measures to Consider

- Expectant management
  ○ Preferred for gestation < 34 weeks
  ○ Bed rest with sedation prn
  ○ Monitoring of BP, weight, reflexes
  ○ Serial fetal surveillance

- ○ Serial preeclampsia labs
- ○ Medications as indicated below
- Active management
  - ○ Expedite delivery
  - ○ Steroids to promote fetal lung maturity
  - ○ IV access and fluids
  - ○ Route of birth dictated by
    - ■ Maternal and fetal condition
      - • Preterm fetus may do best with Cesarean delivery
      - • Prompt delivery is only option in eclamptic mother
      - • $MgSo_4$ may slow labor/induction (ACOG, 2002b)
    - ■ Anesthesia concerns
      - • Prompt C/S may be preferred
      - • Labile BP may contraindicate regional anesthesia
      - • Edema may make endotracheal intubation more difficult
- Medications
  - ○ $MGSO_4$, anticonvulsant
    - ■ 4-6 gm IV bolus followed by 2 g/hour
    - ■ Titrate to renal output, reflexes (ACOG, 2002b)
    - ■ Have calcium gluconate immediately available
  - ○ Oxytocin induction or augmentation of labor as necessary
  - ○ Antihypertensive meds
    - ■ Limited benefit
    - ■ Used to regulate labile BP
      - • 170/110 to 130/90 optimum
      - • Monitor intake and output
        - ○ Hourly I & O
        - ○ NPO
        - ○ Foley catheter
        - ○ IV fluids on pump

Providing Treatment:
Alternative Measures to Consider

- ○ Expectant management
  - ■ Quiet, dark room
  - ■ Rest in left lateral position
  - ■ Support people present or available
  - ■ Provide calm atmosphere of caring and safety
- Homeopathic Rescue Remedy to pulse points
- Prayer

Providing Support:
Education and Support Measures to Consider

- Provide information about
  - ○ Diagnosis
  - ○ Options for care
  - ○ Symptom recognition
  - ○ Anticipated course of events
    - ■ Need for calm and quiet
- Discussion regarding potential for
  - ○ Change in birth plans
  - ○ Medical interventions
  - ○ Initiation of labor
  - ○ Newborn special care
- Address client and family concerns
- Client/family to notify if additional symptoms develop, i.e.
  - ○ Epigastric pain
  - ○ Scotomata
  - ○ Visual disturbance
  - ○ Severe headache

Follow-up Care:
Follow-up Measures to Consider

- Follow vital signs/reflexes/symptoms
  - ○ At least q 2–4 hours

○ Follow for 24–48 hours postpartum

• Repeat preeclampsia or HELLP labs

• Document

Collaborative Practice:
Consider Consultation or Referral

• OB/GYN service

  ○ Suspected or confirmed preeclampsia

  ○ For women requiring transport due to PIH

  ○ For women with PIH who appear unstable

• Pediatric service

  ○ For presence at birth when maternal PIH present

  ○ Nonreassuring fetal status, such as

    ▪ Preterm birth

    ▪ Nonreassuring FHR patterns

• For diagnosis or treatment outside the midwife's scope of practice

Care of the Woman with Preterm Labor

Key Clinical Information

Preterm labor is defined as the onset of regular uterine contractions in a woman who is between 20–37 weeks gestation, who in addition has either spontaneous rupture of the membranes, or progressive cervical change (ACOG, 2003). It is the second leading cause of neonatal mortality in the United States, and occurs in approximately 10% of pregnancies (Tucker, Goldenberg, Davis, Copper, Winkler, & Hauth, 1991; Sinclair, 2004). Many women who have preterm contractions do not in fact go into preterm labor. Differentiation of preterm labor from preterm contractions can be challenging and stressful, especially for the midwife practicing in a rural area where perinatal services are limited or require substantial travel time. The combination of positive fetal fibronectin testing (fFN) and cervical length less than 25 mm is a strong predictor of impending preterm delivery (ACOG, 2003).

Client History:
Components of the History to Consider

• EDC confirmation

  ○ LMP, menstrual cycles

  ○ Ultrasound dating

  ○ β-HCG results

• Determination of labor status

  ○ Signs and symptoms of preterm labor

  ○ Onset and duration of symptoms

  ○ Precipitating factors

    ▪ Sexual activity within 96 hours (see fFN below)

    ▪ Prolonged standing, heavy lifting

    ▪ Stress, trauma

    ▪ Vaginal bleeding

• Signs and symptoms may be vague

  ○ Mild or severe cramping

  ○ Dull backache

  ○ Suprapubic or pelvic pressure

  ○ Loose stools

  ○ Increased or "different" vaginal discharge

• History or symptoms of infection, such as

  ○ Urinary tract infections or asymptomatic bacteriuria

  ○ Vaginal infections or STIs

  ○ Group B strep

• Assess risk factors for preterm birth

  ○ Adolescent pregnancy

  ○ Advanced maternal age

  ○ Prepregnant BMI < 19.8

  ○ Cervical cone biopsy

  ○ Poverty

  ○ Multiple gestation

- ○ Tobacco use
- ○ Prior history of preterm birth
- ○ Intrauterine growth retardation
- ○ Uterine anomalies
- Previous determinations of cervical
  - ○ Length
  - ○ Consistency
  - ○ Funneling

Physical Examination:
Components of the Physical Exam to Consider

- Maternal and fetal vital signs
- Abdominal exam
  - ○ Presence of contractions
  - ○ Uterine tenderness
  - ○ Fetal heart rate
  - ○ Estimated fetal weight for gestational age
  - ○ Fetal presentation, position, lie
  - ○ CVA tenderness
- Pelvic exam
  - ○ Sterile speculum exam for specimen collection
    - ▪ Fetal fibronectin (fFN)
    - ▪ GBS
    - ▪ Wet mount
    - ▪ Chlamydia/gonorrhea
    - ▪ Specimen for ferning
  - ○ Cervical change from baseline
  - ○ Status of membranes
  - ○ Vaginal discharge
- Evaluation for complications of pregnancy which would favor delivery vs. tocolysis

Clinical Impression:
Differential Diagnoses to Consider

- Pregnancy complicated by

- ○ Preterm contractions
- ○ Preterm labor
- ○ Multiple gestation
- ○ Pylonephritis
- ○ Renal calculi or colic
- ○ Abruptio placenta
- ○ Gastritis
- ○ Appendicitis
- ○ SGA fetus/IUGR
- ○ Inaccurate or unknown dates

Diagnostic Testing:
Diagnostic Tests and Procedures to Consider

- Labs
  - ○ Fetal fibronectin fFN
    - ▪ Collect prior to digital exam
    - ▪ Recent sexual activity or blood may affect results
  - ○ GBS
  - ○ Chlamydia
  - ○ Gonorrhea
  - ○ Wet mount
  - ○ Ferning, nitrazine testing if SROM suspected
  - ○ STAT urinalysis, C & S
  - ○ CBC with differential smear
  - ○ Additional labs as indicated by client history and presentation
- Ultrasound—based on symptoms and gestational age
  - ○ Cervical length and funneling
    - ▪ Length > 4 mm low risk
    - ▪ Length 4–26 mm moderate risk
    - ▪ Length <25 mm high risk
  - ○ Determination of approximate gestational age
  - ○ Verify number of fetuses

- Placental location and status
- AFI, biophysical profile
- Guidance for amniocentesis
- Amniocentesis for fetal surfactant and L/S ratio

Providing Treatment:
Therapeutic Measures to Consider

- Rest
  - Stop work, stop lifting
  - Refrain from sexual arousal and intercourse
  - Stop breast feeding or other breast stimulation
- Hydration—IV or po
- Tocolytic medication
  - Use before 34 weeks gestation
  - Dilation less than 4 cms
  - Medications to consider with collaborating physician (ACOG, 2003)
- Calcium channel blockers (Byren & Morrison, 2004; ACOG, 2003)
  - Prolonged pregnancy ≥ 48 hours
  - Less severe side effect profile than ß agonists
    - May cause hypotension
    - Avoid in client with liver disease
  - Nifedipine 5–10 mg SL q 15 minutes (Sinclair, 2004)
    - May repeat x 4 doses
    - Maintenance 10–20 mg po q 4–6 hours
- ß agonists
  - Significant side effect profile
  - Decrease dose for maternal HR ≥ 130 BPM
  - Begin with IV dosing
  - Change to po
    - Labor stopped x 12–24 hours
    - 30 minutes before stopping IV dosing
  - Terbutaline

- IV 2.5 µg /minutes—increase in 2.5 µg increments
  - Increase q 20 minutes based on effect
  - Max dose 20 µg/minute
- SQ dose 0.25 mg q 3 hours
- po dose 2.5–5.0 mg q 4–6 hours
  - Ritodrine
    - IV dose 0.05–0.35 mg/minute
    - po dose 20 mg q 2–4 hours (ACOG, 2003)
- Magnesium Sulfate
  - 40 g in 100–500 ml
  - 4–6 g loading dose
  - 2–4 g/h maintenance
- Indomethacin (Moses, 2004)
  - Only used before 32 weeks
    - May cause premature closure of ductus arteriosis
  - Loading dose 50 mg po
  - Maintenance dose 25 mg po q 4 hours
  - Max dosing period 48 hours
- Corticosteroid use (ACOG, 2002a; National Institute of Health, 2000)
  - Use between 24–34 weeks gestation
  - Maximum benefit 1–7 days postdosing
  - Betamethazone—2 doses
    - 12 mg IM q 24 hours, or
  - Dexamethazone—4 doses
    - 6 mg IM q 12 hours
- Selective Cesarean for very preterm infant(s)

Providing Treatment:
Alternative Measures to Consider

- Observe for preterm contractions vs. preterm labor
- Alternative therapies:
  - False unicorn root tincture

- 5 drops q 5–15 minutes
- Taper as contractions diminish
- Continue for 3–4 days
  ○ Valerian root tincture, *or*
  ○ Skullcap tincture, *or*
  ○ Cramp bark and wild yam tincture (1:1)
    - ½ dropperful 3 x daily (Frye, 1998)
- Assess overall nutritional status, supplement with
  ○ Calcium citrate 1000 mg daily
  ○ Magnesium 500 mg daily

Providing Support: Education and Support Measures to Consider

- Threatened preterm labor
  ○ Limit activity, decrease or stop work, arrange household help
  ○ Avoid sexual arousal or activity
  ○ Call if symptoms resume or increase
  ○ Daily fetal kick counts
  ○ Encourage smoking cessation, improvement of nutrition, etc., as applicable
- Progressive preterm labor
  ○ Discuss
    - Best care in circumstances
    - Anticipated events for preterm birth
    - Neonatal care for gestational age
    - Encourage family and social support involvement

Follow-up Care: Follow-up Measures to Consider

- Document
- Threatened preterm labor
  ○ Negative exam and labs
  ○ Reevaluate within 7 days

○ Sooner if symptoms persist or increase
- Consider serial ultrasound evaluation based on findings
  ○ Fetal surveillance
  ○ Cervical length
- Preterm labor and birth
  ○ Preterm infant care options locally or regionally
  ○ Consider transfer of care to perinatal specialist
- Provide support and reassurance
- Connect with community resources for assistance as indicated
  ○ Breast-feeding support
  ○ "Premie" clothing
  ○ Rides to neonatal special care unit

Collaborative Practice: Criteria to Consider for Consultation or Referral

- OB/GYN service
  ○ For suspected preterm labor
  ○ Confirmed preterm labor
- Consider transfer, as applicable, to
  ○ Hospital care
  ○ Regional perinatal care center
- Pediatric service
  ○ For presence at birth
  ○ For follow-up of "premie" newborn
- Social Service
  ○ Social support services
  ○ Parents of "premies" support groups
  ○ Grief counseling prn
- For diagnosis or treatment outside the midwife's scope of practice

Care of the Woman with Prolonged Latent Phase Labor

Key Clinical Information

The latent phase of labor may be considered prolonged when it exceeds approximately 20 hours in nullipara or 14 hours in multipara from the onset of *regular* contractions to the onset of active labor (3–4 cm dilation). The latent phase of labor is considered to end with the onset of uncomfortable, rhythmic uterine contractions that last 45 seconds or more, and are moderate to strong by palpation. Progressive cervical change is the hallmark of labor; persistent uterine contractions in the absence of cervical change should not be considered labor and should be treated as preparation for labor. Maternal fatigue caused by persistent irregular contractions can have a profound impact on the woman's labor energy levels and may influence the clinician to intervene when labor has not yet begun in earnest.

Client History:
Components of the History to Consider

- LMP, EDC
- G, P
- Previous labor patterns in multipara
- Current contraction pattern
  - Onset of contractions
    - Intermittent contractions
    - Presence of regular contractions
    - Associated cervical change
  - Maternal response to contractions
  - Status of membranes
  - Associated factors and symptoms
    - Increase in vaginal discharge
    - Mucous plug
    - Spotting
    - Recent intercourse or orgasm

- Use of alternative uterotonics
- Maternal and fetal well-being
  - Sleep, rest, and activity
  - Nutrition and fluid intake
  - Fetal activity

Physical Examination:
Components of the Physical Exam to Consider

- Fetal vital signs and well-being
  - FHT
  - Fetal motion
- Maternal well-being
  - Vital signs, including temp
  - Abdominal exam
    - Estimated fetal weight
    - Fetal presentation and position
  - Pelvic exam for progressive changes in
    - Cervical effacement
    - Cervical dilation
    - Descent of presenting part
    - Status of membranes
    - Amniotic fluid volume
    - Pelvimetry
  - Assess hydration
    - Urine output, color, specific gravity
    - Skin turgor
  - Signs of decreased coping ability
    - Excessive anxiety
    - Fear
    - Tension
  - Evaluate for signs of exhaustion

Clinical Impression:
Differential Diagnoses to Consider

- Disordered uterine contractions

- ○ False labor
- ○ Prodromal labor
- ○ Uterine irritability
- Labor complicated by
  - ○ Uterine inertia
  - ○ Desultory labor
  - ○ Malpresentation
  - ○ Asynclitic presentation
  - ○ Persistent occiput posterior
  - ○ Face presentation
  - ○ Breech presentation
  - ○ Obstructed labor

Diagnostic Testing:
Diagnostic Tests and Procedures to Consider

- Fetal evaluation
  - ○ FHR
  - ○ Fetal kick counts
  - ○ Amniotic fluid color if ROM
  - ○ BPP/AFI as indicated
- Maternal evaluation
  - ○ Urine for specific gravity
  - ○ Evaluation of contractions
    - Palpation
    - External electronic monitoring
    - UPC if membranes ruptured
- Pre-op labs if concerned about CPD

Providing Treatment:
Therapeutic Measures to Consider

- Therapeutic rest
  - ○ May stop contractions due to uterine irritability
  - ○ Allows rest and restoration (Hunter & Chern-Hughes, 1996)
    - Benadryl 50 mg po

- Seconal 100 mg po
- Morphine sulfate 10–20 mg IM or SQ (with or without vistaril 50 mg IM)
- Vistaril 50–75 mg IM
- Demerol 25–50 mg IM (with or without phenergan 25 mg)
- Hydration, oral or IV
- Stimulation of labor (Hunter & Chern-Hughes, 1996)
  - ○ Oxytocin stimulation
  - ○ AROM

Providing Treatment:
Alternative Measures to Consider

- Watchful waiting
- Provide safe environment to allow for
  - ○ Rest, including intermittent naps
  - ○ Hydration and adequate nutrition
- Warm bath/hydrotherapy
- Massage
- Strong chamomile or hops tea to facilitate rest (Foster, 1996)
- Position changes to facilitate optimal fetal positioning
- Labor stimulation (Summers, 1997)
  - ○ Nipple stimulation
  - ○ Castor oil
    - 2–4 oz po
    - Repeat in 1–2 hours if necessary
  - ○ Black/blue cohosh tincture
    - 10 gtt q 10–30 minutes
    - Increase dosage prn according to contraction pattern
  - ○ Evening primrose oil
    - Apply directly to the cervix

Providing Support:
Education and Support Measures to Consider

- Listen to maternal concerns
  - Explore fears related to labor, birth, parenting
  - Provide reassurance
- Work to provide a safe-feeling birth environment
- Discuss options with woman and her significant other(s)
  - Review stages of labor
  - Rest
  - Stimulation of contractions
  - Potential change in birth plans
    - Location
    - Provider(s)

Follow-up Care:
Follow-up Measures to Consider

- Document
- Update documentation after each evaluation
- Reevaluate q 1–2 hours for
  - Response to therapy
  - Progressive labor signs
    - Strength and duration of contractions
    - Application of presenting part to cervix
    - Dilation and descent
    - Positioning of fetal vertex
    - Status of membranes (Hunter & Chern-Hughes, 1996)
  - Developing maternal and fetal complications
    - Hourglass membranes
    - Caput formation
    - Swelling of cervix
    - Maternal exhaustion
    - Obstructed labor

- Infection
- Fetal distress
- If therapeutic rest is not successful
  - Consider stimulation of labor
  - Reevaluate potential causes
- If progress does not occur evaluate for evidence of
  - Ineffective uterine contraction
  - Suboptimal fetal presentation or position
  - Fetopelvic disproportion

Collaborative Practice:
Consider Consultation or Referral

- OB/GYN service
  - Diagnosis of prolonged latent phase
  - Lack of successful response to therapy
  - As needed for change of birth location
- For diagnosis or treatment outside the midwife's scope of practice

Care of the Woman with Premature Rupture of the Membranes

Key Clinical Information

Premature rupture of membranes (PROM) is defined as ROM that occurs before the onset of labor. Ninety percent of women with PROM will enter labor by 24 hours post-ROM. When there is greater than 24 hours between ROM and delivery of the infant, prolonged rupture of membranes is said to occur. Preterm premature rupture of the membranes is ROM that occurs before term. Complications of premature rupture of the membranes include complications related to preterm birth following PROM, fetal distress related to cord compression, and fetal infection. Maternal complications include maternal intra-amniotic infection, increased risk of Cesarean delivery, and postpartum endometritis (Varney et al., 2004; ACOG, 1998).

Client History:
Components of the History to Consider

- LMP, EDC, gestational age
- Relevant prenatal and maternity history
  - GBS status
  - Complications of current or previous pregnancy
  - Previous PROM
  - Last pap results
  - STI testing and results
  - New sexual partner(s)
- Current signs and symptoms
  - Onset of symptoms
  - Duration of symptoms
  - Amount, color, consistency of vaginal leakage
  - Last sexual activity
  - Presence of warning signs
    - Fever or chills
    - Palpitations
    - Uterine tenderness
    - Flank tenderness
- Presence of risk factors for PROM (Varney et al., 2004)
  - Nonvertex presentation
  - Previous pregnancy with PROM
  - Chorioamnionitis
  - Polyhydramnios
  - Multiple gestation
  - Vaginal group B strep or other pathogenic vaginal flora
  - Smoking > ½ pack per day
  - Nutritional deficiencies
  - Family history of PROM
  - Cervical conization

Physical Examination:
Components of the Physical Exam to Consider

- VS with temps q 1–2 hours
  - Maternal fever (temp > 32.2°C or 99°F)
  - Maternal or fetal tachycardia (maternal HR > 100, FHR > 160)
- Abdominal exam
  - Amniotic fluid volume/ballottement
  - Presence of contractions
  - Estimated fetal weight
  - Determine fetal presentation, lie
  - Frequent evaluation of fetal FHR
  - Palpation for uterine tenderness
- Sterile speculum exam
  - Visualization of leakage of amniotic fluid
  - Visualization of cervix is possible
  - Collection of specimen(s) for examination
    - Ferning
    - Nitrazine
    - GBS culture or screen
- SVE (defer or limit exams)
  - Cervical dilation
  - Effacement
  - Station
  - Confirm presentation
  - Rule out cord prolapse

Clinical Impression:
Differential Diagnoses to Consider

- Premature rupture of membranes
- Urinary incontinence
  - Physiologic
  - Secondary to urinary tract infection
- Increased vaginal secretions due to
  - Pregnancy

- ○ Vaginitis
- ○ Sexually transmitted infection
- ○ Intercourse
- Cervical cancer

Diagnostic Testing:
Diagnostic Tests and Procedures to Consider

- Vaginal fluid evaluation
  - ○ Nitrazine or pH testing (pH 7.0–7.7)
  - ○ Ferning
  - ○ Wet prep and KOH
- Cultures as indicated
  - ○ If expectant management planned
    - GBS culture of vagina and rectum
    - Chlamydia/gonorrhea status
- Ultrasound evaluation
  - ○ Oligohydramnios/AFI
  - ○ Biophysical profile
  - ○ Guidance for amniocentesis
- Amniocentesis for fetal pulmonary maturity testing
- CBC with differential
  - ○ Maternal leukocytosis (WBC > 16,000 with no labor)
- Urine for UA and C & S
  - ○ Clean catch
  - ○ Straight cath specimen
- Fetal surveillance
  - ○ NST if > 32 weeks gestation
  - ○ Daily fetal movement counts
  - ○ Biophysical profile/AFI

Providing Treatment:
Therapeutic Measures to Consider

- Bed rest recommended for
  - ○ Nonvertex presentation

- ○ Preterm PROM
- Antibiotic prophylaxis (see GBS)
- Expectant management based on gestational age (ACOG, 1998)
  - ○ Term
    - Labor and birth occur within 28 hours in 95% of cases
    - Observation of 24–72 hours acceptable per ACOG
    - Avoid digital exams until labor well established
    - Induction of labor (see Induction)
  - ○ Preterm with no additional complications
    - Conservative management preferred
    - Birth generally occurs within 7 days
    - Glucocorticoids to enhance fetal lung maturity
    - Tocolysis (rarely)
    - Transport to center with newborn special care

Providing Treatment:
Alternative Measures to Consider

- Watchful waiting
  - ○ No internal exams
  - ○ Temps q 2 hours
  - ○ Daily CBC
  - ○ Adequate hydration and nutrition
  - ○ Await onset of labor
- Stimulation of labor with natural remedies (see Induction)

Providing Support:
Education and Support Measures to Consider

- Discuss significance of PROM
  - ○ Anticipated fetal outcome for gestational age
  - ○ Anticipated newborn care

- Risks and benefits of options for care
- Maternal risk with PROM
  - Ascending intrauterine infection
  - Increased incidence of intervention
- Fetal risks with PROM
  - Umbilical cord compression
  - Ascending or preexisting infection
- Potential need for medical care
- Potential for change in
  - Birth plan
  - Location of birth
  - Birth attendant
- Signs and symptoms of
  - Chorioamnionitis
  - Neonatal sepsis
  - Postpartum endometritis

Follow-up Care:
Follow-up Measures to Consider

- Document
- Review results of
  - Maternal testing
  - Fetal surveillance
    - Fetal kick counts
    - NST
    - Biophysical profile
    - Serial AFI
    - FHR
- Intermittent auscultation of FHT
- Continuous fetal monitoring
- Cervical ripening or induction of labor (see Induction of Labor)
  - Essential if amnionitis suspected
  - ROM > 24–72 hrs
- Reassess for signs or symptoms of complications

- Maternal fever
- Abdominal tenderness
- Abnormal FHT patterns
  - Tachycardia
  - Bradycardia
  - Nonreassuring FHR patterns
- Update plan as changes occur
- Expedite birth if
  - Symptoms of infection develop
  - Fetal compromise occurs
  - Maternal preference
- Evaluate postpartum for
  - Endometritis
  - Other infection
  - Newborn sepsis
- Offer time for discussion and processing
  - Labor and birth events
  - Outcomes
  - Potential effect on future pregnancies

Collaborative Practice:
Consider Consultation or Referral

- OB/GYN service
  - Documented PROM with
    - Delay in onset of labor
    - Signs or symptoms of
- Infection
- Cord prolapse
- Fetal compromise
- Pediatric service
  - Onset of labor with fetal or maternal infection
  - For birth as indicated by fetal status
  - Newborn evaluation following prolonged ROM

- For diagnosis or treatment outside the midwife's scope of practice

Care of the Woman with Shoulder Dystocia

Key Clinical Information

Shoulder dystocia occurs when there is difficulty birthing the shoulders after the baby's head has already been born. Nearly half of all shoulder dystocia occurs in babies that weigh less than 4000 grams, so it is not the baby's size alone is that creates the difficulty. Rather it is the fit of this particular baby through the pelvis of this particular mother. Studies have been unable to reliably predict which mothers and babies will be at risk for shoulder dystocia (ACOG, 2002c).

Shoulder dystocia may be anticipated with a long second stage, and the presence of the "turtle sign" after the head emerges. The head extends with difficulty, and the chin remains snug against the perineum. Restitution does not occur. The shoulders may be wedged in the pelvis—"tight shoulders"—or they may be impacted above the pelvic brim. Prompt identification of shoulder dystocia should result in the rapid initiation of systematic maneuvers to deliver the baby. Shoulder dystocia may result in significant damage to the infant, such as brachial plexus injury, fracture of the clavicle, hypoxia, or death. Traction on the baby has been associated with increased risk of newborn injury (Varney et al., 2004).

Client History: Components of the History to Consider

- LMP, EDC, gestational age
- Maternal height/weight
- Documented clinical pelvimetry
- Potential risk factors for shoulder dystocia
  - Maternal diabetes
  - History of large infants
  - Maternal obesity
  - Postdate pregnancy
  - Large fetus, by palpation or ultrasound
  - History of prior difficult delivery
  - CPD (ACOG, 2002c)
  - Desultory labor
  - Prolonged second stage

Physical Examination: Components of the Physical Exam to Consider

- Abdominal exam in labor
  - Fetal presentation and position
  - Flexion of head at pelvic brim
  - Estimate fetal weight with onset of labor
- Pelvic exam(s) during labor
  - Progression of cervical dilation
  - Rate of descent
  - Maternal tissue elasticity
  - Pelvimetry
- At delivery
  - Slow progression of extension
  - Retraction of head ("turtle sign")
  - Failure to restitute
  - Suffusion of infant's face
  - Need for one or more maneuvers to deliver baby

Clinical Impression: Differential Diagnoses to Consider

- Shoulder dystocia
- "Tight" shoulders
- Short cord
- Fetal anomaly that prevents descent

Diagnostic Testing:
Diagnostic Tests and Procedures to Consider

- Ultrasound for EFW
  - Often inaccurate by > 1–2 lbs
  - Size is often not the issue
- Pre-op labs

Providing Treatment:
Therapeutic Measures to Consider

- Engage mother in cooperating
- Mother on back
  - McRobert's maneuver (knees to shoulders)
    - Advantages:
      - Alters angle of inclination of symphysis
      - Flattens sacrum
      - Gives midwife most room to work
      - Reduces amount of traction required to effect birth
        - May decrease traction-related fetal injury
    - Disadvantages:
      - Requires two assistants
  - Request firm suprapubic pressure
- Encourage maternal pushing efforts
- Attempt birth
  - With *gentle* traction on head
  - If descent occurs, assist with birth
    - Fingers on both shoulders
    - Maintain arms in close contact with trunk
- If birth does not occur
  - Stop maternal pushing efforts
  - With dominant hand in vagina check position of shoulders
    - Place hand on infant's back
    - Palpate anterior axillary crease
      - 🔔 Do *not* pull with fingers in axilla

- Use firm traction on the suprascapular bones to
  - Decrease the bisacromial diameter
  - Attempt rotation of anterior shoulder into pelvis
    - Use firm, gentle pressure
    - Rotate baby's back toward symphysis
    - Rotate shoulders into the oblique
  - As anterior shoulder rotates
  - Move client to hands and knees prn
  - Maintain baby's position
  - Use gentle outward traction
  - This should bring posterior shoulder into the pelvis
    - Deliver posterior arm prn
  - Encourage maternal pushing efforts
    - "Walk" shoulders out using both hands
    - Traction on suprascapular bones
    - Keep arms close to body
    - Use gentle, firm outward traction
  - Rotate baby manually from side to side
    - Back always moving anteriorly
    - "Corkscrew" the body out
- Mother on hands and knees for birth
  - Flex legs so belly rests on legs
  - Knees to shoulders
  - Deliver posterior arm first
- Tub birth
  - Have mother stand and lean over tub
    - This may release impaction
  - Assist as you would for mother on hands and knees, or
  - Have mother exit tub
    - Move to hands and knees, or McRobert's
    - Continue as above

- For severe unrelieved shoulder dystocia consider
  - Alternative positioning
  - Call for OB and pediatric assistance
  - Fracture of clavicle
  - Empty bladder with straight catheter
  - Enlarge or cut episiotomy
  - Rule out other causes of dystocia
    - Direct palpation of pelvic contents
    - Fetal anomalies
    - Extremely short cord
  - Zavenelli maneuver (Varney et al., 2004; ACOG, 2002c)
    - Replacement of head in vagina
    - Reverse process of extension
    - Followed with C-section
- Prepare for
  - Full neonatal resuscitation (AAP/AHA, 2000)
  - Immediate postpartum hemorrhage
- Cesarean section for documented macrosomia
  - Not demonstrated to be effective for
    - Infants under 5000 gm in normoglycemic mothers
    - Infants under 4500 gm in diabetic mothers (ACOG, 2002c)

Providing Treatment:
Alternative Measures to Consider

- Gaskin maneuver (Brunner, Drummond, Meenan & Gaskin, 1998)
  - Rotate mother to hands and knees
  - Rotate in direction baby is facing
  - Alters pelvic geometry
  - Advantages
    - Position change may resolve impaction
    - Gravity may facilitate delivery
  - Disadvantages
    - Cannot use suprapubic pressure
    - Limited access to infant
    - May exaggerate impaction
- Squatting
  - Advantages
    - Position change may resolve impaction
    - Results in a wider pubic (outlet) angle
  - Disadvantages
    - Cannot use suprapubic pressure
    - May decrease inlet dimensions
    - Limited access to infant

Providing Support:
Education and Support Measures to Consider

- Discuss potential for difficult birth with mother who has
  - Documented macrosomia
  - EFW more than 1 lb larger than largest previous infant
- Follow-up after birth with discussion
  - Regarding care given
  - Infant well-being
  - Maternal feelings about
    - Complications
    - Interventions
    - Outcomes
    - Labor and birth
- Review signs of
  - Postpartum endometritis
  - Postpartum depression

Follow-up Care:
Follow-up Measures to Consider

- Immediately after birth
  - Provide newborn resuscitation as necessary
  - Evaluate infant for birth injury

- Observe for PPH following delivery
- Evaluate for maternal injury
- Document
  - 🔔 Birth details in delivery note
  - Physical findings at birth
    - Identification of shoulder dystocia
    - Maneuvers used and their effects
    - Noted injury to mother or infant
  - Consultations requested during birth
- Seek opportunity for peer support
  - Peer review (nondiscoverable)
  - Case presentation or discussion
  - Informal support

Collaborative Practice:
Consider Consultation or Referral (Varney et al., 2004; Sinclair, 2004; Wood, 1994)

- OB/GYN service
  - Potential for shoulder dystocia anticipated
  - Diagnosis of shoulder dystocia
- Pediatric service
  - In anticipation of neonatal resuscitation
  - For newborn evaluation after difficult birth
- For diagnosis or treatment outside the midwife's scope of practice

Care of the Woman Undergoing Vacuum-Assisted Birth

Key Clinical Information

Vacuum-assisted birth carries with it significant risks to mother and baby (ACOG, 2000). The benefits of using the vacuum extractor to aid in the birth of the baby should clearly outweigh the potential risks associated with this procedure. Midwives who assist with birth using outlet vacuum extraction should be educated and trained in indications and contraindications, techniques, and complications associated with the use of the device.

Client History:
Components of the History to Consider

- Verify LMP, EDC, and term gestation
- Relevant prenatal and OB history
  - Progress of labor, including second stage
  - Fetal and maternal response to labor
  - Review pelvimetry
- Presence of any contraindications to vacuum assisted birth (Sweet, 1997)
  - Weak or infrequent uterine contraction
  - Vertex not well engaged
  - CPD
  - Premature infant (< 37 weeks)
  - Suspected macrosomia
  - Nonvertex presentation
  - Uncooperative client
  - Poor expulsive effort
- Indications for vacuum-assisted birth (ACOG, 2000a)
  - Prolonged second stage
    - > 3 hours for nullip
    - > 2 hours for multip
  - Fetal distress
  - Maternal exhaustion

Physical Examination:
Components of the Physical Exam to Consider

- Abdominal exam
  - Fetal lie, presentation, position
  - Estimated fetal weight (EFW)
  - Presence of adequate, effective regular contractions
- Pelvic exam
  - Dilation must be complete
  - Station
    - +2 station = midforceps delivery

- Physician management recommended
- Vacuum extraction vs. forceps vs. C/S
  - Vertex visible at introitus = outlet delivery
  - Presence of caput or marked molding
    - Increases risk of fetal trauma
  - Assess fetal presentation and position

Clinical Impression: Differential Diagnoses to Consider

- Vacuum-assisted birth for
  - Maternal fatigue
  - Prolonged second stage
  - Fetal distress

Diagnostic Testing: Diagnostic Tests and Procedures to Consider

- Pre-op labs
- Evaluate effectiveness of uterine contractions
  - Palpation
  - Electronic fetal monitoring
- Evaluate fetal response via FHR
  - Auscultation
  - Electronic fetal monitoring

Providing Treatment: Therapeutic Measures to Consider

- Oxytocin stimulation to improve contractions
- Vacuum-assisted birth
  - Empty bladder and rectum
  - Consider local anesthesia
  - Consider episiotomy
    - May increase risk of third- or fourth-degree laceration
    - Mediolateral episiotomy may give more room
  - Verify position of vertex

- Apply vacuum cup to posterior fontanel
- Verify that no maternal tissues are under cup rim
  - Request suction
    - 4 in Hg or 100 mm Hg between contractions
    - 15–23 in Hg or 500 mm Hg with contractions
  - *Do not allow vacuum to remain at maximum levels for more than 10 accrued minutes*
- Apply gentle steady traction
  - With contractions only
  - Follow curve of Carus
- Discontinue attempts to assist birth with vacuum if
  - Cup disengages 3 times
  - Scalp trauma visible after cup disengages
  - No progress following 3 attempts at traction
  - 15–30 minutes with no success
  - Birth has not occurred within 10 *accrued* minutes of maximum suction

Providing Treatment: Alternative Measures to Consider

- Assess for maternal and fetal well-being
  - Be patient
  - Allow rest period
  - Provide for adequate hydration and nutrition
- Continue maternal pushing efforts
  - Encourage voiding
  - Push only with urge
- Vigilant assessment of maternal and fetal status
  - Vital signs
  - Fetal descent
- Position changes
  - Side-lying
  - McRobert's position

  ○ Lithotomy with leg support

    ▪ Feet should push against fixed object

    ▪ Arms should pull

    ▪ Back should be as flat as possible

    ▪ Use of squatting bar helpful

  ○ Squatting

  ○ Birthing stool

  ○ Hand and knees

  ○ Floating in birthing tub

Providing Support:
Education and Support Measures to Consider

• Discuss with client and family

  ○ Concerns related to slow progress

  ○ Options for care

  ○ Recommendations and indications

• Vacuum-assisted birth procedure

  ○ Discuss risks and benefits with client

    ▪ Risk of fetal trauma

      • Cephalohematoma

      • Intracranial trauma

      • Shoulder dystocia

      • Ecchymosis, abrasions (ACOG, 2000a)

  ○ Risk of maternal trauma

    ▪ Third- or fourth-degree laceration

    ▪ Sulcus tears

    ▪ Possible need for Cesarean birth

  ○ Benefits

    ▪ Vaginal birth of infant

    ▪ Faster than forceps or C-section

    ▪ Less risk of fetal trauma than forceps

• Depends on skill of operator and force used

    ▪ May decrease need for C-section

Follow-up Care:
Follow-up Measures to Consider

• Prepare for potential

  ○ Shoulder dystocia

  ○ Postpartum hemorrhage

  ○ Third- or fourth-degree laceration

  ○ Newborn injury

  ○ Newborn resuscitation

• Document (see Procedure Note)

• Evaluate for maternal or neonatal injury

  ○ Examine vagina carefully for lacerations

  ○ Examine infant carefully for injury

• Discuss birth with mother and family

  ○ Allow exploration of feelings

  ○ Review indications for assisted birth

Collaborative Practice:
Criteria to Consider for Consultation or Referral

• OB/GYN service

  ○ Indications for vacuum extraction

  ○ Maternal indications, C-section may be necessary

• Pediatric service

  ○ Fetal distress

  ○ Fetal injury

  ○ For fetal observation of delayed signs of injury

• For diagnosis or treatment outside the midwife's scope of practice

Care of the Woman During Vaginal Birth After Cesarean

Key Clinical Information

Vaginal birth after Cesarean (VBAC) provides carefully selected women with an alternative to surgical delivery of the infant. A scarred uterus is at greater risk of rupturing than an unscarred uterus. Many factors contribute to scar integrity. Among the factors are the type of closure (e.g., 1 layer versus 2 layers), adequate tissue nutrition and oxygenation to support wound healing, an intact and functioning immune system, and minimal stress on the wound during and immediately following wound healing (Bujold, Bujold, Hamilton, Harel & Gauthier, 2002).

Uterine ruptures occur at a documented rate of approximately 0.5–1%. This rate is increased in women with a single-layer uterine closure, two or more previous Cesarean births, an interdelivery interval of 24 months or less, history of postoperative fever or infection, and women who have their labor augmented or induced with oxytocin (Shipp, 1999). When uterine rupture does occur, outcomes are improved with the immediate availability of skilled surgical services.

Client History:
Components of the History to Consider

- Obtain operative records for previous C-section
  - Indication for primary C-section
  - Gestational age with prior C/S
  - Type of uterine incision
  - Type of uterine closure
  - Postoperative course (Ethicon, 2004)
- Review current pregnancy course
- Positive factors for the VBAC candidate
  - Nonrepeating cause
  - Client motivated for vaginal birth
  - Previous vaginal birth
  - Vertex presentation
  - Two-layer uterine closure
  - No history of post-op fever or infection
  - Maternal age < 30
  - 24+ months since previous C/S
  - Spontaneous onset of labor
  - Progressive labor
- Negative factors for the VBAC candidate

  - Classical or midline uterine incision
  - Documented CPD
  - Nonvertex presentation of baby
  - Two or more previous Cesareans
  - Single-layer uterine closure
  - Maternal age > 30
  - Less than 18 months since previous C/S
  - Nonprogressive labor (ACOG, 2004a)

Physical Examination:
Components of the Physical Exam to Consider

- Comprehensive labor evaluation
  - Clinical pelvimetry with history of CPD or FTP
  - EFW
  - Presentation, position, engagement
  - Maternal and fetal vital signs
- Reevaluate progress at frequent intervals
- Maternal and fetal response to labor
  - Contraction pattern
  - Cervical change
  - Fetal decent
- Signs of uterine rupture
  - Fetal bradycardia or non-reassuring FHR
  - Maternal tachycardia
  - Abdominal pain may or may not be present (ACOG, 2004a)

Clinical Impression:
Differential Diagnoses to Consider

- Potential VBAC candidate
  - Nonrepeating condition
  - Appropriate candidate per practice
  - Client preference for labor and vaginal birth
  - Access to surgical support
  - Informed choice and consent

- Repeat C/S candidate
  - Repeating cause for C/S
  - Client preference
  - Nonprogressive labor
  - Informed choice and consent
- Uterine scar dehiscence or rupture

Diagnostic Testing:
Diagnostic Tests and Procedures to Consider

- Pre-op labs
  - CBC
  - Type and screen
- Continuous observation of maternal and fetal status
  - 1:1 nurse or midwife care with auscultation *or*
  - External fetal monitor *or*
  - Internal fetal monitor

Providing Treatment:
Therapeutic Measures to Consider

- Evaluate for onset of progressive labor
- Provide a supportive labor and birthing environment
- Limit invasive exams or procedures
- Oral intake
  - NPO
  - Ice chips
  - Clear liquids
- IV access
  - Saline lock
  - IV at KVO
- Maternal and fetal evaluation of well-being
- Medications
  - Cytotec contraindicated for use with scarred uterus

- Oxytocin as indicated
  - May facilitate vaginal birth due to uterine inertia
  - Overstimulation may increase risk of rupture (ACOG, 2004a)
- Pain relief as needed (see First Stage Labor)

Providing Treatment:
Alternative Measures to Consider

- Facilitate physiologic labor
  - Ambulation
  - Hydrotherapy
  - Positioning
  - Doula support
  - Adequate hydration and nutrition
- Foster maternal autonomy
  - Provide a supportive labor environment

Providing Support:
Education and Support Measures to Consider

- Discuss options with client and family
  - VBAC versus repeat C-section
  - Surgical coverage options
  - Location(s) for birth
  - Options for labor care and support
- Obtain informed consent
  - Success rate 60–80% (ACOG, 2004a)
  - Risk of catastrophic uterine rupture
    - Low transverse uterine incision 0.19–0.8% (Varney et al., 2004)
    - Higher with any other type of incision
    - Risk of maternal or fetal death with catastrophic rupture
  - Risks, benefits, and alternatives to VBAC
  - Discussion regarding facility/practice parameters for VBAC

- Anticipated care of VBAC women in labor
  - Labor procedures, e.g., IV, labs, etc.
  - Average length of time for urgent C/S
    - At facility
    - If transport required

Follow-up Care:
Follow-up Measures to Consider

- Consult OB/GYN of client choice prenatally
- Uterine scar dehiscence or rupture
  - May result in fetal and/or maternal death
  - May occur in labor or during birth
  - Access surgical services STAT
  - Assure IV access
    - Provide fluid replacement
    - Order blood
  - Treat shock
- Document 👐
  - Review of previous C/S operative notes
  - Discussions with client and family
  - Client preference
  - Informed choice and consent
  - Treatment of complications
  - Consultations
- Update notes frequently, especially in labor

Collaborative Practice:
Criteria to Consider for Consultation or Referral

- OB/GYN service
  - Previous incision that is not low transverse
  - Planned repeat C-section
  - Planned VBAC
  - STAT for client in labor with
    - Symptoms of uterine rupture

- Evidence of developing dystocia or obstruction
- Demand for repeat C/S
- Pediatric service
  - Non-reassuring FHR
- For diagnosis or treatment outside the midwife's scope of practice

References

American College of Nurse-Midwives [ACNM]. (1998). *Position statement: The certified nurse-midwife/certified midwife as first assistant at surgery.* Washington, DC: Author.

ACNM Clinical Bulletin No. 2. (Jan. 1997). Early-onset group B strep infection in newborns: Prevention and prophylaxis. *Journal of Nurse-Midwifery, 42,* 403–408.

American College of Obstetricians and Gynecologists [ACOG]. (1995). Technical bulletin #207: Fetal heart rate patterns: Monitoring, interpretation, and management. In *2002 compendium of selected publications.* Washington, DC: Author.

ACOG. (1998a). Practice bulletin #1: Premature rupture of membranes. In *2005 compendium of selected publications.* Washington, DC: Author.

ACOG. (1998b). Education bulletin #253: Special problems of multiple gestation. In *2005 compendium of selected publications.* Washington, DC: Author.

ACOG. (2000a). Practice bulletin #17: Operative vaginal delivery. In *2005 compendium of selected publications.* Washington, DC: Author.

ACOG. (2000b). Practice bulletin #13: External cephalic version. In *2002 compendium of selected publications.* Washington, DC: Author.

ACOG. (2001). Committee opinion #265: Mode of singleton breech delivery. In *2005 compendium of selected publications.* Washington, DC: Author.

ACOG. (2002a). Committee opinion #273: Antenatal corticosteroid therapy for fetal maturation. In *2005 compendium of selected publications.* Washington, DC: Author.

ACOG (2002b). Practice bulletin #33: Diagnosis and management of pre-eclampsia and eclampsia. In *2005 compendium of selected publications.* Washington, DC: Author.

ACOG. (2002c). Practice bulletin #40: Shoulder dystocia. In *2005 compendium of selected publications*. Washington, DC: Author.

ACOG. (2003). Practice bulletin #43: Management of preterm labor. In *2005 compendium of selected publications*. Washington, DC: Author.

ACOG. (2004a). Practice bulletin #54: Vaginal birth after cesarean. In *2005 compendium of selected publications*. Washington, DC: Author.

ACOG. (2004b). Practice Bulletin #55: Management of post-term pregnancy. In *2005 compendium of selected publications*. Washington, DC: Author.

American Academy of Pediatrics/American Heart Association [AAP/AHA]. (2000). *Textbook of neonatal resuscitation* (4th ed.). Elk Grove, IL: American Academy of Pediatrics.

Antenatal corticosteroids revisited: Repeat courses. *NIH Consensus statement 2000, 17*, 1–10.

Bishop, E. H. (1964). Pelvic scoring for elective induction. *Obstetrics and Gynecology, 24*, 267.

Brucker, M. C. (2001). Management of the third stage of labor: An evidence-based approach. *Journal of Midwifery and Women's Health, 46*, 381–392.

Bruner, J., Drummond, S., Meenan, A. L., & Gaskin, I. M. (1998). The all fours maneuver for reducing shoulder dystocia. *Journal of Reproductive Medicine, 43*, 439–443.

Bujold, E., Bujold, C., Hamilton, E. F., Harel, F., & Gauthier, R. J. (2002). The impact of single-layer or double-layer closure on uterine rupture. *American Journal of Obstetrics and Gynecology, 186*, 1326–1330.

Byrne, B., & Morrison, J. (2004). Preterm birth. In F. Godlee (Ed.), *Clinical evidence concise* (pp. 392–394). London: BMJ.

Centers for Disease Control and Prevention [CDC]. (2002). *Perinatal group B streptococcal disease: Background, epidemiology, and overview of revised CDC prevention guidelines*. Retrieved October 19, 2005, from http://www.cdc.gov/groupbstrep/docs/GBS.slideset.DEC2.forweb.ppt.

Chandrasekhar, S., & Datta, S. (2002). Anesthetic management of the pre-eclamptic parturient. In *Current reviews for nurse anesthetists*. Fort Lauderdale, FL: Frank Moya Continuing Education Programs.

El Halta, V. (1996). Normalizing the breech delivery. *Midwifery Today, 38*, 22–24, 41.

Ethicon. (2004). *Wound closure manual*. Retrieved February 13, 2005 from http://www.jnjgateway.com/public/USENG/Ethicon_WCM_Feb2004.pdf.

Falcao, R. (n.d.). *Non-pharmaceudical induction*. Retrieved February 2, 2005, from http://www.gentlebirth.org/archives/natinduc.html#Herbal.

Foster, S. (1996). *Herbs for your health*. Loveland, CO: Interweave Press.

Frigoletto, F. D. Jr, Lieberman, E., Lang, J. M., Cohen, A., Barss, V., Ringer, S., et al. (1995). A clinical trial of active management of labor. *New England Journal of Medicine, 333*, 745–50.

Frye, A. (1998). *Holistic midwifery*. Portland, OR: Labrys Press.

Frye, A. (1997). *Understanding diagnostic tests in the childbearing year* (6th ed.). Portland, OR: Labrys Press.

Hannah, M. E., & Hannah, W. J. (2000). Planned cesarean section versus planned vaginal birth for breech presentation at term: A randomized multicenter trial. *Lancet, 356*, 1375–1383.

Hargitaib B., Marton, T., & Cox, P. M. (2004). *BEST PRACTICE NO 178*: Examination of the human placenta. *Journal of Clinical Pathology 57*, 785–792.

Hart, G. (2002). Induction and circular logic. *Midwifery Today, 63*, 24–26, 66.

Hernandez, C., Little, B. B., Dax, J. S., Gilstrap, L. C., & Rosenfield, C. R. (1993). Prediction of the severity of meconium aspiration syndrome. *American Journal of Obstetrics and Gynecology, 169*, 61–70.

Hofmeyr, G. J. (2004a). Amnioinfusion for meconium-stained liquor in labour. In *The Cochrane Library*, Issue 2, 2004. Chichester, UK: John Wiley & Sons.

Hofmeyr, G. J. (2004b). Amnioinfusion for preterm rupture of membranes. In *The Cochrane Library*, Issue 2, 2004. Chichester, UK: John Wiley & Sons.

Hofmeyr, G. J. (2004c). Amnioinfusion for umbilical cord compression in labour. In *The Cochrane Library*, Issue 2, 2004. Chichester, UK: John Wiley & Sons.

Hunter, L. P., Chern-Hughes, B. (1996). Management of prolonged latent phase labor. *Journal of Nurse-Midwifery, 41*, 383–388.

Institute for Clinical Systems Improvement. (2004). *Prevention, diagnosis and treatment of failure to progress in obstetrical labor*. Bloomington, MN: Institute for Clinical Systems Improvement.

Jolivet, R. R. (2002). Early-onset neonatal group B streptococcal infection: 2002 guidelines for prevention. *Journal of Midwifery & Women's Health, 47*, 435–446.

Katz. V. L., Farmer, R., & Kuller, J. A. (2000). Preeclampsia into eclampsia: Toward a new paradigm.

American Journal of Obstetrics & Gynecology, 182, 1389–1396.

Langston, C., Kaplan, C., Macpherson, T., Manci, E., Peevy, K., Clark, B., Murtagh, C., Cox, S., & Glenn, G. (1997). Practice guideline for examination of the placenta: Developed by the Placental Pathology Practice Guideline Development Task Force of the College of American Pathologists. *Archives of Pathology and Laboratory Medicine, 121,* 449-76.

Livingston, J. C., Livingston, L. W., Ramsey, R., Mabie, B. C., & Sibai, B. M. (2003). Magnesium sulfate in women with mild pre-eclampsia: A randomized controlled trial. *Obstetrics & Gynecology, 101,* 217–226.

Lokugamage, A. U., Sullivan, K. R., Niculescu, I., Tigere, P., Onyangunga, F., El Refaey, H., et al. (2001). A randomized study comparing rectally administered misoprostol versus syntometrine combined with an oxytocin infusion for the cessation of primary post partum hemorrhage. *Acta Obstetricia et Gynecologica Scandinavica, 80,* 835–839.

Long, P. (2001). Safe management of third stage labor: A technical report based on review of the current literature. In Farley, C. L. (Ed.), Final Projects Database. (Available from Philadelphia University, Graduate Midwifery Programs, 222 Hayward Hall, Schoolhouse Lane and Henry Avenue, Philadelphia, PA 19144.)

Martin, J. N., Jr., Rinehart, B. K., May, W. L., Magann, E. F., Terrone, D. A., & Blake, P. G. (1999). The spectrum of severe pre-eclampsia: A comparative analysis of HELLP syndrome classification. *American Journal of Obstetrics & Gynecology, 180,* 1373–1384.

Mehl-Medrona, L., & Medrona, M. M. (1997). Physician- and midwife-attended home births: Effects of breech, twin, and post-dates outcome data on mortality rates. *Journal of Nurse-Midwifery, 42,* 91–98.

Mercer, J. S., & Skovgaard, R. L. (2002). Delayed cord clamping. Neonatal transitional physiology: A new paradigm. *Journal of Perinatal & Neonatal Nursing, 15,* 56–75.

Miller, S., Lester, F., Hensleigh, P. (2004). Prevention & treatment of PP hemorrhage: New advances for low-resource settings. *Journal of Midwifery & Women's Health, 49,* 283–292.

Moses, S. (2004). Indomethacin. Retrieved February, 2, 2005, from http://www.fpnotebook.com/PHA37.htm

Murphy, J. L. (Ed.). (2004). *Nurse practitioner's prescribing reference.* New York: Prescribing Reference.

Nothnagle, M., & Taylor, J. S. (2003). Should active management of the third stage of labor be routine? *American Family Physician 67,* 2119–2120.

Paszkowski, T. (1994). Amnioinfusion: A review. *The Journal of Reproductive Medicine, 39,* 588–594.

Peaceman, A. M., & Socol, M. L. (1996). Active management of labor. *American Journal of Obstetrics & Gynecology, 175,* 363–368.

Phelan, J. P. (1997, October). *Intrauterine fetal resuscitation; Betamimetics and amnioinfusion.* Presented at Issues and Controversies in Perinatal Practice Conference, Bangor, ME.

Prendiville, W.J., Elbourne, D., & McDonald, S. (2004). Active versus expectant management in the third stage of labour. In *The Cochrane Library,* Issue 4. Chichester, UK: John Wiley & Sons.

Roberts, J. (1994). Current perspectives on pre-eclampsia. *Journal of Nurse-Midwifery, 39,* 70–90.

Roberts, J. (2002). The push for evidence: Management of the second stage. *Journal of Midwifery & Women's Health, 47,* 2–15.

Rothrock, J. C. (1993). *The RN first assistant* (2nd ed.). Philadelphia: J.P. Lippincott.

Rx Med. (n.d.). *Cytotec.* Retrieved March 13, 2005, from http://www.rxmed.com/b.main/b2.pharmaceutical/ b2.1.monographs/CPS-%20Monographs/CPS-%20 (General%20Monographs-%20C)/CYTOTEC.html.

Schuchat, A (1998). Epidemiology of group B streptococcal disease in the United States: Shifting paradigms. *Clinical Microbiology Reviews, 11,* 497–513.

Shipp, T. D. (1999). Intrapartum rupture and dehiscence in patients with prior lower uterine segments vertical and transverse incisions. *Obstetrics & Gynecology, 94,* 735–740.

Sinclair, C. (2004) *A midwife's handbook.* St. Louis, MO: Saunders.

Soule, D. (1996). *The roots of healing.* Secaucus, NJ: Citadel Press.

Summers, L. (1997). Methods of cervical ripening and labor induction. *Journal of Nurse-Midwifery, 42,* 71–83.

Sweet, B. R. (Ed.). (1997). *Mayes' midwifery* (12th ed.) London: Bailliere Tindall.

Tucker, J. M., Goldenberg, R. L., Davis, R. O., Copper, R. L., Winkler, C. L., & Hauth, J. C. (1991). Etiologies of preterm birth in an indigent population: Is prevention a logical expectation? *Obstetrics & Gynecology, 77,* 343–348.

Tucker, M. (2004, July 1). Expert opinion backs two indications for amnoinfusion. *OB-GYN News.*

Varney, H., Kriebs, J. M., & Gegor, C. L. (2004). *Varney's midwifery* (4th ed.). Sudbury, MA: Jones and Bartlett.

Walraven, G., Dampha Y., Bittaye, B., Sowe, M., & Hofmeyr, J. (2004). Misoprostol in the treatment of postpartum haemorrhage in addition to routine management: A placebo randomised controlled trial. *British Journal of Obstetrics & Gynaecology, 111,* 1014–1017.

Weed, S. (1985). *Wise woman herbal for the childbearing year.* Woodstock, NY: Ashtree.

Weismiller, D. G., (1998). Transcervical amnioinfusion. *American Family Physician, 57,* 504–512.

Wiswell, T. E., Gannon, C. M., Jacob, J., Goldsmith, L., Szyld, E., Weiss, L., et al. (2000). Delivery room management of the apparently vigorous meconium-stained neonate: Results of the multicenter, international collaborative trial. *Pediatrics, 105,* 1–7.

Wood, C. L. (1994). Meconium-stained amniotic fluid. *Journal of Nurse-Midwifery, 39,* 106s–109s.

World Health Organization [WHO]. (1988) *Care of the umbilical cord: A review of the evidence.* Retrieved March 4, 2005, from http://www.who.int/reproductive-health/publications/MSM_98_4/MSM_98_4_chapter4.en.html.

WHO. (1996). *Care in normal birth: A practical guide.* Report of a Technical Working Group. WHO/FRH/MSM/96.24, Geneva, Switzerland.

Yoder, B. (1994). Meconium-stained amniotic fluid and respiratory complications: Impact of selective tracheal suction. *Obstetrics & Gynecology, 83,* 77–84.

Care of the Mother and Baby After Birth

6

The baby's birth signals a time of immense transition when both mother and infant are particularly vulnerable to disruption.

Fostering mother–baby bonding is an integral part of midwifery practice. Continued supportive care allows the mother and baby to focus on each other as they adapt to their respective changes under the watchful eye of the skilled midwife. Evaluation for postpartum depression, effective infant feeding, and variations from the norm allows early intervention to reduce sequelae of potential complications that may result in harm to mother or baby.

The postpartum period highlights cultural practices and beliefs about birth and the newborn. For the midwife practicing in a multicultural environment it provides a wonderful opportunity to explore nurturing in its many forms. Infant feeding and bonding influence each woman's self-image and her view of herself as competent to the tasks that parenting brings. Changes in intimate relationships are common, as the baby takes up time and physical as well as emotional energy. Concerns about fertility resurface, providing another opportunity to explore women's health within the context of individual women's lives.

Postpartum Care, Week 1

Key Clinical Information

During the postpartum period each woman rapidly undergoes vast changes as her body returns to the nonpregnant state and she adapts emotionally to the changes in her family with the birth of her child. While the physiologic process is much the same in each individual, every woman responds differently to the birth of a child and will have specific and distinct personal needs to be met.

Client History:
Components of the History to Consider

- Age, gravity, and parity
- Review of pregnancy, labor, and birth
  - Prenatal course
  - Labor and birth information
    - Length of labor
    - Complicating factors for labor and/or birth
    - Manner of birth
    - Lacerations or episiotomy
- Infant well-being since birth
  - Feeding
  - Sleeping
  - Activity
- Inquire as to general well-being
  - Pain
    - Location
    - Severity
    - Relief measures used and results
  - Sleep/rest
  - Appetite
  - Flow
  - Breasts
  - Other symptoms
- ROS
- Adaptation to postpartum status
  - Maternal emotional response to
    - Labor and birth
    - Changes postpartum
    - Changes in family dynamics
  - Observe interaction with infant
    - Feeding
    - Bonding
    - Caretaking

Physical Examination:
Components of the Physical Exam to Consider

- Vital signs: BP, T, P
- Chest
  - Heart and lungs
  - CVA tenderness
- Breasts and nipples
  - Cracks or fissures
  - Engorgement
  - Colostrum or milk
- Abdomen
  - Fundus: Location, consistency, tenderness
  - Muscle tone: Diastasis, hernia
  - Incision: Dressing, redness, erythema, exudate
  - Bladder: Distention, tenderness
  - Bowel sounds
- Lochia
  - Type, amount, odor
- Perineum and rectum
  - Approximation of tissues
  - Bruising, inflammation, hematoma
  - Edema
  - Hemorrhoids
- Extremities
  - Edema
  - Reflexes
  - Homan's sign
  - Redness, heat, or pain
  - Varicosities

Clinical Impression:
Differential Diagnoses to Consider

- Postpartum, vaginal birth
  - With or without episiotomy or laceration

- Spontaneous vaginal birth
- Assisted vaginal birth
- Postpartum, Cesarean birth
- Post-op tubal ligation
- Postpartum or postoperative course with complicating factors, such as
  - Preeclampsia
  - Anemia
  - Puerperal infection

Diagnostic Testing:
Diagnostic Tests and Procedures to Consider

- H & H or CBC 1st or 2nd pp day
- Rh studies
- As indicated for complications of
  - Pregnancy
  - Postpartum
  - Medical condition

Providing Treatment:
Therapeutic Measures to Consider

- Laxatives
  - Colace
  - Senokot
  - Milk of magnesia
- Urinary system
  - Encourage frequent voiding
  - Catheterize prn for urinary retention
  - Insert Foley catheter if unable to void x 2
- Heavy lochia and/or uterine atony
  - Methergine 0.2 mg po q 4 h x 6 doses
- Pain management (Varney et al., 2004)
  - Ibuprofen 400–800 mg q 12 hours
  - Percocet 1–2 tabs q 6 h prn
  - Darvocet-N 100: 1 po q 4 hours prn

- Empirin #3: 1–2 tabs q 4 hours prn
- Tylenol #3: 1–2 tabs q 4 hours prn
- Sleep (Murphy, 2004)
  - Ambien 5–10 mg at HS
  - Dalmane 30 mg at HS
  - Nembutal sodium 50–100 mg at HS
- Immune status
  - Rh immune globulin IM
  - Rubella vaccine SC

Providing Treatment:
Alternative Measures to Consider

- Bowel care
  - Encourage fiber and fluids
    - Psyllium seed
    - Prune juice
    - Dried fruits
- Perineal care
  - Comfrey compresses
  - Homeopathic arnica montana po
  - Sitz baths, plain or herbal
- Urinary care
  - Encourage frequent voiding
  - Urinary retention
    - Oil of peppermint drops in toilet
- Uterine care
  - Heavy lochia and/or uterine atony
    - Blue cohosh
    - Shepherd's purse
- Afterpains
  - Hot pack to abdomen
  - Nurse frequently
  - Void frequently
- Sleep
  - Encourage frequent rest periods

◦ Chamomile tea to promote rest

Providing Support:
Education and Support Measures to Consider

- Active listening
  - ◦ Birth experience
  - ◦ Maternal and family response to baby
  - ◦ Feeding
  - ◦ Feelings
- Provide information about
  - ◦ Continued care of infant
  - ◦ Return to fertility
  - ◦ Contraception options, prn
- Medication instructions
  - ◦ Prenatal vitamins
  - ◦ $FeSo_4$
  - ◦ Other medications as indicated
- When to return for care
  - ◦ Postpartum visit schedule
  - ◦ Signs and symptoms of postpartum complications
  - ◦ When and how to access midwife

Follow-up Care:
Follow-up Measures to Consider

- Document
- 2 week recheck
  - ◦ New mothers
  - ◦ Complicated prenatal or postpartum course
  - ◦ Wound check post-Cesarean
  - ◦ Initiate hormonal contraceptives
  - ◦ Screen for postpartum depression
- 4–6 week postpartum exam
  - ◦ Involution
  - ◦ Lactation

- ◦ Perineum
- ◦ Bowel and bladder function
- ◦ Sleep patterns
- ◦ Family adaptation
- ◦ Concerns and questions
- 8 weeks for
  - ◦ IUD insertion
  - ◦ Diaphragm or cervical cap fitting

Collaborative Practice:
Criteria to Consider for Consultation or Referral

- OB/GYN service
  - ◦ Evidence of maternal complications postpartum
    - ▪ Infection
    - ▪ Acute urinary retention
    - ▪ Subinvolution of the uterus
    - ▪ Thrombophlebitis
    - ▪ Hematoma
    - ▪ Pulmonary embolism
- Social services
  - ◦ WIC, AFDC
  - ◦ Support groups

Postpartum Care, Weeks 1–6

Key Clinical Information

It is astonishing how rapidly most women adjust following the birth of a baby. By 4–6 weeks after the birth most women are returning to usual functioning, and adapting to the changes that the baby has brought into the family's life. Maternal evaluation at this time is directed toward determining the presence of any complications or concerns and addressing any need for birth control information or supplies. Support for the woman's new role, especially with first-time mothers, fosters a positive self-image and feelings of capability as she cares for her infant.

Women who have difficulty with postpartum adjustment may benefit from referrals to local resources, such as parenting groups or classes, breast-feeding groups, play groups, and other support services. Isolation during this time is not uncommon, and many women need to be actively directed (given permission) toward participation in activities other than newborn care.

Client History: Components of the History to Consider

- Review
  - Labor and birth events and outcomes
  - Initial postpartum course
  - GYN history
  - Medical/surgical history
  - Social history
- Physical return to nonpregnant status
  - Amount, color, and consistency of lochia
  - Breasts, status of lactation
  - Perineal or abdominal discomfort
  - Voiding and stooling
  - Activity and sleep patterns
- Emotional adaptation
  - Adjustment to parenting
  - Satisfaction with parenting
  - Interactions and support of family/significant others
  - Signs or symptoms of depression
  - Interactions with infant
- Infant feeding
- Sexual activity
- Preference for contraception as indicated
- Review of systems

Physical Examination: Components of the Physical Exam to Consider

- Exam components will vary based on
  - Timing of visit
  - Indication for visit
  - Client history
- Vital signs including temp
- Thyroid
- Thorax
  - Heart
  - Lungs
  - CVA tenderness
  - Breast exam
    - Lactation
    - Nipple integrity
    - Masses
    - Axilla
- Abdominal exam
  - Diastasis
  - Muscle tone
  - C-section or tubal ligation incision
- Pelvic exam
  - External genitalia for status of perineum/lacerations
  - Speculum exam
    - Appearance of cervix
    - Specimen collection
- Bimanual exam
  - Uterine involution
  - Vaginal muscle tone
  - Presence of cystocele or rectocele
- Rectal exam
- Extremities
  - Edema
  - Varicosities
  - Phlebitis

○ Reflexes

Clinical Impression: Differential Diagnoses to Consider

- Normal postpartum course
- Undesired fertility
- Postpartum complications, such as
  ○ Subinvolution of the uterus
  ○ Endometritis
  ○ Breast-feeding difficulties
  ○ Mastitis
  ○ Postpartum depression
  ○ Maternal adaptation problems
- Postpartum follow-up of complications, such as
  ○ Gestational diabetes
  ○ Preeclampsia
  ○ Post-op wound infection

Diagnostic Testing: Diagnostic Tests and Procedures to Consider

- Pap smear
- STI screen as indicated by history
- Labs
  ○ H & H, CBC
  ○ FBS for gestational diabetics
  ○ TSH
  ○ Other labs as indicated by history

Providing Treatment: Therapeutic Measures to Consider

- Initiation of birth control, as desired (see Chapter 7)
  ○ Natural family planning
  ○ Nonprescription methods
  ○ Prescription methods

- Postpartum depression screening
- Vitamin and mineral supplementation
  ○ $FeSo_4$ replacement
  ○ Calcium
  ○ Multivitamin

Providing Treatment: Alternative Measures to Consider

- Nutritional support
  ○ Increased fiber to stimulate regular bowel function
  ○ Whole foods diet
  ○ Adequate fluid intake
  ○ Increased nutritional needs to promote healing and foster general well-being

Providing Support: Education and Support Measures to Consider

- Encourage social support
  ○ Assistance and caring from family and friends
  ○ Midwife or nurse home visit
- Provide information about
  ○ Recommended diet
  ○ Anticipated weight changes postpartum
  ○ Potential decrease in libido
    ▪ Postpartum
    ▪ With breast-feeding
  ○ Initiation of physical activity
  ○ Birth control options
- Resources in the area for specific needs
  ○ Play or support groups for new mothers
  ○ Mothers of twins
  ○ La Leche League
  ○ Parenting skills classes
  ○ Teen parent groups

Follow-up Care:
Follow-up Measures to Consider

- Document
- Return visit in 12 months or as indicated by visit, e.g.,
  - Postpartum depression screening
  - Birth control
  - STI treatment or screening
  - Subinvolution
- Call with questions or concerns

Collaborative Practice:
Consider Consultation or Referral

- Psychotherapist or psychiatrist
  - Significant postpartum depression
  - Poor maternal adaptation
- OB/GYN service
  - For poor wound healing or infection
- Medical service, problems such as
  - Diagnosis of diabetes or glucose intolerance
  - Essential hypertension
  - Thyroid disorder
- Social service
  - WIC/AFDC
  - Housing
  - Drug rehabilitation
  - Child welfare
- For diagnosis or treatment outside the midwife's scope of practice

Postpartum Depression

Key Clinical Information

Postpartum depression may range from "the blues" to significant depression or postpartum psychosis. Depression may occur within 3–6 months after giving birth. Screening of every woman following birth facilitates early identification of women who require more than simple support to cope with their emotional changes during the postpartum period.

Many women may feel reluctant to divulge negative feelings about themselves or their baby. A supportive, nonjudgmental environment, where active listening is consistently demonstrated, fosters the trust many women need to talk about their feelings. Postpartum depression affects up to 12% of women who give birth (Righetti-Velterna, Conne-Perreard, Bousquet, & Manzano, 1998) with as many as 50% of women experiencing postpartum blues. Postpartum depression occurs in 26–32% of adolescent women who give birth and is more common in women with history of mood disorder.

Client History:
Components of the History to Consider

- Age, parity
- Birth and postpartum history
  - Labor and birth experience
  - Perception of postpartum period
  - Baby's age
  - Method of infant feeding
  - Sleep patterns and amounts
  - Hormone intake
  - Onset and type of symptoms (present > 2 weeks) (Miller, 1996)
- Risk factors for postpartum depression
  - Adolescent women
  - History of mood disorder
  - Postpartum for up to 6–18 months
  - Family history of mood disorder
  - Feeling unloved, especially by infant or father of child
  - Unplanned and/or unwanted pregnancy
  - Single or separated with minimal support
- Indicators of postpartum depression

- Presence of sleep disorder
- Thoughts of harming infant
- Feelings of inadequacy
- Extreme fatigue
- Crying
- Anxiety
- Appetite changes
- Irritability/mood changes (Righetti-Velterna et al., 1998)
- Identify
  - Stressors
  - Sleep/wake patterns
  - Social support
    - Housing needs or issues
    - Financial issues
    - Support systems
    - Perceived resources
  - Attitude toward
    - Self
    - Partner
    - Child(ren)
  - Potential for harming self or infant

Physical Examination: Components of the Physical Exam to Consider

- Vital signs, including temp
- Signs or symptoms of
  - Postpartum thyroidosis
  - Anemia
  - Infection
- Evaluate for
  - Sleep deprivation
  - Changes in personal appearance
  - Lethargy
  - Apathy

Clinical Impression: Differential Diagnoses to Consider

- Postpartum depression
  - Mild/Moderate
  - Severe/risk of suicide or infanticide
- Preexisting depression exacerbated by birth
- Severe sleep deprivation
- Psychosis
- Medical illness, such as
  - Thyroid dysfunction

Diagnostic Testing: Diagnostic Tests and Procedures to Consider

- Thyroid profile
- Urinalysis
- CBC with differential

Providing Treatment Therapeutic Measures to Consider

- Consider trial of antidepressant (Clark & Paine, 1996)
  - Medication choice based on
    - Symptom type and severity
    - Method of infant feeding (Leopold & Zoschnick, 1997)
- Consider trial of estrogen therapy
  - Mild symptoms with early onset
  - Estrogen patch 0.05 or 0.1 mg
  - Use 3–6 months if improvement noted (Gregoire et al., 1996)
- Combination hormonal contraceptives
  - May improve or exacerbate depression

Providing Treatment: Alternative Measures to Consider

- Herbal remedies

- Saint-John's wort 300 mg tid
- Lemon balm tea, 2 cups daily
- Blessed thistle
  - Infusion 1 cup daily
  - Tincture 10–20 drops 3–4 times daily
- Adequate nutrition
  - Whole foods
  - Adequate fluids
  - Avoid caffeine, alcohol, and cigarettes
- Support groups
- Light therapy
- Time away from baby
- Time scheduled for
  - Sleep
  - Personal care
  - Daily walking or activity
  - Personal time
  - Favorite activities
  - Intimate time with partner
- 🜍 Alternative therapies should not be a substitute for supervised psychiatric care for the women who threatens, or appears at risk, to harm herself or her family.

Providing Support:
Education and Support Measures to Consider

- Prenatal education
  - Normalcy of feelings associated with postpartum blues
  - Signs and symptoms of postpartum depression
  - Screening process at postpartum visit
- Local resources
  - Support groups
  - La Leche league
  - Parenting organizations

- Crisis hotline number
- Mental health professionals
- After birth
  - Review resources
  - Encourage
    - Family support
    - Rest with baby
    - Avoid isolation
    - Maintain nutrition
  - Signs and symptoms of pp depression
  - How to access help and support

Follow-up Care:
Follow-up Measures to Consider

- Document
- Midwife contact
  - Telephone contact within 24–48 hours
  - Weekly visits (home or office) while acute
  - As needed for titration of medication
- Update plan as condition changes

Collaborative Practice:
Criteria to Consider for Consultation or Referral

- Mental health or psychiatric service
  - For psychotherapy, counseling, education with a mental health professional
  - For medication, as indicated by client need and midwife scope of practice
  - Clients who do not respond to therapy within 7–14 days
  - If client or infant is perceived to be at risk for harm
  - Presence of psychotic symptoms
  - For any client who is suicidal or homicidal
  - Rejection of, or physical aggression (threatened or actual) against infant

- Social services
  - Assistance with social issues
    - Housing
    - Food
    - Finances
    - Childcare
- Medical service
  - Suspected or confirmed medical condition
- For diagnosis or treatment outside the midwife's scope of practice

Endometritis

Key Clinical Information

Endometritis indicates an infection of the uterus, or endometrium. Endometritis is more common following Cesarean birth; however, it can occur in any postpartum woman. Bacteria, such as strep, staph, and *E. coli*, typically ascend from the lower genital tract. Infection may extend into the fallopian tubes and pelvic peritoneum. Other potential sites of postpartum infection include episiotomy or laceration sites and areas of bruising or hematoma formation. Prompt recognition and treatment is required to prevent onset of systemic infection or localized tissue necrosis.

Postpartum infection is indicated by two temperature elevations to 38°C/100.4°F more than 24 hours after birth or a temperature of 38.7°C/101.5°F at any time. Prompt evaluation should be made to determine the location of the infection. Postpartum endometritis usually presents on second to seventh postpartum day (Varney et al., 2004).

Client History: Components of the History to Consider

- Length of time since birth
- Onset, duration, and severity of symptoms
  - Fever and chills

- Malaise
- Presence and location of pain
- Odor of lochia
- Wound exudate
- Redness and inflammation at wound site
- Other associated symptoms
- General well-being
  - Appetite
  - Urinary function
  - Respiratory function
- Prenatal risk factors
  - Anemia
  - Poor nutrition
  - Diabetes or GDM
  - GBS +
  - Bacterial vaginitis
  - STI diagnosis or treatment
  - Complications of labor or birth
    - Prolonged labor
    - Prolonged rupture of membranes
    - More than 4–6 internal exams
    - Breaks in aseptic technique
    - Excessive blood loss
    - Uterine or cervical manipulation
    - Cesarean section
    - Retained placental fragments
  - Medical/surgical history
    - Appendicitis
    - Diverticular disease
    - Immunocompromised condition
  - ROS

Physical Examination: Components of the Physical Exam to Consider

- Vital signs, BP, T, P, R

- Cardiopulmonary system
  - Color
  - Breath sounds
  - Rales
  - Respiratory effort
- Breast exam
  - Redness
  - Mass
  - Pain
- Abdominal exam
  - Uterine size
  - Location of pain
  - Guarding
  - Rebound tenderness
  - Referred pain
  - Tenderness with uterine motion
- Wound or laceration exam
  - Exudate
  - Redness
  - Swelling
- Evaluation of lochia
  - Odor
  - Amount
- Extremities
  - Edema
  - Homan's sign
  - Femoral and pedal pulses

Clinical Impression:
Differential Diagnoses to Consider

- Genital tract
  - Uterine infection
  - Wound infection
    - Surgical incision
    - Episiotomy
    - Laceration
    - Pelvic hematoma
- Breast infection
- Urinary tract
  - Infection
  - Renal calculi
- Cardiopulmonary system
  - Respiratory infection
  - Deep vein thrombosis
  - Pulmonary embolus
- Appendicitis
- Drug reaction

Diagnostic Testing:
Diagnostic Tests and Procedures to Consider

- CBC w/differential
- Urinalysis
- O_2 saturation
- Cultures as indicated
  - Urine
  - Blood
  - Wound
- Radiology studies as indicated
  - Chest X-ray
  - Ultrasound/CT scan
    - Pelvic
      - Hematoma
      - Retained placental fragments
      - Appendix
    - Abdominal
      - Appendix
      - KUB
    - Extremities

Providing Treatment:
Therapeutic Measures to Consider

- Hydration
  - po fluids
  - IV therapy
- Prevention of DVT
  - Antiembolitic stockings
  - Isometric exercises
- Antimicrobial therapy
  - IV antibiotic therapy is indicated for serious infection, such as
  - Cefotetan 1–2 g IV q 12 hours
  - Mezlocillin 4 g IV q 4–6 hours
  - Ticarcillin/clavaniculate 3.1 g IV q 6 hours
  - Ampicillin/sulbactam 3 g IV q 4–6 hours
  - Gentamycin 1.5 mg/kg load, then 1 mg/kg q 8 h, *plus* Clindamycin 900 mg IV q 6 hours (Murphy, 2004)

Providing Treatment:
Alternative Measures to Consider

- Rescue remedy to pulse points
- Hot pack to abdomen
- Echinacea tea or tincture
- Homeopathic arnica for soft tissue injury
- ⏱ Alternative remedies are not a substitute for prompt medical care
  - Inadequately treated local infection may become systemic
  - Systemic infection can rapidly lead to death

Providing Support:
Education and Support Measures to Consider

- Supportive measures
  - Rest
  - Adequate nutrition
  - Emotional support
  - Provision for infant care
- Discuss with client and family
  - Working diagnosis
  - Urgency of condition
  - Need for diagnostic testing
- Potential need for
  - Medical evaluation
  - Hospitalization
  - Treatment
- Compatibility of medications with breast-feeding, prn
- Provide emotional support
  - Listen
- Update information as situation demands

Follow-up Care:
Follow-up Measures to Consider

- Anticipate response to medication within 48 hours
- Consider abscess or hematoma if minimal or no response
- Document
- Update notes frequently and with any changes

Collaborative Practice:
Criteria to Consider for Consultation or Referral

- OB/GYN service
  - Evaluation or treatment of postpartum infection
  - Transfer of care from home or birth center for hospitalization
  - Medical complications of the postpartum period that require medical evaluation and care
- For diagnosis or treatment outside the midwife's scope of practice

Hemorrhoids

Key Clinical Information

Hemorrhoids are varicosities of the veins that line the anal canal. They are a common finding in the postpartum period. Hemorrhoids may be swollen and painful, or they may become thrombosed and require incision and drainage. Prompt treatment of hemorrhoids postpartum may prevent thrombosis of external hemorrhoids that have become trapped by the anal sphincter.

Client History:
Components of the History to Consider

- Length and positions used during second-stage labor
- Prior history of hemorrhoids
- Relief measures used and their effects
- Usual bowel function
- Presence of rectal bleeding

Physical Examination:
Components of the Physical Exam to Consider

- Perineal evaluation
  - Approximation of repair, if any
  - Edema
  - Hemorrhoids
    - May be single or rosette
    - Note
      - Size
      - Location
      - Edema
      - Redness
- Palpation to verify presence of thrombosed hemorrhoid
  - Firm clot felt within vein
  - Exquisitely painful to touch
- Rectal examination for
  - Thrombosis
  - Abscess
  - Anal fissure or lesions
  - Undiagnosed third- or fourth-degree laceration

Clinical Impression:
Differential Diagnoses to Consider

- Hemorrhoids
  - Hemorrhoids, NOS
  - Hemorrhoids, thrombosed
- Anal abscess or mass
- Anal fissure
- Rectovaginal hematoma
- Undiagnosed third- or fourth-degree laceration

Diagnostic Testing:
Diagnostic Tests and Procedures to Consider

- Anoscopy

Providing Treatment:
Therapeutic Measures to Consider

- Manually reduce hemorrhoids as necessary
- Incise and drain thrombosed hemorrhoids
- Topical analgesics
  - Americaine spray
  - Nupercainal ointment or suppositories
- Hemorrhoidal preparations
  - Steroid preparations indicated for
    - Bleeding
    - Severe inflammation
  - Anusol cream
  - Anusol-HC suppositories
  - Preparation H
  - Proctocort

- ○ Proctofoam
- ○ Proctofoam-HC (Murphy, 2004)
- Relieve and/or prevent constipation
  - ○ Stool softeners
    - ■ Colace—50–200 mg daily
    - ■ Surfac—240 mg po daily until normal
  - ○ Laxatives
    - ■ Peri-colace (softener + stimulant)
      - • 1–2 capsules hs
    - ■ Perdiem (fiber + stimulant)
      - • 1–2 tsp in 8 oz water hs or in AM
    - ■ Senocot (senna stimulant)
      - • 2 tabs q hs
    - ■ Fiber supplements
      - • Citrucel—1 TBS in 8 oz water 1–3 x daily
      - • Metamucil—1 packet or 1 tsp in 8 oz water 1–3 x daily
    - ■ Gylcerine suppositories
    - ■ Enemas
      - • Fleet enema
      - • Soapsuds enema
- Severe hemorrhoids, no thrombosis
  - ○ Rectal packing
    - ■ Provides counterpressure
    - ■ Lubricate with hemorrhoid cream
    - ■ Remove after 12–24 hours

Providing Treatment:
Alternative Measures to Consider

- Sitz baths
  - ○ Warm water
  - ○ Herbal infusions
    - ■ Comfrey
    - ■ Red clover
    - ■ Nettle
- Ice packs

- Witch hazel compresses
- Adequate dietary fiber and fluids
- Knees-to-chest position to drain hemorrhoids
  - ○ Hands and knees
  - ○ Head on pillow
  - ○ Bottom elevated
- Measures to speed soft tissue healing
  - ○ Aloe vera gel
  - ○ Comfrey compresses used tid
- Homeopathics
  - ○ Arnica 30x 2 tabs qid
  - ○ Hamamelis 30C (Smith, 1984)

Providing Support:
Education and Support Measures to Consider

- Diet adequate in fluids and fiber
  - ○ Dried fruit
  - ○ Psyllium seed
  - ○ Prune juice
  - ○ Rhubarb
  - ○ Blueberries
- Treatment options and instructions
  - ○ Avoidance of
    - ■ Straining
    - ■ Prolonged sitting on toilet
    - ■ Holding stool
  - ○ When to call
    - ■ Bleeding
    - ■ Increasing pain

Follow-up Care:
Follow-up Measures to Consider

- Document
- Reevaluate hemorrhoids
  - ○ 12–24 hours after treatment

- 1 week
- Persistent rectal bleeding

Collaborative Practice: Consider Consultation or Referral

- OB/GYN Service
  - Thrombosed hemorrhoids for I & D
  - Suspected third- or fourth-degree laceration
  - Rectal
    - Abscess
    - Anal fissure
    - Hematoma
    - Bleeding
- For diagnosis or treatment outside the midwife's scope of practice

Mastitis

Key Clinical Information

Mastitis may occur in the early or late postpartum period. Early identification and prompt treatment at the first signs may prevent the need for antibiotic treatment. Delay in treatment may result in abscess formation or systemic infection. All breast-feeding women should be aware of the presenting signs and symptoms of mastitis, preventive measures, when and how to contact their midwife for evaluation, and possible treatment.

Client History: Components of the History to Consider

- Breast-feeding history
  - Duration of breast-feeding
  - Infant feeding style
  - Recent changes to nursing patterns
  - Usual breast care
- Previous history of breast problems
  - Mastitis

- Abscess
- Breast biopsies
- Breast reduction or implants
- Onset, duration, and severity of symptoms
  - Painful breast(s), worse when nursing
  - Redness of breast
  - Induration of breast
  - Fever and/or chills
  - Malaise or flulike symptoms
  - Headache (Varney et al., 2004)
- Self-help measures used and effectiveness

Physical Examination: Components of the Physical Exam to Consider

- Vital signs, especially temperature and pulse
- General well-being
- Breast exam
  - Engorgement
  - Tenderness, redness, swelling
  - Induration
  - Warmth, generalized or local
  - Cracks or fissures in nipples
  - Masses
    - Firm or soft
    - Fixed or mobile
    - Tender or nontender
  - Axillary exam
    - Engorgement
    - Lymph nodes
- Additional components as indicated by history and physical

Clinical Impression Differential Diagnoses to Consider

- Simple mastitis

- Breast abscess
- Severe mastitis with systemic involvement
- Breast cancer

Diagnostic Testing:
Diagnostic Tests and Procedures to Consider

- CBC
- Breast ultrasound for mass
  - Abscess suspected
  - Differentiate solid vs. cystic
- Culture of breast milk for pathogen
  - Unresponsive to therapy
  - Systemic involvement
- Mammograms not recommended during lactation

Providing Treatment:
Therapeutic Measures to Consider

- Fever
  - Acetaminophen
  - Ibuprofen
  - Aspirin
- Antibiotic therapy for infection, such as
  - Dicloxacillin 250 mg qid x 10 days
  - Keflex 500 mg po bid x 10 days
  - Erythromycin
    - Eryc 250 mg po q 6 hours x 10 days
    - Ery-tab 400 mg q 6 hours x 10 days, *or* 333 mg q 8 hours, *or* 500 mg q 12 hours
    - EES 1.6 g/day in 2, 3, or 4 evenly divided doses
  - Nafcillin 250–500 mg po q 4–6 hours x 10 days (or other penicillinase-resistant penicillin) (Varney et al., 2004; Murphy, 2004)

Providing Treatment:
Alternative Measures to Consider

- Adequate hydration and nutrition
- Rest with baby at breast
- For rest
  - Hops infusion
  - Skullcap tincture (Weed, 1985)
- For fever, infusion of
  - Echinacea
  - Yarrow
  - Peppermint
- Echinacea tea or tincture
- Comfrey compresses to affected area
- Homeopathics (Davis, 1997)
  - Arnica 30C
  - Bryonia 30C
  - Phytolacca 30C
  - Belladonna 30 C

Providing Support:
Education and Support Measures to Consider

- Careful hand washing and breast care
  - Warm compresses to affected area
  - *Gentle* massage toward nipple
  - Frequent nursing and/or pumping
- Change infant's suckling positions
  - Cradle
  - Side-lying
  - Football
  - Belly to belly
- Increase fluid intake
- Rest, rest, rest
- Request assistance with
  - Housekeeping
  - Childcare

- ○ Promoting rest
- Provide medication instructions
  - ○ Take as directed until medication is gone
  - ○ Baby may get diarrhea or GI upset
  - ○ Continue to nurse unless contraindicated by
    - ▪ Medication used
    - ▪ Significant side effects in baby
    - ▪ Serious illness of mother
  - ○ Pumping is an option, not as effective as nursing
- Instructions for when and how to contact
  - ○ Fever ≥ 100.4°F
  - ○ Chills
  - ○ Malaise
  - ○ Worsening symptoms

Follow-up Care:
Follow-up Measures to Consider

- Document
- Reassess within 24 hours
  - ○ To confirm effectiveness of therapy
  - ○ For evaluation if no improvement
- Consider hospitalization
  - ○ Persistent fever
  - ○ Systemic symptoms
  - ○ IV antibiotic therapy

Collaborative Practice:
Consider Consultation or Referral

- OB/GYN service
  - ○ For mastitis unresponsive to therapy
  - ○ For breast abscess
- Lactation consultant
  - ○ Mastitis preventive instruction
  - ○ Breast care and feeding during illness
    - ▪ Infant positioning
    - ▪ Massage techniques
    - ▪ Recommendations and support
  - ○ Assistance with supplements if needed
- Social service
  - ○ Home help
  - ○ Visiting nurse
  - ○ Other support services
- Pediatric service
  - ○ As indicated by infant response to medication
- For diagnosis or treatment outside the midwife's scope of practice

Newborn Resuscitation
Key Clinical Information

Most term babies make the transition at birth without needing anything more than gentle supportive care. Occasionally, however, some newly born infants do not begin to breathe as anticipated and need intervention to assist them. Maintaining an intact cord fosters a gentle transition for the baby, and as long as the cord is pulsing, provides a secondary source of oxygen to the baby, as well as volume expansion (Mercer & Skovaard, 2002). Palpation of the cord may cause the cord to spasm and eliminate this secondary oxygen source. The most effective method of obtaining the newborn pulse is by auscultation of the infant's chest. Breath sounds can be assessed at the same time.

To maintain the skills required for newborn resuscitation, the midwife must practice on a regular basis. Mock resuscitation drills should be performed regularly and documented in the midwife's continuing education log.

Client History:
Components of the History to Consider

- Presence of risk factors for fetal asphyxia

- Cord factors, such as
  - Cord prolapse
  - Cord compression
- Placental factors, such as
  - Placental abruption
  - Placental insufficiency
  - Placenta previa
- Maternal factors, such as
  - Vascular disease
  - Hypoxia
  - Hypertension
  - Hypotension
  - Uterine hyperstimulation
  - Maternal narcotic use in labor
- Fetal factors, such as
  - Prematurity
  - Fetal isoimmunization
  - Meconium-stained amniotic fluid
  - Traumatic delivery
    - Instrumentation
    - Malpresentation
    - Shoulder dystocia
- Causes of respiratory distress include
  - Hyaline membrane disease
  - Persistent pulmonary hypertension
  - Sepsis
  - Meconium aspiration
  - Choanal atresia
  - Diaphragmatic hernia

Physical Examination: Components of the Physical Exam to Consider

- Evaluate for
  - Gestational age
  - Presence of meconium
- Respirations
- Heart rate
- Color
- Muscle tone (AAP/AHA, 2000)
- Basic steps, no meconium
  - Prevent heat loss
  - Place on warm surface
    - Maternal abdomen
    - Radiant warmer
  - Dry
    - Remove wet linen
  - Position
    - Open airway
  - Suction as needed
    - Gently use bulb suction
    - Avoid causing vagal response
  - Tactile stimulation
    - Flick or tap soles
    - Rub back
- Evaluate respirations
  - Normal rate 40–60/minutes
  - May be irregular
  - No abdominal retractions
  - No grunting, gasping, or wheezing
- Evaluate heart rate
  - Normal rate 120–160 BPM
  - Regular rate and rhythm
- Evaluate color
  - Should pink easily with respirations
  - Cyanosis of hands and feet is common
  - Pallor indicates poor perfusion due to
    - Volume depletion, *or*
    - Inadequate blood pressure
  - Central cyanosis indicates
    - Current adequate perfusion, *with*

- Hypoxia
- Meconium present
  - Assess vigor
    - Muscle tone
    - Respirations
    - Heart rate
  - Nonvigorous infant
    - Suction before any stimulation
    - Use method appropriate for scope of practice
    - Proceed with ventilation as needed

Clinical Impression:
Differential Diagnoses to Consider

- Infant condition
  - Primary apnea
  - Secondary apnea
  - Respiratory distress
- Resuscitation measures
  - Basic steps only
  - Free-flow oxygen
  - Assisted ventilation
    - < 30 min
    - > 30 min
  - Chest compressions
  - Endotracheal intubation
    - For suctioning
    - For ventilation
    - For medication
  - Insertion of
    - Orogastric tube
    - Oral airway

Diagnostic Testing:
Diagnostic Tests and Procedures to Consider

- Endotracheal intubation
  - Nonvigorous infant, with meconium
    - Evaluate for meconium below cords
  - For ventilation and medication administration
- Chest X-ray
  - Placement of ET tube
  - Pneumothorax
  - Pneumonia
  - Meconium aspiration
  - Respiratory distress

Providing Treatment:
Therapeutic Measures to Consider

- Nonvigorous infant with meconium
  - Use meconium aspirator on perineum to suction
    - Mouth
    - Nares
    - Pharynx
  - Endotracheal intubation to suction meconium
- 100% O_2 via bag and mask or ET tube
  - Infants with absent or weak respiratory efforts
  - Heart rate less than 100
- Chest compressions (CC)
  - After 30 seconds positive pressure ventilation
  - Infants with heart rate under 60
- Free flow O_2 as indicated by
  - Respiratory effort
  - Color
- Epinephrine 1:10,000
  - Use for HR < 60 BPM, *after*
    - 30 seconds PPV, *and*
    - 30 seconds PPV and CC

- Stimulates cardiac contraction and rate
- Causes peripheral vasoconstriction
- Dose: 0.1–0.3 ml/kg
- Route: ET tube or IV
- Give rapidly
- HR should improve within 30 seconds

Providing Treatment:
Alternative Measures to Consider

- Maintain cord intact
  - If cord is pulsing, baby is getting oxygen
  - Cord pulses with baby's heart rate
  - Do not put traction or pressure on cord
  - Resuscitate baby with cord intact
- Application of homeopathic remedies (e.g., Rescue Remedy) to pulse points is considered safe
  - 🧨 Oral administration of any medication, homeopathic, or herbal remedy may cause aspiration and further compromise infant; use with caution
- Head down position to facilitate drainage of fluids
- Patience for baby with
  - Spontaneous breathing
  - HR > 100
- Prayer, talk to baby, physical touch
- PPV using room air only (Davis et al, 2004)

Providing Support:
Education and Support Measures to Consider

- Discuss care of infant as time allows
- Provide information about
  - Ongoing infant care
  - Tests or treatments
  - Specialty care
- Listen to parents' concerns and fears

- Provide information about support groups or services as indicated

Follow-up Care:
Follow-up Measures to Consider

- Document resuscitation events
- Notify appropriate personnel that infant required resuscitation
  - Infant should be evaluated promptly based on
    - Resuscitation measures required
    - Condition following resuscitation
    - Parent or midwife preferences
- Close observation
  - Baby who required resuscitation
  - Evaluate q 1–4 hours x 24 hours
    - Vital signs
    - Color
    - Activity
- Transport of baby, as indicated, from
  - Community hospital
  - Birth center
  - Home birth

Collaborative Practice:
Consider Consultation or Referral

- OB/GYN service
  - As indicated for labor and birth
- Pediatric service
  - For anticipated need of neonatal resuscitation
  - For infant who
    - Does not improve after 30 seconds O_2 therapy
    - Requires chest compressions
  - Infant with signs or symptoms such as
    - Respiratory distress

- Meconium aspiration syndrome
- Difficulty with temperature regulation
- Persistent cyanosis or pallor
- Vital signs outside of accepted range
- For diagnosis or treatment outside the midwife's scope of practice

Initial Examination and Evaluation of the Newborn

Key Clinical Information

Every midwife should be skilled in examination of the newly born baby. The initial examination serves to determine if the baby is making a successful transition to the outside world from the total support provided within the womb. Babies vary tremendously, and the midwife must evaluate which variations require additional expertise in newborn care.

Client History: Components of the History to Consider

- Brief birth information
  - Apparent gestational age
  - Labor and birth events
  - Need for resuscitation
- Significant events or findings since birth
  - General well-being
  - Vital signs
  - Activity
  - Feeding
  - Voiding/stooling
- Family history
  - Genetic disorders
  - Maternal medical conditions, such as
    - Sickle cell
    - Hepatitis
    - HIV
    - STIs

  - Thyroid
  - Diabetes
- Contributing obstetrical history
  - Prenatal factors
    - Onset of prenatal care
    - Use of drugs, tobacco, and/or alcohol
    - Pregnancy complications
  - Labor and birth factors
    - Duration of pregnancy
    - Duration of labor
    - Use of medications in labor
    - Complications of labor and/or birth
    - Cesarean birth
    - Vacuum extractor
    - Fetal distress
    - Meconium-stained fluid
    - Other (McHugh, 2004a)

Physical Examination: Components of the Physical Exam to Consider

- Apgar scores at 1 and 5 minutes
- Vital signs
- Vital statistics
  - Weight
  - Head circumference
  - Length
  - Chest circumference
- Evaluation of gestational age
- Skin
  - Color
  - Vernix
  - Cracking
  - Presence of lesions
  - Evidence of birth trauma
- Head

- Molding
- Caput
- Cephalhematoma
- Fontanels
- Eyes
  - Red reflex
  - Position, size, shape of orbits
  - Color of iris and sclera
  - Subconjunctival hemorrhage
  - Conjunctivitis
- Ears
  - Position and shape
  - Presence of periauricular sinus or skin tags
  - Hearing testing
- Nose
  - Patency
  - Flaring
- Mouth
  - Lips
  - Gums
  - Palates
  - Tongue
  - Suck
- Back and spine
  - Breath sounds
  - Presence of anomalies
  - Curvature of spine
  - Pilonidal sinus
  - Spinal bifida
  - Patency of anus
- Chest
  - Respiratory effort and breath sounds
  - Heart rate and rhythm
  - Shape
  - Nipples and breast buds

- Abdomen
  - Number of cord vessels
  - Presence of bowel sounds (> 1 hour after birth)
  - Palpation of kidneys, liver margin, presence of masses
- Femoral pulses
- Genitalia
  - Male
    - Position of urinary meatus
    - Descent of testes in scrotum
  - Female
    - Configuration
    - Edema
    - Discharge
- Extremities
  - Range of motion
  - Congenital hip dislocation
  - Extra digits
- Reflexes
  - Rooting
  - Moro reflex (McHugh, 2004a)

Clinical Impression: Differential Diagnoses to Consider

- Normal newborn
- Newborn course complicated by
  - Pregnancy factors
  - Labor and/or birth factors
  - Congenital factors
  - Other conditions (list)

Diagnostic Testing: Diagnostic Tests and Procedures to Consider

- Glucose, heelstick (normal value > 45 mg/dl)
- Cord blood studies

- Metabolic screening tests
- Consider additional testing for
  - Cord blood gases
  - Anemia (HCT normal value 45–65%)
  - Hyperbilirubinemia (normal value < 13 mg/dl)
  - Syphilis
  - HIV
  - Sickle cell anemia
  - Hepatitis B
  - Gram stain of eye exudate
  - Culture of eye exudate for GC/CT

Providing Treatment: Therapeutic Measures to Consider

- Vitamin K
  - Injection: AquaMEPHYTON (Phytonadione)
    - 0.5–1 mg IM within 1 hour of birth
  - Oral: Konakion MM, mixed micellular preparation (Clark & James, 1995)
    - 2 mg po within 1 hour of birth, *followed by*
    - Additional dose at 7 and 30 days of age
- Prophylactic ophthalmic treatment
  - Erythromycin ophthalmic ointment
    - 0.5% x 1 dose
  - Tetracycline ophthalmic ointment
    - 1% x 1 dose
  - Silver nitrate, aqueous solution
    - 1% as single application
- Neonatal conjunctivitis
  - Ceftriaxone 25–50 mg/kg IV or IM
  - Single dose
  - Max dose 125 mg
- Hepatitis B
  - Vaccine prophylaxis

- Begin soon after birth
- Three dose series: 0, 1, 6 months
- May delay with negative mother
  - HBIG (see Hepatitis)
- Phototherapy for hyperbilirubinemia

Providing Treatment: Alternative Measures to Consider

- Defer vitamin K
  - Incidence of hemorrhagic disease without vitamin K ranges from 0.25–0.50%
  - Greatest incidence in breastfed infants who did not receive vitamin K
  - Vitamin K is concentrated in colostrum and hind milk
  - Formula-fed infants get significant vitamin K from cow's milk formula
- Defer erythromycin ophthalmic ointment
  - Negative GC/CT results
  - Culture and treat if conjunctivitis occurs
  - Use plain water wash, prn

Providing Support: Education and Support Measures to Consider

- Discuss physical findings
  - Range of normal
  - Potential or actual concerns
  - Signs and symptoms to watch for
- Discuss purpose of testing and/or medications
  - Encourage questions
  - Engage parents in decision making
- Discuss potential options for care
  - Well-baby care providers
  - Recommended treatments
    - Anticipated results/benefits
    - Risks/side effects

- Alternatives
- Anticipatory guidance for parenting of newborn
  - Expected feeding and activity levels
  - Evaluation of adequate hydration
  - Common patterns of voiding and stooling
  - Warning signs
    - Poor feeding
    - Lethargy
    - Irritability
    - Jaundice
    - Dehydration
    - Fever
    - Poor color
    - Vomiting (McHugh, 2004b)
- Follow-up plans for well-baby care
  - When to contact
  - How to contact

Follow-up Care: Follow-up Measures to Consider

- Document
- Daily evaluation first 2 to 3 days of life
- Weight check at 1 to 2 weeks
- Observation of feeding
  - Determine suck/swallow
  - Note latch if breast-feeding
  - Maternal–infant interaction
- Recheck variations promptly

Collaborative Practice: Consider Consultation or Referral

- Pediatric service
  - Newborn evaluation is not included in midwife's practice
  - Variations, such as

- Presence of anomalies
- Evidence of infection
- Hyperbilirubinemia
- Other conditions not within the range of normal or expected findings (McHugh, 2004b)

- Lactation consultant
  - Breast-feeding difficulties
- For diagnosis or treatment outside the midwife's scope of practice

Care of the Infant Undergoing Circumcision

Key Clinical Information

Circumcision is the surgical removal of part or all of the foreskin of the penis. There is no clear medical indication for routine newborn circumcision. More often it is performed for cultural, social, or religious reasons. The American College of Obstetricians and Gynecologists (ACOG) recommends that parents be provided with "accurate and impartial information" as part of the informed choice process for circumcision (ACOG, 2001). Prenatal discussion allows parents time to reflect whether circumcision is right for their child. Parents whose son is intact may need education regarding genital hygiene, especially if circumcision has previously been the norm for children in the family.

The midwife who plans to include circumcision in her or his practice should learn the skills needed from an experienced midwife, physician, or mohel/mohelet and perform the procedure under expert guidance until skilled at the procedure. Analgesia and/or local anesthesia is recommended to minimize the stress to the baby from the procedure (ACOG, 2001).

Client History:
Components of the History to Consider

- Neonatal course since birth
  - Vitamin K administration
    - Oral vitamin K requires up to three doses before full effectiveness
  - Demonstrated voiding since birth
  - Review infant record
    - Physical exam
    - Lab tests
    - Temperature stability
    - Feeding and voiding since birth
- Contraindications to circumcision
  - Hypospadias
  - Abnormality of the penis
  - Medically unstable infant
  - Parents decline procedure (Lowenstein, 2004)

Physical Examination:
Components of the Physical Exam to Consider

- Vital signs including temperature
- Examination of the penis
  - Evaluate for hypospadias prior to procedure
  - Identify landmarks for penile block if used

Clinical Impression:
Differential Diagnoses to Consider

- Normal male neonatal genitalia
- Elective circumcision

Diagnostic Testing:
Diagnostic Tests and Procedures to Consider

- As indicated to ensure infant's stability prior to procedure

Providing Treatment:
Therapeutic Measures to Consider

- Prepare equipment
  - Gomco clamp
  - Plastibell clamp
  - Mogen clamp
- Provide for pain relief
  - EMLA cream
  - Dorsal penile block
  - Subcutaneous ring block
  - Parental presence
  - Swaddling
  - Analgesics
- Procedure using Gomco clamp (Lowenstein, 2004)
  - Use strict aseptic technique
    - Sterile gloves
    - Mask
    - Antimicrobial prep
    - Sterile drape for genital area
  - Create dorsal slit
  - Identify preputial ring
    - Lift clear of the glans
    - Apply curved hemostats to edge of preputial ring (grasp 2–3 mm of tissue)
  - Remove adhesions
    - Insert straight hemostat or probe dorsally under foreskin
    - Free adhesions to level of corona
    - Avoid trauma to posterior frenulum or meatus
  - Spread hemostat and free foreskin off dorsal side of the glans
  - Insert one blade of open straight hemostat along dorsal foreskin
  - Lift foreskin away from glans and meatus

- Clamp 1 cm of foreskin in the midline
  - Clamp slowly
  - Allow clamp to remain for 60 seconds
  - Crush line should be blanched and thin
- Inset blunt-tipped scissors and carefully cut the crush line
- Application of the clamp
  - Free inner preputial tissue from glans to expose glans and coronal sulcus
  - Using gentle traction on curved hemostats, pull the foreskin over the glans
  - Insert the bell dorsally to completely cover the glans
  - Place straight hemostat through hole on base plate and grasp edges of foreskin to close margins of dorsal slit before fitting hole over glans
  - Carefully maneuver tip of cone to work it through bevel hole, working the base plate down over the secured foreskin until the bell is seated
  - Swing the top plate over and lift the arms onto the yoke
- Note: The apex of the dorsal slit should be completely visible
- Excision of the tissue
  - Ensure top plate is aligned in notch
  - Tighten the nut to crimp foreskin between base plate and bell
  - Carefully excise foreskin with scalpel at the junction of the base plate and bell
- Loosen the nut and gently loosen tissue from bell
- Retract remaining foreskin to below the glans
- Observe for active bleeding
  - Apply pressure, prn
  - Use epinephrine 1:1000 on gauze, prn
- Apply petroleum jelly gauze or other nonadherent dressing
- Comfort baby and return to mother and family

Providing Treatment: Alternative Measures to Consider

- Maintain intact foreskin
- Remove only very tip of foreskin
- Circumcise later in life when and if indicated

Providing Support: Education and Support Measures to Consider

- Provide informed consent
  - Potential benefits of circumcision
    - Decreased incidence of urinary tract infections
    - Small reduction in risk of penile cancer
  - Risks
    - Pain
    - Bleeding
    - Infection
    - Injury
- Provide education to parents who opt for circumcision regarding postprocedure care of the penis
  - Crying is common with first voids postcircumcision
  - Appearance
    - Head of penis may be quite red
    - Swelling just under the glans is normal
    - A blood clot may form at incision site
    - Pink or yellow serous drainage may occur
  - Care of circumcised penis
    - Keep area clean
    - Wash hands before diaper change
    - Change diaper frequently

- Apply petroleum jelly on gauze with each diaper change until healing occurs
- If gauze sticks, soak with warm water to loosen
- Call with signs or symptoms of complications
- Active bleeding: Apply direct pressure to area
- Pus, foul odor, or increased redness or swelling at incision site
- Fever
- Lack of urination within 12–24 hours after circumcision
- Provide education regarding the care of the uncircumcised penis to parents who opt not for circumcision (Sinclair, 2004)
  - Do not retract the foreskin
  - Clean external structures
    - Daily and prn
    - When exposed to stool
  - If redness or irritation occurs
    - Flush area with clear water
    - Allow to air-dry if possible
    - Apply diaper ointment to glans

Follow-up Care:
Follow-up Measures to Consider

- Document (see Procedure Note)
- Observe for potential complications
  - 12–24 hours following procedure
  - Bleeding
  - Infection
  - Removal of excessive foreskin
  - Amputation of distal glans
  - Sepsis
- Release from care
  - Infant stable and feeding
  - Bleeding minimal

- Voiding has occurred

Collaborative Practice:
Consider Consultation or Referral

- Mohel/mohelet
  - For information and opinion about circumcision
  - To perform circumcision
- Pediatric service
  - Infant with congenital defects of the genitals
  - To perform circumcision
- OB/GYN service
  - To perform circumcision
- For diagnosis or treatment outside the midwife's scope of practice

Assessment of the Newborn for Deviations from Normal

Key Clinical Information

Every baby is unique, and the midwife must be able to assess whether variations from the expected simply represent the wide range of normal or indicate the presence of a condition that requires additional assessment and possibly treatment. Although the vast majority of babies born to healthy mothers are themselves healthy, the hallmark of midwifery is improving the heath and well-being of all mothers and babies. This includes being observant for subtle signs and symptoms that may indicate a need for support, gentle intervention, or for skilled medical care.

Client History:
Components of the History to Consider

- Family history
  - Genetic history
  - Congenital anomalies
  - Pregnancy losses

- ○ Social factors
- Pregnancy history
  - ○ Complications of pregnancy
  - ○ Maternal disease or illness
    - ▪ GBS
    - ▪ Herpes
    - ▪ Diabetes
    - ▪ Epilepsy
    - ▪ HIV
    - ▪ Drug, alcohol, or tobacco use
- Labor and birth events
  - ○ Abnormal fetal heart rate patterns
  - ○ Resuscitation
  - ○ Complications at birth, such as
    - ▪ Presence of meconium
    - ▪ Endotracheal intubation or suctioning
    - ▪ Instrument or surgical birth
    - ▪ Shoulder dystocia
    - ▪ Evidence of birth trauma
- Review initial assessment
  - ○ Gestational age
  - ○ Congenital anomalies
  - ○ Lab tests
  - ○ Unusual findings
- Presence of symptoms since birth
  - ○ Type of symptom(s)
  - ○ Onset
  - ○ Duration
  - ○ Severity
  - ○ Treatments tried and infant response

Physical Examination:
Components of the Physical Exam to Consider

- Arrange for or perform comprehensive newborn assessment
  - ○ Within 24 hours of age

- ○ For any evidence of problems
- Vital signs
  - ○ Temperature
  - ○ Respiratory rate, volume, and effort
  - ○ Presence of apnea
  - ○ Heart rate and rhythm
- Reflexes
- Observe for signs and symptoms suggesting need for further evaluation
  - ○ Respirations
    - ▪ Grunting or gasping
    - ▪ Rate < 30 or > 60
  - ○ Heart rate
    - ▪ Bradycardia < 100 BPM
    - ▪ Tachycardia > 170 BPM
    - ▪ Cardiac instability
  - ○ Temperature instability
  - ○ Color
    - ▪ Pallor
    - ▪ Cyanosis
    - ▪ Rubor
    - ▪ Jaundice
- Before 24 hours—most likely pathologic
- After 24 hours—most likely physiologic
  - ○ Muscle tone
    - ▪ Flaccid
    - ▪ Hypotonia
  - ○ Activity level
    - ▪ Lethargy
    - ▪ Irritability
    - ▪ Hyperactivity
    - ▪ Convulsions
- Failure to feed well
- Failure to move an extremity
- GI adaptation
  - ○ Vomiting

- ◦ Diarrhea
- ◦ Abdominal distention
- Presence of congenital anomalies
- Presence of birth-related injuries
  - ◦ Cephalohematoma
  - ◦ Brachial plexus injury
  - ◦ Pneumothorax
  - ◦ Fractured ribs
  - ◦ Subgaleal hemorrhage postvacuum extraction (McHugh, 2004b)

Clinical Impression:
Differential Diagnoses to Consider

- Term or preterm infant with
  - ◦ Respiratory distress
  - ◦ Birth trauma or injury
  - ◦ Physiologic jaundice
  - ◦ Hyperbilirubinemia
  - ◦ Genetic disorders
  - ◦ Group B strep
  - ◦ Congenital anomalies
  - ◦ Drug withdrawal
  - ◦ Other conditions or illnesses

Diagnostic Testing:
Diagnostic Tests and Procedures to Consider

- Total bilirubin
- Blood cultures
- Other tests
  - ◦ As indicated by infant presentation, *and*
  - ◦ Appropriate for midwife's scope of practice

Providing Treatment:
Therapeutic Measures to Consider

- Provide neutral thermal environment

- ◦ Skin to skin on mother
- ◦ On warmed resuscitation unit
- ◦ With hot water bottle for transport
- Provide O_2 for cyanosis
  - ◦ Blowby
  - ◦ Mask
  - ◦ Positive pressure ventilation
- As indicated by diagnosis such as
  - ◦ Phototherapy
  - ◦ Antibiotics

Providing Treatment:
Alternative Measures to Consider

- Home phototherapy: Lights or sunlight
- Homeopathic: Rescue Remedy to pulse points
- Prayer and acceptance of baby as perfect being
- Other remedies as indicated by baby's condition or presentation

Providing Support:
Education and Support Measures to Consider

- At discharge, or following home birth, provide information regarding
  - ◦ Signs and symptoms of illness or injury
  - ◦ Who to contact if symptoms develop
  - ◦ How to contact infant's health care professional
- For ill infant
  - ◦ Provide information about
    - ▪ Diagnosis, if known
    - ▪ Evaluation plan if diagnosis unknown
  - ◦ Provide support to parents during
    - ▪ Newborn workup
    - ▪ Diagnosis
    - ▪ Treatment

Follow-up Care:
Follow-up Measures to Consider

- Reevaluate infant
  - To establish baseline or note change
  - If uncertain regarding normalcy of condition
- Document

Collaborative Practice:
Consider Consultation or Referral

- Pediatric service
  - Neonate with signs or symptoms of
    - Illness
    - Injury
    - Anomaly
    - Unusual behavior or findings
  - Newborn transport or transfer care of infant as indicated by problem
- For diagnosis or treatment outside the midwife's scope of practice

Well-Baby Care

Key Clinical Information

The newborn infant may be cared for by a wide variety of health professionals, including midwives. The midwife who includes care of the infant after the immediate newborn period must develop working relationships with other infant care professionals who may provide care during times of illness, injury or other deviations from the norm. Developing a working relationship with parents by providing information, education, and support is vital to providing best care for the baby. Well-baby care may include evaluation of growth and development, administration of immunizations, and treatment of minor health problems.

Client History:
Components of the History to Consider

- Indication for present evaluation
  - Routine care
  - Problem-oriented care
- Significant maternal history (McHugh, 2004a)
  - Medical history
    - Chronic illness
    - STI
    - Substance abuse
    - Isoimmunization
  - Pregnancy history
    - Onset and duration of prenatal care
    - Pregnancy complications
    - Perinatal complications
- Course of labor and delivery and baby's response
  - Gestational age at birth
  - Interventions during labor or birth
  - Infant Apgar scores
  - Resuscitative efforts and infant response
- Significant findings or events since birth
  - Activity patterns
  - Voiding and stooling patterns
  - Feeding method and efforts
  - Weight loss or gain
  - Developmental milestones
  - Reflex responses
  - Parental observations and concerns
- Observation of parent–child interaction
  - Eye contact
  - Comfort seeking
  - Tone of voice
- Variations from expected newborn course
  - Signs and symptoms of
    - Infection

- Injury
- Neurologic disease
- Birth defects
- Drug addiction

Physical Examination:
Components of the Physical Exam to Consider

- Vital signs
- Growth parameters
  - Head circumference
  - Chest circumference
  - Height
  - Weight
  - Growth pattern
- Observation
  - Muscle tone and activity
  - Feeding
  - Response to environment
- Skin
  - Color and turgor
  - Rashes or lesions
  - Bruises or signs of abuse
- HEENT
  - Fontanels
  - Size and shape
  - Tracking movements of eyes
  - Suck and swallow
  - Tympanic membranes
  - Alertness
- Chest and back
  - Heart rate and rhythm
  - Breath sounds
  - Chest configuration
- Abdomen
  - Consistency

- Bowel sounds
- Extremities
  - Configuration
  - Range of motion
- Genitalia
- Assessment for signs of illness (McHugh, 2004b)
  - Skin tone variations
    - Pallor
    - Cyanosis
    - Ruddiness
    - Jaundice
  - Tachycardia (HR > 170 BPM)
  - Tachypnea (RR > 60 RPM)
  - Jitteriness or irritability
  - Poor muscle tone
  - Bulging or sunken fontanels
  - Hip clicks or laxity
  - Absence of voiding or stooling
  - Unusual sounding cry
  - Feeding difficulties

Clinical Impression:
Differential Diagnoses to Consider

- Well infant
- Infant with signs or symptoms of
  - Infection, such as
    - Conjunctivitis
    - Otitis media
    - Thrush
  - Injury
  - Neurologic disease
  - Birth defects
  - Drug addiction
  - Weight loss
  - Hearing or visual deficits

- ○ Failure to thrive
- ○ Developmental delay
- ○ Allergies

Diagnostic Testing:
Diagnostic Tests and Procedures to Consider

- • Glucose
- • Bilirubin
- • Other labs or tests as indicated by the infant's condition

Providing Treatment:
Therapeutic Measures to Consider

- • Nutritional
  - ○ Supplements as needed
  - ○ Specialty diets
    - ▪ Low phenolalinine
- • Phototherapy for hyperbilirubinemia
- • Childhood immunizations
  - ○ Hepatitis B immunization
  - ○ Diphtheria, pertussis, tetanus (DPT)
  - ○ Oral polio/inactivated polio vaccine (OPV/IPV)
  - ○ Measles, mumps, rubella (MMR)
  - ○ Haemophilus influenza Type b
  - ○ Varicella
  - ○ Pneumococcal
  - ○ Hepatitis A
  - ○ Influenza
- • Treatment for underlying disease or illness
  - ○ Antibiotics
  - ○ Antiretroviral medications
  - ○ Thyroid replacement
- • Other treatments as indicated

Providing Treatment:
Alternative Measures to Consider

- • Nutritional supplementation
  - ○ Soy-based formula
  - ○ Lact-aid if breast-feeding
- • Immunizations
  - ○ Delay in onset of immunizations
  - ○ Lower initial doses of immunizations
  - ○ No immunizations

Providing Support:
Education and Support Measures to Consider

- • Provide information on
  - ○ Anticipated well child
    - ▪ Growth and development
    - ▪ Behaviors
    - ▪ Developmental milestones
  - ○ Diet and nutrition recommendations
    - ▪ Breast-feeding
    - ▪ Formulas
- • Primary feeding method
- • Supplementation
  - ▪ Solid foods
  - ○ Signs and symptoms of concern
    - ▪ Warning signs
    - ▪ When to call with concerns
    - ▪ How to call in off-hours
  - ○ Routine for well-infant care
  - ○ Immunization recommendations
- • Encourage parental participation in decision making
  - ○ Provide rationale for recommendations
  - ○ Discuss alternatives
  - ○ Provide access to additional resources as needed

Follow-up Care:
Follow-up Measures to Consider

- Document all findings, especially any variations from normal

- Weight check at 1–2 weeks of age

- Follow-up oral vitamin K at 1 and 4 week visits

- Common well-child exam schedule
  - q months to 6 months
  - q 3 months 6–18 months
  - q 6 months 18–24 months
  - Annually 2–5 years

Collaborative Practice:
Consider Consultation or Referral

- Pediatric service
  - For well-child care outside the scope of the midwife's practice
  - In the presence of
    - Variations from normal
    - Illness
    - Injury
- For diagnosis or treatment outside the midwife's scope of practice

References

American College of Obstetricians and Gynecologists [ACOG]. (2001). Committee opinion #260: Circumcision. In *2002 Compendium of selected publications.* Washington, DC: Author.

American Academy of Pediatrics/American Heart Association [AAP/AHA]. (2000). *Textbook of neonatal resuscitation.* Elk Grove Village, IL: Author.

Clark, C., & Paine, L. L. (1996). Psychopharmacologic management of women with common mental health problems. *Journal of Nurse-Midwifery, 42,* 254–274.

Clark, F. I., & James, E. J. (1995). Twenty-seven years of experience with oral vitamin K1 therapy in neonates. *Journal of Pediatrics, 127,* 301–304.

Davis, E. (1997). *Hearts and hands: A midwife's guide to pregnancy & birth.* Berkeley, CA: Celestial Arts.

Davis, P. G., Tan, A., O'Donnell, C. P., Schulze, A. (2004). Resuscitation of newborn infants with 100% oxygen or air: A systematic review and meta-analysis. *Lancet, 364,* 1329–1333.

Gregoire, A. J., Kumar, R., Everitt, B., Henderson, A. F., & Studd, J. W. (1996) Transdermal oestrogen for treatment of severe postnatal depression. *Lancet, 347,* 930–933.

Leopold, K., & Zoschnick, L. (1997). Postpartum depression. *The Female Patient, (OB/GYN Edition), 22*(8), 40–49.

Lowenstein, V. (2004). Circumcision. In H. Varney, J. M. Kriebs, & C. L. Gegor (Eds.), *Varney's midwifery* (4th ed., pp. 1313–1326). Sudbury, MA: Jones and Bartlett.

McHugh, M. K., (2004a). Examination of the newborn. In H. Varney, J. M. Kriebs, & C. L. Gegor (Eds.), *Varney's midwifery* (4th ed., pp. 999–1010). Sudbury, MA: Jones and Bartlett.

McHugh, M. K., (2004b). Recognition and immediate care of sick newborns. In H. Varney, J. M. Kriebs, & C. L. Gegor (Eds.), *Varney's midwifery* (4th ed., pp. 1029–1040). Sudbury, MA: Jones and Bartlett.

Mercer, J., & Skovaard, R. (2002). Neonatal transition physiology: A new paradigm. *Journal of Neonatal and Perinatal Nursing, 15,* 56–75.

Miller, L. (1996, April). Beyond "The Blues": Postpartum reactivity and the biology of attachment. *Primary Psychiatry,* 35–38.

Murphy, J. L. (Ed.). (2004). *Nurse practitioner's prescribing reference.* New York: Prescribing Reference.

Righetti-Velterna, M., Conne-Perreard, P., Bousquet, A., & Manzano, J. (1998). Risk factors and predictive signs of postpartum depression. *Journal of Affective Disorders, 49,* 167–180.

Sinclair, C. (2004). *A midwife's handbook.* St. Louis, MO: W. B. Saunders.

Smith, T. (1984). *A woman's guide to homeopathic medicine.* New York: Thorsons.

Swartz, M. H. (1994). *Textbook of physical diagnosis: History and examination.* (2nd ed.). Philadelphia: W. B. Saunders.

Varney, H., Kriebs, J. M., & Gegor, C. L. (2004). *Varney's midwifery* (4th ed.). Sudbury, MA: Jones and Bartlett.

Weed, S. (1985). *Wise woman herbal for the childbearing year.* Woodstock, NY: Ashtree.

Bibliography

Bachmann, G. A. (1993). Estrogen-androgen therapy for sexual and emotional well-being. *The Female Patient, 18,* 15–24.

Behrman, R. E., Kleigman, R. M., & Arvin, A. M., (1996). *Nelson textbook of pediatrics* (15th ed.). Philadelphia: W.B. Saunders.

Barger, M. K. (Ed.). (1988). *Protocols for gynecologic and obstetric health care.* Philadelphia: W. B. Saunders.

Briggs, G.G., Freeman, R. K., & Yaffe, S. J. (1998) *Drugs in pregnancy and lactation* (5th ed.). Philadelphia: Williams & Wilkins.

Foster, S. (1996). *Herbs for your health.* Loveland, CO: Interweave Press.

Frye, A. (1998). *Holistic midwifery.* Portland, OR: Labrys Press.

Gelbaum, I. (1993) Circumcision: Refining a traditional surgical technique. *Journal of Nurse-Midwifery, 38*(Suppl.), 18S–30S.

Graves, B. W. (1992). Newborn resuscitation revisited. *Journal of Nurse-Midwifery, 37*(Suppl.), 36S–42S.

Scott, J. R., DiSaia, P. J., Hammond, C. B., Gordon J. D., & Spellacy W. N. (1996). *Danforth's handbook of obstetrics and gynecology.* Philadelphia: Lippincott-Raven.

Sinclair, C. (2004). *A midwife's handbook.* St. Louis, MO: W. B. Saunders.

Smith, T. (1984). *A woman's guide to homeopathic medicine.* New York: Thorsons

Swartz, M. H. (1994). *Textbook of physical diagnosis: History and examination.* (2nd ed.). Philadelphia: W. B. Saunders.

Varney, H., Kriebs, J. M., & Gegor, C. L. (2004). *Varney's midwifery* (4th ed.). Sudbury, MA: Jones and Bartlett.

Weed, S. (1985). *Wise woman herbal for the childbearing year.* Woodstock, NY: Ashtree.

Care of the Woman with Reproductive Health Needs: Care of the Well Woman

7

Midwives are women's health care specialists. By providing women's health care in an environment of support and understanding, midwives foster a woman's ability to care for herself.

In nearly every culture, women have a history of meeting others' needs before attending to their own. This may be due to social conventions, lack of knowledge about women's health needs, or limited resources such as communication barriers, transportation issues, or a lack of funds with which to pay for services. In our fragmented American society, many women may not know how to access services, or may be unable to navigate the complex health care system in a manner that meets their basic needs.

Midwives are needed to reach out to women in the communities where they live and practice to bridge this chasm. Community midwifery may range from home-based care, to a local clinic, to a complex service that functions within the confines of a tertiary care hospital. No matter what the setting, each individual midwife can make a difference.

Listening to women is an essential component of midwifery care. The process of active listening includes validating women's experiences, offering nonjudgmental support, and considering how the information disclosed affects this woman, as a person, within her family and her community.

Opportunities for midwifery include providing grassroots encouragement for women to develop support networks within their own neighborhood, cultural enclave, or ethnic group. Many midwives offer women's health education as a community service. Where opportunities to offer birth care are limited or unavailable, midwives provide gynecologic or primary care services. A commitment to women and an inquiring mind are all that is necessary to begin the adventure of improving the health of women using the midwifery model of care.

Women may come to their midwife for care that includes reproductive health screening and assessment, college- or employment-related evaluations, diagnostic testing, and health maintenance. For many women, the annual reproductive health exam is their one planned preventive health visit. The midwife must be diligent in assessing all body systems, and not focusing exclusively on reproductive health care.

The Well-Woman Exam

Key Clinical Information

The well-woman exam is an opportunity for women to learn about their bodies while at the same time caring for themselves. Each visit offers both the woman and the midwife a chance to develop a partnership in which to address the client's unique concerns. During the initial visit the client history required will be quite comprehensive, while on repeat visits, especially in a community where the midwife provides ongoing care to the same women, a brief update of the history may be all that is required.

Midwives caring for young women may be asked to perform a sports or college entry examination during the annual well woman visit. Education in the additional components of these exams is easily obtained through continuing professional education programs.

Client History: Components of the History to Consider

- Reason for visit
- Last menstrual period (LMP)
- Obstetrical history
  - Gravity, parity
  - Infertility or losses
  - Problems, concerns
  - Plans for future pregnancies
- Gynecological history
  - Menstrual patterns
  - Length of flow
  - Amount of flow

- Pain, clots, etc.
- Sexual history
  - Sexual orientation
  - New or change in partners
  - Method of birth control if applicable
- Concerns
- Medical/surgical history
  - Allergies
  - Medications and remedies
    - Over the counter
    - Prescription
    - Herbal/homeopathic remedies
  - Current immunization status
  - Diseases, conditions, or problems
  - Surgeries
  - ⊛ BCG vaccine or positive PPD
- Current health care
  - Primary care provider
  - Specialist care
  - Diagnostic testing
  - Treatments
- Health philosophy and care
  - Survival
  - Medically oriented
  - Alternative
- Social history
  - ⊛ Cultural influences on health care
  - Use of alcohol, tobacco, drugs
  - Family community support systems
  - Domestic violence screen
  - Emotional well-being screen
  - Diet and physical activity
- Family history
  - Medical conditions
  - Hereditary conditions

- Review of systems (ROS)
  - Client impression of her health
  - Physical
  - Emotional
  - Changes in weight or appetite
  - Bowel and bladder function
  - Weakness, fatigue, malaise
  - Shortness of breath/palpitations
  - Other symptoms by body system
    - HEENT
    - Cardiopulmonary
    - Gastrointestinal
    - Neurologic
    - Reproductive
    - Musculoskeletal
    - Endocrine
    - Integumentary

Physical Examination: Components of the Physical Exam to Consider

- Vital signs
  - Height, weight, BMI
  - Blood pressure, pulse, respirations
- Skin
  - Lesions
  - Scars
  - Bruises
- Head, eyes, ears, nose, and throat
  - Eyes
    - Visual acuity
    - Ophthalmic exam
    - Nystagmus
  - Ears
    - Hearing
    - Canals
    - Tympanic membranes
  - Mouth
    - Lesions
    - Condition of teeth and gums
    - Tonsils
  - Thyroid
    - Symmetry
    - Size
    - Masses or nodules
  - Lymph nodes
- Back and Chest
  - Lesions
  - Configuration, symmetry
  - CVA tenderness
  - Scoliosis, kyphosis
  - Lungs
    - Rate, rhythm, and depth of respirations
    - Breath sounds
    - Changes with percussion
  - Heart
    - Rate and rhythm
    - Extra or unusual sounds
- Murmurs
- Whistles or clicks
  - Breasts
    - Shape and symmetry
    - Presence of masses
    - Nipple discharge
    - Axillary nodes
- Abdomen
  - Configuration
  - Masses, pain
  - Diastasis recti
  - Bowel sounds
- Extremities

- ○ Range of motion
- ○ Reflexes
- ○ Symmetry
- ○ Strength
- ○ Joint stability or mobility
- Pelvic exam
  - ○ External genitalia and rectum
    - ▪ Bartholin's, urethra, Skene's (BUS)
    - ▪ Configuration
    - ▪ Lesions, discharge
    - ▪ Hemorrhoids
  - ○ Speculum exam
    - ▪ Vagina
- Lesions
- Discharge
- Odor
  - ▪ Cervix
- Discharge
- Lesions
- Configuration
  - ▪ Specimen collection
- Bimanual exam
  - ○ Uterine position
  - ○ Size and shape
  - ○ Pain on cervical motion
  - ○ Adnexal
    - ▪ Masses
    - ▪ Pain
    - ▪ Mobility
- Rectal exam
  - ○ Hemorrhoids
  - ○ Masses
  - ○ Bleeding
  - ○ Specimen collection

Clinical Impression: Differential Diagnoses to Consider

- Well-woman preventive health exam, NOS
- Well-woman preventive health exam with
  - ○ Preparticipation sports evaluation
  - ○ College-entry evaluation
  - ○ Preemployment screening
- Well-woman exam with significant findings, such as
  - ○ Reproductive health issues
    - ▪ Undesired fertility
    - ▪ Sexually transmitted infection
    - ▪ Infertility
    - ▪ Pregnancy
  - ○ General health issues
    - ▪ Thyroid disorder
    - ▪ Rectal bleeding
    - ▪ Infection
    - ▪ Asthma

Diagnostic Testing: Diagnostic Tests and Procedures to Consider

- Testing performed or collected during visit
  - ○ Dip urinalysis
  - ○ Pregnancy testing
  - ○ Fingerstick Hct or Hgb
  - ○ Pap smear
  - ○ STI testing
  - ○ Wet prep for BV or Trich
  - ○ Stool for occult blood
  - ○ Mantoux test for TB
- Lab testing
  - ○ CBC or H & H
  - ○ Hepatitis profile
  - ○ HIV testing

- Q-β HCG
- Sickle cell prep
- Fasting blood sugar
- Urinalysis and/or culture
- Thyroid screening
- Cultures
  - Throat
  - Skin lesions
- Radiology
  - Ultrasound
  - Mammogram
  - Chest X-ray for positive+ PPD, BCG vaccine

Providing Treatment:
Therapeutic Measures to Consider

- Provide immunizations as indicated (CDC, 2002)
  - Tetanus, diphtheria
  - Hepatitis B
  - Measles, mumps, rubella
  - Varicella
  - Influenza (over 50)
  - Pneumococcal vaccine (over 65)
- Provide treatment based on diagnosis

Providing Treatment:
Alternative Measures to Consider

- Provide treatment based on diagnosis

Providing Support:
Education and Support Measures to Consider

- Address client concerns
- Preventive health recommendations
  - Diet
  - Physical activity

- Weight management
- Smoking cessation
- Substance abuse treatment
- Notification process for results
- Recommendations for ongoing care

Follow-up Care:
Follow-up Measures to Consider

- Document
- Return for reading of Mantoux, prn
- Notify clients of test results
- Report adverse reactions to vaccines
  - Vaccine Adverse Event Reporting System
    - www.vaers.org
    - 800-822-7967

Collaborative Practice:
Consider Consultation or Referral

- OB/GYN service
  - Abnormal pap smears
  - Abnormal breast exam
  - Other GYN problem
- Medical service, by specialty
  - Confirmed occult blood in stool
  - Rectal mass
  - Orthopedic problems
  - New diagnosis of illness, such as
    - HIV
    - Hepatitis
    - Thyroid disorder
    - Diabetes
    - Hypertension
    - Heart disease
- Social service
  - Transportation services

- ○ Mental health services
- ○ Drug and alcohol rehab services
- ○ Homeless shelters
- ○ Abused women's services
- • For diagnosis or treatment outside the midwife's scope of practice

Preconception Evaluation

Key Clinical Information

Preconception counseling provides an opportunity to address health needs that may affect pregnancy before the pregnancy occurs. Midwife-initiated discussions may spark awareness and interest in modifying health behaviors as a prelude to a planned pregnancy, or foster correct use of birth control for pregnancy prevention.

Client History: Components of the History to Consider

- • Age
- • Previous OB/GYN history
  - ○ G, P
    - ▪ Result of previous pregnancies
  - ○ STIs, HIV status
  - ○ Abnormal pap smears, cervical treatment
  - ○ Types of birth control used
  - ○ Infertility
- • Medical and surgical history
  - ○ Current medical problems
  - ○ Previous surgery
  - ○ Medications
- • Social history
  - ○ Physical activity patterns
  - ○ Mental well-being
  - ○ Nutrition
    - ▪ Eating disorders

- ▪ Overweight, or underweight
- ▪ Pica
- ○ Substance abuse
- ○ Physical abuse
- ○ Partner/family support
- ○ Occupational hazards
- • Family history: client and partner
  - ○ Birth defects
  - ○ Genetic disorders
  - ○ Multiple births
  - ○ Losses (Scherger, 1993)
- • Personal concerns
  - ○ Readiness (self and partner)
  - ○ Financial concerns
  - ○ Spouse and/or family concerns
  - ○ Cultural considerations for childbearing
- • Review of systems (ROS)

Physical Examination: Components of the Physical Exam to Consider

- • Complete physical exam as indicated by
  - ○ History
  - ○ Interval since last physical
- • Primary focus on
  - ○ Thyroid
  - ○ Breast exam
  - ○ Pelvic exam

Clinical Impression: Differential Diagnoses to Consider

- • Preconception reproductive health care
- • Screening for health risks related to pregnancy
- • Preconception counseling related to risk factors, such as
  - ○ Diabetes

- Hypertension
- Genetic disorders
- Neural tube defects
- Advanced maternal age
- HIV infection
- Substance abuse (Scherger, 1993)

Diagnostic Testing:
Diagnostic Tests and Procedures to Consider

- TB testing
  - PPD or Mantoux testing
  - Chest X-ray
- Cervicovaginal screening
  - Pap smear
  - Wet mount for BV
  - GBS
  - Chlamydia
  - Gonorrhea
- Blood tests
  - Rubella and hepatitis B titers
  - Blood type and Rh
  - H & H or CBC
  - TSH or thyroid screen
  - Toxoplasmosis screen
  - HIV testing
- Mammogram
- Other as indicated by history

Providing Treatment:
Therapeutic Measures to Consider

- Treat medical conditions
  - Adjust medications according to drug pregnancy category
- Vitamin and mineral supplement
  - Folic acid 0.4 mg/400mcg po daily

- Begin at least 4 weeks prior to planned conception
- Continue through at least 13 weeks gestation
- Consider multivitamin with or without iron
- Update immunization status
  - Rubella
  - Hepatitis B
  - Tetanus, diphtheria
  - Varicella
  - Avoid pregnancy for 3 months following live virus immunization (Sweet, 1999)

Providing Treatment:
Alternative Measures to Consider

- Whole foods diet
- Mineral and folic acid from food sources
- Fertility awareness methods for determining ovulation

Providing Support:
Education and Support Measures to Consider

- Fertility awareness
  - Menstrual cycle and ovulation
  - Signs of fertility
  - Fertility charting
  - Signs of conception
  - Early embryonic development
- Health Promotion
  - Counsel regarding pertinent issues as determined by history
  - Encourage dental work prior to conception
  - Encourage regular physical exercise
  - Provide nutrition information and recommendations
  - Avoidance of cigarettes, alcohol, recreational drugs

- Environmental concerns
  - Workplace hazards
  - Toxic chemicals
  - Radiation contamination
- Health concerns
  - Effects of health problems on developing fetus
  - Recommendations for optimal care
- Provide pregnancy information and inform about resources in the community
- Address birth options, locations, and services

Follow-up Care:
Follow-up Measures to Consider

- Document
- Provide test results
- Return for
  - Reading of Mantoux test
  - Follow-up of recommendations
  - Review of fertility charts
  - Onset of amenorrhea for HCG testing
  - No pregnancy within 6–12 months
  - Questions or concerns

Collaborative Practice:
Consider Consultation or Referral

- OB/GYN service
  - Genetic counseling
  - Abnormal preconception labs
  - Infertility evaluation or treatment
  - High risk pregnancy
- Social services
  - Substance abuse centers
  - Nutritional risk assessment by dietician
  - Physical abuse
  - Psychosocial issues

- Medical service
  - Management of disease or illness, such as
    - Diabetes
    - Hypertension
- For diagnosis or treatment outside the midwife's scope of practice

Smoking Cessation
Key Clinical Information

Smoking is an addiction that is both physical as well as psychological. To successfully stop smoking there must be desire to quit, a method to address the physical symptoms of nicotine withdrawal, and exploration and cultivation of more positive coping skills and habits. Midwives can provide a supportive environment for the woman who is motivated to stop smoking.

Client History:
Components of the History to Consider

- Age
- Medical and surgical history
- Current medical problems
  - Diabetes
  - Heart disease
    - Coronary artery disease
    - Elevated cholesterol
    - Hypertension
  - Respiratory disorders
    - Asthma
    - Chronic cough
    - Bronchitis
    - COPD
    - Emphysema
  - Mental health disorders
    - Eating disorders
    - Depression

- Bipolar disease
- Psychosis
  - Medications, including
    - Antihypertensive medications
    - Estrogen products
- Oral contraceptives
- Hormone replacement therapy
  - Antidepressants
- Wellbutrin (same as Zyban)
- MAO Inhibitors
- Social history
  - Partner/family support
  - Stress levels
  - Work environment
  - Other smokers in family
- Fagerstrom tobacco addiction assessment (Heatherton, Kozlowski, Frecker, & Fagerstrom, 1991)
  - How soon after waking is first cigarette smoked?
    - Time less than 5 minutes: 3 points
    - Time 5 to 30 minutes: 2 points
    - Time 31 to 60 minutes: 1 point
  - How many cigarettes are smoked per day?
    - More than 30 per day: 3 points
    - 21 to 30 per day: 2 points
    - 11 to 20 per day: 1 point
  - Interpretation
    - Heavy nicotine dependence: 5–6 points
      - Consider 21 mg nicotine patch
    - Moderate nicotine dependence: 3–4 points
      - Consider 14 mg patch
    - Light nicotine dependence: 0–2 points
      - Consider 7 mg patch or no patch
- Personal concerns
  - Readiness, motivation

- Previous attempts to stop smoking
- Coping skills
- Weight gain
- Family medical history
  - Diabetes
  - Heart disease
    - Coronary artery disease
    - Elevated cholesterol
    - Hypertension
    - Stroke
- Review of systems

Physical Examination: Components of the Physical Exam to Consider

- Vital signs
- Height, weight, BMI
- As indicated by
  - History and ROS
  - Interval since last exam
- Cardiopulmonary system
  - BP, carotid pulses
  - Heart rate and rhythm
  - Evaluation of heart sounds
  - Lung fields

Clinical Impression: Differential Diagnoses to Consider

- Smoking cessation

Diagnostic Testing: Diagnostic Tests and Procedures to Consider

- Lipid profile
- ECG

Providing Treatment: Therapeutic Measures to Consider

- Nicotine-containing medications (Murphy, 2004)
  - Pregnancy category D
    - Risk may outweigh benefit
    - Provide informed consent
  - Nicoderm or Habitrol
    - 7 mg/24 hours, 14 mg/24 hours, or 21 mg/24 hours
    - Begin with 21 or 14 mg patch
    - Use 2–6 weeks then decrease dose
    - Repeat with decreased dose
  - Nicotrol step-down patch (transdermal)
    - 5–15 mg/16 hour patch, or
    - Use during waking hours
  - Nicorette gum
    - 2 mg, 4 mg strength
    - Use 2 mg if < 1 pack per day smoker
    - Max 24 pieces/day
  - Nicotrol NS, inhaler
    - 0.5 mg/spray, 10 mg/cartridge inhaler
    - 1–2 doses/hour
- Nonnicotine medication (Murphy, 2004)
  - Bupropion HCL (Zyban)
    - 150 mg po x 3 days
    - 150 bid with 8 hours between doses
    - Stop smoking within 1–2 weeks of initiation
    - May use with nicotine medications
    - Pregnancy category B
    - Not for use in those with
      - Eating disorders
      - Seizures
      - Wellbutrin or MAOIs
  - Nortriptyline (deCosta, Younes, & Lorenco, 2002; Hall et al., 2002)

- Usual dose 75 mg daily
- Titrate to serum level 50–150 ng/ml
- As effective as Bupropion

Providing Treatment: Alternative Measures to Consider

- Decrease cigarette use by 1–2 cig/week
- Learn new coping skills
- Avoid situations that increase desire to smoke
- Keep gum or healthy finger food available for oral satisfaction
- Increase physical activity

Providing Support: Education and Support Measures to Consider

- Provide clear medication instructions
  - Nicotine-containing medications
    - Stop smoking with prior to or with onset of use
    - Use lower dose with
      - Cardiac history
      - Pregnancy
      - Body weight < 100 lbs
    - Patches
      - Apply new patch daily to nonhairy skin
        - Upper torso or arm
      - Do not reuse skin sites for at least 1 week
      - New patch applied each 24 hours
  - Bupropion HCL
    - Take as instructed
    - May decrease appetite
    - May cause medication interactions
  - Nortriptyline
    - May treat concomitant depression
    - May cause
      - Dry mouth

- Sedation
- Cardiac arrhythmias
- Counsel as determined by history
  - Encourage regular physical exercise
  - Provide nutrition information
  - Provide information regarding
    - Local resources for developing healthy coping mechanisms
    - Smoking support groups

Follow-up Care:
Follow-up Measures to Consider

- Document
- Revisit two weeks after beginning smoking cessation
  - Client support and counseling
  - Evaluation of
    - Current smoking patterns
    - BP, WT changes
    - Symptoms or side effects of medication
- Register pregnant clients on bupropion HCL by calling Glaxo (800) 336-2176

Collaborative Practice:
Consider Consultation or Referral

- Medical service
  - Cardiac history
  - Adverse medication reaction
  - Onset of cardiac symptoms with use of nicotine-containing medications
- Mental health service
  - Exacerbation of depression symptoms
- Social service
  - Smoking cessation support services
  - Other services as necessary to reduce stress

- For diagnosis or treatment outside the midwife's scope of practice

Fertility Awareness
Key Clinical Information

Fertility awareness charting can be easily incorporated into midwifery practice. It offers women a means to become more attuned to the functioning of their reproductive system and its impact on overall health and well-being. Fertility awareness can be used as an effective method of birth control for the couple that is attentive to the nuances of the female cycle. This requires an openness to discussion, acceptance of life cycles, and compromise. This process fosters development of an emotionally intimate relationship and places sex at the periphery rather than at the center of the union (Singer, 2004).

Documentation of changes through the cycle can be useful in recognizing ovulation, identifying menstrual problems, and understanding the changes of the perimenopause. Every woman can benefit from an increased awareness and understanding of her body's functioning throughout her life. Teaching fertility awareness to adolescent women provides a wonderful outreach opportunity for midwives, and it can be instrumental in delaying onset of sexual activity.

Client History:
Components of the History to Consider

- OB/GYN history
- Menstrual history
  - LMP
  - Frequency of menses
  - Duration of menses
  - Midcycle pain, discharge
- Sexual history
  - Age of onset of sexual activity
  - Safe sex practices
    - Abstinence

- STI testing

- Condom use

- Monogamy

  ○ Sexual relationships

  - Long-term monogamy

  - Serial monogamy

  - Multiple partners

  - Same sex and/or opposite sex partner(s)

- Current method of birth control, if any

- Goals of learning fertility awareness

- Medical, surgical history

Physical Examination:
Components of the Physical Exam to Consider

- Exam not necessary to teach fertility awareness

- Weight, height, BMI

- Physical exam components as indicated by

  ○ Age and health status

  ○ History and client interview

Clinical Impression:
Differential Diagnoses to Consider

- Education and counseling

- Contraceptive management

Diagnostic Testing:
Diagnostic Tests and Procedures to Consider

- Pap

- STI testing

- Thyroid

- Ovulation predictor tests

  ○ Test for leutenizing hormone

  ○ www.birthcontrol.com

Providing Treatment:
Therapeutic Measures to Consider

- Prescription methods of birth control

- Hormone replacement therapy

- Hormonal treatment of menstrual irregularities

Providing Treatment:
Alternative Measures to Consider

- Fertility awareness charting (Singer, 2004; Kass-Annese & Danzer, 2003)

  ○ Appropriate for women

  - From menarche through menopause

  - During breastfeeding

  - With menstrual irregularities

- Nonpharmacologic methods of birth control

- Natural family planning using fertility awareness

- Abstinence

- Periodic abstinence (rhythm method)

  ○ Avoid intercourse during fertile times

- Withdrawal

  ○ May work for some couples

  ○ There may or may not be sperm in preejaculatory fluid

  ○ May or may not interrupt sexual satisfaction

- Natural spermicides (see Barrier Methods)

- Outercourse (Weinstein, 1994)

  ○ Hugging and kissing

  ○ Holding and fondling

  ○ Sexual activity that does not include penetration

Providing Support:
Education and Support Measures to Consider

- Provide information and resources about (Singer, 2004)

  ○ Changes throughout the menstrual cycle

  ○ Primary fertility signals

- Basal body temperature
- Cervical fluid
- Cervical changes
  - Secondary fertility signals
    - Midcyle pain
    - Ferning of salivary fluid
    - Spotting
    - Breast tenderness
    - Libido changes
  - Resources for fertility awareness
    - Charts
      - www.fertilityawareness.net
      - Couple to Couple League
    - Couple to Couple League International
      - Catholic organization
      - Natural family planning materials
      - www.ccli.org
      - Phone (513) 471-2000
    - Ovulation microscopes
      - www.fertile-focus.com
      - www.ovulation-predictor.com
- When using fertility awareness for birth control
  - Discussion regarding best method for couple
  - Option to add barrier methods or spermicide at midcycle
- Engage partner in discussions

Follow-up Care:
Follow-up Measures to Consider

- Document
- Return for care
  - For fertility chart review
  - As recommended by age and sexual activity
  - For Pap and STI testing
  - With pregnancy

Collaborative Practice:
Consider Consultation or Referral

- For diagnosis or treatment outside the midwife's scope of practice

Barrier Methods of Birth Control
Key Clinical Information

Barrier methods provide not only contraception, but also may provide some protection from sexually transmitted infections. Use of barrier methods requires that couples take the time to learn to use their method correctly and then use it consistently. Effectiveness of barrier methods is related to the method type, use of spermicide, parity of the woman, and actual use patterns. Efficacy ranges from a low of 3% failure to as high as 40%. Multiparous women tend to have higher failure rates than nulliparous women. Barrier methods may be used as an adjunct to other methods, or used alone. More information on barrier methods is available at www.birthcontrol.com.

Client History:
Components of the History to Consider

- Allergies
- Medications
- OB/GYN history
  - LMP—normal menstrual pattern
  - G,P
  - Last exam, pap, and STI testing, as applicable
  - History of STIs—diagnosis and treatment
  - History of abnormal pap smears—diagnosis and treatment
- Past and current medical and surgical history
- Social history
  - Cigarette smoking, drug, and/or alcohol use
  - Living situation and resources
  - Sexual partner support for method of birth control

- Method-related considerations
  - Assess ability to learn and use method reliably
  - Assess impact of unplanned pregnancy
  - Previous reaction to spermicide

Physical Examination: Components of the Physical Exam to Consider

- Well-woman exam, with focus on
  - Vaginal, cervical anatomy and position
  - Fit of diaphragm or cap
  - Woman's ability to insert/remove device

Clinical Impression: Differential Diagnoses to Consider

- Contraceptive management
  - Diaphragm fitting
  - Cervical cap fitting
  - Contraceptive education
    - Condoms
    - Spermicide
    - Options

Diagnostic Testing: Diagnostic Tests and Procedures to Consider

- Pap smear
- Urinalysis
- STI screening
- Other screening tests according to age and health history

Providing Treatment: Therapeutic Measures to Consider

- Diaphragm
  - Not recommended for patients with history of UTIs

- Female superior position decreases effectiveness
  - Must be used with spermicide
- Cervical cap
  - May cause increased rate of cervical erosion
  - Recommended to be used with spermicide
  - Prentif cavity rim cervical cap
    - 4 sizes
    - Latex
    - Requires fitting
  - FemCap
    - 3 sizes based on parity
    - Nonlatex
  - Lea shield
    - 1 size
    - Available from Canada
    - Nonlatex
  - Oves cap
    - Disposable cap
    - Requires fitting
    - Medical grade silicone
    - 3 sizes
- Male condom
  - Provides some measure of protection against STIs
  - May contribute to latex allergy
  - Requires male cooperation to use effectively
- Contraceptive sponge
  - Today sponge
  - Nonoxyl-9
  - 89–91% effective
- Protectaid
  - Available in Canada
  - F5 gel
  - 90% effective
- Pharmatex sponge

- ○ Available in Canada
- ○ Benzalkonium chloride
- ○ 83% effective
- Reality female condom
  - ○ Allows female control for STI protection and contraception
  - ○ Greater protection than male condom

Providing Treatment:
Alternative Measures to Consider

- Fertility awareness
- Abstinence
- Withdrawal
- Natural spermicide (Trapani, 1984)
  - ○ For use with cervical cap or diaphragm (Use instead of nonoxyl-9)
  - ○ 1 cup water
  - ○ 1 teaspoon fresh lemon juice
  - ○ 5 teaspoons table salt
  - ○ 10 teaspoons cornstarch
  - ○ 10 teaspoons glycerin
  - ○ Mix solids, add liquids while stirring, cook over low heat until thick. Store in sealed containers. Discard unused portions after 30 days.

Providing Support:
Education and Support Measures to Consider

- Instruct in proper use, cleaning, and care of reusable devices
- Have client perform a return demonstration of insertion and removal of diaphragm or cervical cap
- Review effectiveness of chosen method
- Review other birth control methods and their effectiveness
- Condoms are recommended to protect against STIs

Follow-up Care:
Follow-up Measures to Consider

- Document discussions regarding
- Call or return for care
  - ○ 2 weeks evaluation of diaphragm or cervical cap
  - ○ 3–4 months repeat pap smear for cap users
  - ○ Annual well-woman visit
  - ○ Method-related problems
  - ○ Amenorrhea
  - ○ Positive pregnancy test

Collaborative Practice:
Consider Consultation or Referral

- OB/GYN service
  - ○ For diagnosis or treatment outside the midwife's scope of practice

Emergency Contraception

Key Clinical Information

Emergency contraception is most effective as soon as possible after unprotected intercourse. Emergency contraceptive pills (ECP) must be taken within 72 hours after unprotected sexual exposure, while the Copper-T IUD may be placed up to 7 days after unprotected intercourse. ECP is not recommended for regular use as contraception. When prescribed as Preven, the emergency contraceptive kit includes a pregnancy test. Both Preven and Plan B include detailed client instructions. Side effects may include nausea and vomiting, and a prescription for an antiemetic may be helpful (Program for Appropriate Technology in Health, 1997). Clients may access the Emergency Contraceptive Hotline by calling (888) NOT-2-Late (668-2528-3). Providers may be listed on the hotline by calling the same number.

Client History:
Components of the History to Consider

- Allergies
- Medications
- Number of hours since unprotected intercourse
- OB/GYN history
  - LMP—normal menstrual pattern
  - G, P
  - Current or recent use of contraception
  - Last exam, Pap smear, and STI testing if applicable
  - History of STIs
  - History of abnormal Pap smears
- Contraindications to ECP use
  - Pregnancy
  - Undiagnosed genital bleeding
- Contraindications to IUD insertion (see Intrauterine Device)
- Assess
  - Ability to use ECP as directed
  - Potential unplanned pregnancy
  - Reasons for unprotected sexual exposure
  - Plans for long-term birth control
- Social history
  - Date rape or sexual assault/abuse
  - Judgment altered by substance abuse

Physical Examination:
Components of the Physical Exam to Consider

- Not required for ECP, but may be useful when
  - History is unclear
  - STI testing indicated
  - Other symptoms are present
- No exam within past 12 months
  - Limited exam
  - Complete well-woman exam

Clinical Impression:
Differential Diagnoses to Consider

- Contraceptive management following unprotected sexual exposure
  - Emergency contraceptive pills
  - Copper-T IUD insertion

Diagnostic Testing:
Diagnostic Tests and Procedures to Consider

- Pregnancy testing
  - If menstrual history is uncertain or unclear
- STI screening
- Other screening tests
  - According to age and health history

Providing Treatment:
Therapeutic Measures to Consider

- Provide antiemetic 1 hour before first ECP dose (ACOG, 2001b)
  - Compazine
    - 5–10 mg tablet q 6–8 hours prn
    - 15 mg spansule q 24 hours x 2
  - Phenergan
    - 25 mg tablet or suppository
      - q 8–12 hours prn
    - Benadryl 25–50 mg po
      - q 4–6 hours prn
- Emergency contraceptive pills (ECP) (Program for Appropriate Technology in Health, 1997)
  - First dose ASAP but at least within 72 hours
  - Second dose 12 hours after first dose
  - Plan B
    - Progestin only
    - May cause less nausea
    - 0.75 mg levonorgestrel per dose
    - 1 tab per dose, 2 doses

- Preven (ECP Kit)
  - Estrogen/progestin
  - 0.05 mg ethinyl estradiol/0.25 mg levonorgestel
  - 2 tabs, 2 doses (Murphy, 2004)
- Lo/Ovral
  - 0.03 mg ethinyl estradiol/0.30 mg levonorgestrel
  - 4 tabs, 2 doses
- Levelen/Nordette (light orange pills)
  - 0.03 mg ethinyl estradiol/0.15 mg levonorgestrel
  - 4 tabs, 2 doses
- Tri-Levelen/Triphasil (yellow pills)
  - 0.03 mg ethinyl estradiol/0.125 mg levonorgestrel
  - 4 tabs, 2 doses
- Copper-T IUD insertion (see Intrauterine Device)

Providing Treatment:
Alternative Measures to Consider

- Nausea
  - Seabands
  - Ginger tea
- Herbs that foster onset of menstruation
  - Blue cohosh
  - Angelica root
  - Dong quai
  - Vitex or chasteberry
  - Black cohosh (Soule, 1996)
  - Evening primrose oil
- Homeopathic remedies that foster onset of menstruation (Smith, 1984)
  - Pulsatilla
  - Sepia
  - Caulophyllum
  - Calcarea carb.
- For additional information about herbal remedies to prevent or avoid pregnancy see
  - *A Difficult Decision: A Compassionate Book About Abortion* by Joy Gardner
  - *The Roots of Healing* by Deb Soule

Providing Support:
Education and Support Measures to Consider

- Verify client does not want to become pregnant
- ECP
  - Explain how to use ECPs correctly
  - Emphasize that ECPs are for emergency use only
  - Counseling regarding common side effects
    - Nausea and vomiting
    - Breast tenderness
    - Menses
      - May be earlier or later than usual
      - Within 21 days of ECP
  - Return for care if no menses within 21 days
- Discuss
  - Safe sexual practices
  - Pregnancy and STI prevention
  - Other contraceptive options
- Options if ECP is not effective
  - Not teratogenic
- ECP more likely to be used with provider visit for
  - Information
  - Counseling
  - Prescription

Follow-up Care:
Follow-up Measures to Consider

- Document

- Have client return for care with
  - Symptoms suggesting complications
  - Amenorrhea that continues over 21 days after ECP
  - For initiation of regular contraception
  - Client requires further information or counseling or care regarding STIs or pregnancy prevention

Collaborative Practice: Criteria to Consider for Consultation or Referral

- OB/GYN service
  - If ECP not effective for termination of pregnancy per client choice
  - For diagnosis or treatment outside the midwife's scope of practice

Hormonal Contraceptives: Pills, Patches, Rings, and Injections

Key Clinical Information

Hormonal contraceptives are now available in a wide array of delivery methods. Contraceptive pills, patches, rings, and injections offer reliable pregnancy prevention and the potential for improved compliance. Birth control pills offer a well-established woman-controlled method of hormonal birth control. They may result in a decrease in ovarian cancer risk, a decrease in the rate of endometrial cancer, allow women to suffer less dysmenorrhea, and result in a lighter menstrual flow. Rings and patches provide contraceptive hormones on a continual basis, avoiding the peaks and valleys of oral administration. Depo provera and Lunelle contraceptive injections offer a hormonal method of birth control for women who cannot reliably use other hormonal methods. While there may be a prompt return to fertility after the injection, there may also be a significant delay in return to fertility. Some women report PMS-like symptoms while on Depo provera, which is a progestin-only medication. The

Mirena and the Progestasert IUDs include a progestin component: to aid in pregnancy prevention via thickening of cervical mucous to limit entry of sperm into the uterus (see Intrauterine Device). All hormones may pass through breast milk. While estrogen has been demonstrated to decrease milk production, long-term effects of estrogen and progesterone on the newborn are not well documented.

Client History: Components of the History to Consider

- Allergies
- Medications
- OB/GYN history
  - LMP—normal menstrual pattern
  - G, P—date of most recent birth if postpartum
  - Last exam, Pap smear, and STI testing if applicable
  - STIs—diagnosis and treatment
  - Abnormal pap smears—diagnosis and treatment
  - Breast, mammogram abnormalities—diagnosis and treatment
- Risk factors for osteoporosis
  - Low Ca+ diet
  - Sedentary
  - Small frame
  - Family history
  - Duration of injectable contraceptive use
- Past and current medical and surgical history
  - Depression or mental health disorder
  - Liver dysfunction or disease
  - Gallbladder disease
  - Heart disease
    - Hyperlipemia
    - Hypertension

- Thrombophlebitis
- Social history
  - Cigarette smoking
  - Drug and/or alcohol use
  - Living situation and resources
  - Sexual partner support for method of birth control
  - Risk factors for STIs
- Family history
  - Gallbladder disease
  - Coronary artery disease before age 50
  - Stroke before age 50
- Contraindications to injectable contraceptive use
  - Pregnancy
  - History of breast cancer
  - Undiagnosed genital bleeding
  - Inability to return for injections as scheduled
- Contraindications to oral contraceptive use (ACOG, 2000)
  - Pregnancy
  - Liver disease
  - Undiagnosed abnormal genital bleeding
  - Thrombophlebitis or thromboembolitic disease
  - Coronary heart disease or cerebrovascular disease
  - Cancer of the reproductive organs
  - Relative contraindications
    - Women who smoke and are > 35 years old
    - BP 140/90 or greater
    - Diabetes
    - Asthma
    - Kidney disease
    - Gallbladder disease

- Lupus
- Depression
- Assess the woman's ability and motivation to use client-regulated hormonal contraception (Reider & Coupey, 2000)
  - Daily routine for pill taking
  - Weekly routine for patch
  - 3-week cycle for ring
  - Ability to cope with side effects while adjusting to hormones
  - Motivation to prevent pregnancy

Physical Examination: Components of the Physical Exam to Consider

- BP
- Height, weight, BMI
- Complete physical exam
  - Focus on reproductive system
  - Thyroid
  - Breasts
  - Pelvic
    - Speculum exam
    - Bimanual exam

Clinical Impression: Differential Diagnoses to Consider

- Contraceptive management
  - Hormonal contraceptive use
    - Oral contraceptives
- Progesterone only pills (POP)
- Monophasic OC
- Biphasic OC
- Triphasic OC
- 90-day OC
    - Contraceptive patch
    - Contraceptive vaginal ring

- Injectable contraceptive
- Hormonal IUD
  - Hormonal contraceptive use complicated by
    - Hypertension
    - Hyperlipidemia
    - Noncompliance
    - Intermenstrual bleeding
    - Mood changes
    - Depression
    - Pregnancy

Diagnostic Testing: Diagnostic Tests and Procedures to Consider

- Pap smear
- Urinalysis
- STI screening
- Screening tests according to age and health history
  - Lipid profile
    - Family history of CAD
    - Smoker on OC
  - Fasting blood sugar
  - TSH
  - Pregnancy testing

Providing Treatment: Therapeutic Measures to Consider

- Progestin only pills (POP)
  - Micronor
  - Nor-QD
  - Ovrette
  - Must take same time each day
  - Breakthrough bleeding common
  - Reduced effectiveness with
    - TB medications

- Anticonvulsants
- Barbiturates
- Combination OCs
  - May decrease breast milk production
  - Very low dose birth control pills
    - Alesse
    - Levlite
    - Lo-Estrin 1/20
    - Nordette
    - Contain both estrogen and progestin
    - May have improved side effect profile than regular dose OC
  - Low-dose birth control pills
    - Tri-Levelen
    - Demulen
    - Jenest
    - Necon
    - Slightly higher dose
    - Often less menstrual irregularity
    - May have increased side effects
  - 90-day pills (Seasonale)
    - Monophasic OC
    - Take for 84 days continuously
    - Initial high rate of BTB
    - Take for 4 periods/year
  - Recommended OC use
    - Lowest effective dose
    - Higher doses available for specific indications
- Transdermal patch: Ortho Evra
  - Combination patch
  - Effectiveness approx 99%
  - Decreased effectiveness in women > 198 lbs.
- NuvaRing Contraceptive Vaginal Ring
  - Combination ring
  - Lower dose of medication is needed

- ○ Effectiveness approx 98–99%
- Injectable contraceptives
  - ○ Progesterone only
    - ▪ Amenorrhea common
    - ▪ May be delay in return to fertility
    - ▪ May contribute to osteoporosis
  - ○ Initial injection must be given *only*
    - ▪ Within first 5 days of normal menses
    - ▪ Within first 5 days postpartum if not breast-feeding
    - ▪ At 4–6 weeks postpartum if breast-feeding
  - ○ Lunelle
    - ▪ 0.5 mg IM
    - ▪ Repeat q 28–30 days
  - ○ Depo-Provera
    - ▪ 150 mg IM
    - ▪ Repeat q 12–13 weeks
- Hormonal IUD (see Intrauterine Device)
  - ○ Insert per manufacturer's recommendations
  - ○ Lighter menses common

Providing Treatment: Alternative Measures to Consider

- Fertility awareness
- Outercourse
- Abstinence
- Withdrawal
- Natural spermicides

Providing Support: Education and Support Measures to Consider

- Information and instruction
  - ○ Use of hormonal contraceptives
  - ○ Effectiveness
  - ○ Side effects

- ○ Warning signs
- ○ Return schedule
- Pills
  - ○ Barrier or alternate method recommended x 2–3 weeks of first cycle
  - ○ Condoms recommended to protect against STIs
  - ○ Breakthrough bleeding is common in first cycles
  - ○ Take pill daily at same time
  - ○ Take pills ASAP if forgotten
  - ○ Use backup method if more than two pills are missed
- Patches
  - ○ Applied every 7 days x 3 weeks
  - ○ Apply to clean, dry skin of the
    - ▪ Buttocks
    - ▪ Upper outer arm
    - ▪ Lower abdomen
    - ▪ Upper torso
  - ○ 1 week off patch
  - ○ Use additional method or abstinence during first week of use
  - ○ Replace if full or partial detachment occurs
  - ○ Side effects same as with OC
- Ring
  - ○ Insert into vagina
    - ▪ Leave in place for 3 weeks
    - ▪ No ring for 1 week
  - ○ Side effects same as OC
- All methods: Call if the following occur
  - ○ Amenorrhea
  - ○ Persistent intermenstrual bleeding
  - ○ Chest pain or shortness of breath
  - ○ Numbness or tingling of arms or legs
  - ○ Severe headaches

- Depression
- Visual disturbances

- Potential health benefits
  - Regulation of menses
  - Decreased cramping and flow
  - Protection against uterine and ovarian cancer
  - Decreased risk of bone loss
  - Decrease in risk of pelvic infections
- Potential risks
  - Nausea
  - Irregular menses
  - Pregnancy
  - Stroke
  - Osteoporosis

Follow-up Care:
Follow-up Measures to Consider

- Document
- Return for care
  - Evaluation of contraceptive use
    - BP and weight
    - Review of correct hormone use
    - Satisfaction with method
  - Injectable contraceptive administration
  - Questions or concerns
  - Side effects or warning signs
  - Well-woman care

Collaborative Practice:
Criteria to Consider for Consultation or Referral

- OB/GYN service
  - Clients with relative contraindications to hormonal contraceptives who wish to try this method
  - Development of complication(s) of hormonal contraceptive use

- For diagnosis or treatment outside the midwife's scope of practice

The Intrauterine Device
Key Clinical Information

The IUD is a highly effective reversible method of birth control that may be hormonal or nonhormonal. The Para-Guard IUD is impregnated with copper, and is effective for 10 years. The hormonal IUDs include the Mirena which releases the progestin levonorgestrel and is effective for 5 years, and the Progestasert, which releases progesterone and is effective for 1 year (Advocates for Youth, n.d.). Like any method of birth control, careful evaluation to determine who is an appropriate candidate for this method is essential. Benefits of IUD use include its effectiveness (99+%), and ease of use. The common IUD side effect of heavy bleeding has been minimized by the Mirena; the progestin thins the lining of the uterus, and menses tend to be light. Risks include uterine perforation, pelvic infection, ectopic pregnancy, and expulsion (Varney et al., 2004).

Client History:
Components of the History to Consider

- Age
- G, P
- Allergies
- Medications
- Medical/surgical history
- Verify
  - LMP or date of delivery
  - Contraceptive history and current use
  - Last Pap/GYN exam
    - Pap results
    - STI test results
  - No history of fibroids or unusual configuration of uterus

- The ideal history for IUD insertions includes
  - No history of PID
  - Mutually monogamous long-term relationship
  - One or more full-term pregnancies
  - Negative history of heavy menses
  - Negative history of severe dysmenorrhea
  - Comfortable with the thought of an IUD in her uterus
  - Does not want a pregnancy for 3–10 years
  - Is able to check for the IUD string
- Contraindications to IUD insertion (Varney et al., 2004)
  - Pregnancy
  - Abnormalities of the uterus
  - PID past or present
  - Uterine or cervical malignancy
  - Copper allergy or Wilson's disease (copper IUD)
  - Previous ectopic pregnancy
  - Valvular heart disease
  - Unresolved abnormal Pap or cervical cancer
  - Decreased immune response
  - Acute liver disease (hormonal IUD)
  - Current DVT (hormonal IUD)
- Prior to removal determine
  - Indication for removal
  - Birth control method desired, if any

Physical Examination:
Components of the Physical Exam to Consider

- Physical exam as indicated by client history
- Prior to insertion
  - Obtain Pap smear and STI testing prn
    - Obtain results prior to IUD insertion
  - Bimanual exam to determine

- Uterine size and contour
- Uterine position
- Involution if postpartum
  - Speculum exam
    - Sound uterus (6–9 cm is recommended)
- Prior to removal
  - Speculum exam for visualization of strings
  - Based on indication for removal

Clinical Impression:
Differential Diagnoses to Consider

- Contraceptive management
  - IUD insertion
  - IUD removal
- Complications of IUD insertion/use
  - Vasovagal syncope
  - Perforation of the uterus
  - Expelled IUD
  - Lost IUD
  - Intermenstrual bleeding
  - Pregnancy with IUD in situ

Diagnostic Testing:
Diagnostic Tests and Procedures to Consider

- Pap smear
- Chlamydia and gonorrhea testing
- Hepatitis profile
- HIV testing
- Other labs as indicated by health status

Providing Treatment:
Therapeutic Measures to Consider

- Ibuprofen or naproxen 1 hour before procedure
- Have atropine sulfate available for vagal response

- May give IM when IV route not available
- 0.4–0.5 mg IM for bradycardia (Varney et al., 2004)

- Antibiotic prophylaxis not indicated (ACOG, 2001a)
- Procedure for insertion
  - Read manufacturer's instructions
  - Obtain informed consent (see Client Education)
- Timing of insertion
  - 4–8 weeks postpartum
  - During menses
  - As emergency contraception
  - Any time, as long as pregnancy is ruled out
- Use sterile technique
- Swab cervix with antiseptic solution (e.g., betadine prep)
- Position tenaculum gently
  - Close slowly to decrease cramping
  - Position on anterior lip for anteverted cervix
  - Position on posterior lip for retroverted uterus
  - Avoid vessels at 3 and 9 o'clock positions (Varney et al., 2004)
- Sound uterus prior to insertion
  - Apply traction to tenaculum
  - Gently insert sterile sound until slight resistance is felt
  - Do not use force
  - Note depth of sound
  - Use sound to prepare IUD insertion device for correct uterine size
- Load IUD into insertion device using sterile technique
- Use traction on tenaculum to straighten uterine curvature

- Gently insert IUD according to manufacturer's instructions
- Remove insertion device
- Remove tenaculum
- Obtain hemostasis
  - Apply pressure to bleeding sites
  - Apply silver nitrate to bleeding sites (may cause cramping)
- Trim strings to approximately 1.5–2 inches in length
- Observe for vagal response prior to discharge
  - Trendelenburg's position
  - Smelling salts
  - Atropine sulfate 0.4–0.5 mg IM (Varney et al., 2004)
- Procedure for removal
  - Grasp strings and pull gently but firmly
  - If strings not visible at os
    - Palpate cervical canal with sterile forceps
    - Grasp string or IUD if felt and pull gently
  - If unable to palpate IUD
    - Evaluate for presence of IUD with ultrasound
    - Removal under anesthesia may be required

Providing Treatment: Alternative Measures to Consider

- Fertility awareness
- Abstinence
- Withdrawal
- Natural spermicides

Providing Support: Education and Support Measures to Consider

- Review history with client, and spouse if needed

- Review all birth control options appropriate for this woman
- Discuss risks, benefits, effectiveness of IUD
- Provide information about
  - Preprocedure preparation
  - IUD cost
  - Details of insertion procedure
  - Potential side effects
    - Signs and symptoms
    - When to call
  - How to call during off hours
- Teach client to feel strings
  - After insertion
  - Before intercourse for first cycle
  - After menses or monthly

Follow-up Care:
Follow-up Measures to Consider

- Document (see Procedure Note)
- Return for care
  - 2–6 weeks postinsertion or after next menses
  - With onset of
    - Fever, pain, or heavy bleeding
    - Pregnancy
    - Missing strings
  - For planned return to fertility
  - For schedule replacement
    - 1 year for Progestasert
    - 5 year for Mirena
    - 10 year for Para-Guard

Collaborative Practice:
Criteria to Consider for Consultation or Referral

- OB/GYN service
  - Relative contraindications for IUD insertion

- Uterine anomalies
- History of postpartum endometritis or PID in past 3 months
  - Client desire for paracervical block for insertion
  - For complications of IUD insertion
    - Difficulty sounding uterus
    - Perforation of uterus
  - Complications of IUD use
    - IUD string not visible or palpated and removal is desired
    - Pregnancy with IUD in situ
    - PID with IUD in situ
  - For diagnosis or treatment outside the midwife's scope of practice

Norplant Contraceptive Implant

Key Clinical Information

The Norplant System is a subdermal contraceptive implant that consists of six Silastic capsules filled with a time release form of levonorgestrel. The Norplant System is not currently being marketed in the United States due to difficulty with consistency in hormonal release. However, there still may be numerous women with the system in place, and the system is still approved by the FDA. Another implant, Jadelle, consists of two capsules and is available to women in other countries.

Client History:
Components of the History to Consider

- Allergies
- Medications
- G, P, LMP
- Date of insertion of Norplant
- Symptoms
  - Pregnancy

- ○ Complications of Norplant
- Contraindications for Norplant use (Wyeth, 2003)
  - ○ Pregnancy
  - ○ Active thrombophlebitis or thromboembolitic disease
  - ○ Undiagnosed genital bleeding
  - ○ Acute liver disease
  - ○ Benign or malignant liver tumors
  - ○ Known or suspected breast cancer
- Assess client desire for birth control

Physical Examination:
Components of the Physical Exam to Consider

- Palpation of Norplant insertion site
  - ○ Depth and spacing of capsules
  - ○ Scar tissue
  - ○ Evaluation for removal technique
- Palpation of liver margins

Clinical Impression:
Differential Diagnoses to Consider

- Contraceptive management
  - ○ Contraceptive implant removal
- Complications of contraceptive implants
  - ○ Unplanned pregnancy
  - ○ Infection at insertion site
  - ○ Intermenstrual bleeding
  - ○ Headaches
  - ○ Unacceptable weight gain
  - ○ Difficult removal

Diagnostic Testing:
Diagnostic Tests and Procedures to Consider

- Testing as indicated by history and physical

Providing Treatment:
Therapeutic Measures to Consider

- Ibuprofen 800 mg
  - ○ Take 1–2 hours prior to procedure
  - ○ Use tid x 2 days for pain
- Have atropine sulfate available
  - ○ Use for vagal response, bradycardia
  - ○ 0.4–0.5 mg IM
- Obtain informed consent
- Use sterile technique
- Prep removal site
- Provide local anesthesia using 1–2% lidocaine with epinephrine
  - ○ Consider buffering lidocaine with 7.5% sodium bicarbonate to reduce stinging (Family Practice Notebook, 2000)
  - ○ 10:1 lidocaine:bicarb
  - ○ Mix well before injecting
- Removal techniques vary
  - ○ May need larger incision than for insertion
  - ○ Capsules will be covered by fibrous sheath
  - ○ Allow 30+ minutes for removal
- One removal technique
  - ○ Make 2 cm incision over capsules
  - ○ Palpate capsule
    - Using digital pressure, push capsule toward wound
  - ○ Grasp capsule with fine-tipped clamp
    - Pull end of capsule into wound
    - Abrade fibrous sheath from capsule end
  - ○ Grasp exposed capsule with second clamp
    - Release first clamp
    - Pull capsule from wound
  - ○ Repeat for additional capsules
- May need return visit for removal of all capsules

- Close incision
  - 4-0 vicryl or nylon skin suture
  - Steri-strips
- Apply sterile dressing
- Wrap site with pressure dressing

Providing Treatment:
Alternative Measures to Consider

- Norplant may be left in place provided there are no contraindications present

Providing Support:
Education and Support Measures to Consider

- Counseling regarding removal
  - More complex procedure for removal
  - May leave in situ indefinitely
  - Bruising and tenderness at site
- Postremoval care
  - Intermittent ice x 24 hours
  - Elevate x 24 hours
  - Keep dry x 3 days
  - Call with symptoms of infection
- Provide information regarding birth control options

Follow-up Care:
Follow-up Measures to Consider

- Document (see Procedure Note)
- Ice and elevate x 2 hours to decrease bruising
- Return to for care
  - 1–2 weeks for
    - Removal site check
    - Stitch removal
  - For signs and symptoms of infection
  - Well-woman care, prn

Collaborative Practice:
Criteria to Consider for Consultation or Referral

- OB/GYN service
  - Difficult removal
  - For diagnosis or treatment outside the midwife's scope of practice

Unplanned Pregnancy

Key Clinical Information

Unplanned or unwanted pregnancies result from sexual assault, birth control failures, or limited foresight stemming from a multitude of factors. Many women, with support, opt to continue their pregnancy. They may care for the infant or relinquish the baby for adoption after birth. Other women opt for early termination of the pregnancy. Women often have long-term emotional consequences related to the decision to continue or terminate a pregnancy. The role of the midwife is to provide sound information and supportive, nonjudgmental care so that each woman can make an informed personal decision when confronted with this difficult situation.

Adoptions may range from traditional "closed record" adoptions, where the baby is typically whisked away immediately after birth, to "open adoption" where the birth mother may meet prospective parent(s) to determine if she deems them suitable as parent(s) for her child. During open adoptions the adoptive parents may be present for the birth, or may receive the infant shortly after birth. A postadoption waiting period is common to allow the birth mother an opportunity to review her choice before it becomes legally binding.

Medical or surgical termination of pregnancy offers women another option for the unplanned pregnancy, or one in which there are significant fetal anomalies. Medical abortion is successful approximately 95–99% of the time when initiated *before* 8 weeks gestation. When pregnancy is complicated or beyond 8 weeks gestation, surgical abortion is more effective.

Client History:
Components of the History to Consider

- Age
- Obstetric history
  - G, P
  - Current pregnancy
    - LMP, cycle history
    - Date of conception, if known
    - Current or prior method of birth control
    - Date of pregnancy test
    - Signs and symptoms of pregnancy
    - Dating ultrasound results
    - Alpha fetal protein or triple screen results
    - Amniocentesis or level II ultrasound results
    - Blood type and Rh factor if known
- GYN History
  - Last pap and exam
  - STI screening and results
- Medical/surgical history
  - Allergies
  - History of genetic disorders
  - Medical conditions
  - Prior surgery
- Social issues
  - Feelings about pregnancy
  - Personal support systems
  - Financial concerns regarding pregnancy options
  - 🌀 Cultural considerations affecting decision
  - Other social issues
    - Drug, alcohol, and tobacco use
    - Domestic violence

- Mental health concerns
- Contraindications to medical abortion (Varney et al., 2004)
  - Abnormal pelvic exam, potential for ectopic pregnancy
  - IUD in situ
  - Potential for noncompliance with required follow-up
  - Presence of significant medical problems
    - Cardiopulmonary
    - Endocrine
    - Hepatic
    - Hematologic
  - Refusal to follow-up with definitive surgical treatment if medical treatment fails
- Assess resources for emotional support

Physical Examination:
Components of the Physical Exam to Consider

- Vital signs
- Pelvic exam for sizing of pregnancy

Clinical Impression:
Differential Diagnoses to Consider

- Unplanned pregnancy
  - Adoption planned
  - For medical abortion
  - For surgical abortion, first trimester
  - For surgical abortion, second trimester
- Pregnancy, complicated by
  - Fetal anomalies
  - Abnormal genetic testing

Diagnostic Testing:
Diagnostic Tests and Procedures to Consider

- Blood type, Rh, and antibody screen

- Serum or urine HCG
- CBC, or H & H
- Pelvic ultrasound
  - Vaginal or abdominal
  - Rule out ectopic pregnancy
  - Estimate gestational age

Providing Treatment: Therapeutic Measures to Consider

- Medical abortion (Mackenzie & Yeo, 1997)
  - Verify surgical coverage
    - Client preferences
    - Retained products of conception
- Obtain informed consent
- Mifepristone (Mifeprex)
  - Dose: 600 mg po in presence of provider
  - Observation x 30 minutes
  - Provide for pain relief
    - Acetaminophen
    - Acetaminophen with codeine
    - NSAIDS
      - Compatible with mifepristone
      - Provide significant pain relief
  - Return visit scheduled for 36–48 hours
    - 40 mg misoprostol po
    - Observe for +/- 4 hours (expulsion of products of conception occurs during this time in 60% of clients)
  - Rh immune globulin 1 dose (full or mini) for Rh negative women post-abortion

Providing Treatment: Alternative Measures to Consider

- Herbal remedied to foster interruption of pregnancy (see Emergency Contraception)

- Remedies to support the reproductive system during medical or surgical abortion
  - Herbals
    - Red raspberry leaf
    - Dong quai
    - Vitex
    - Lemon balm
    - Alfalfa leaf
    - Nettle leaf (Soule, 1996)
  - Homeopathic
    - Arnica
    - Sabina
    - Pulsatilla (Smith, 1984)
    - Rescue Remedy

Providing Support: Education and Support Measures to Consider

- Provide factual, unbiased information during options counseling
- Available options may be based upon
  - Age of client
  - Availability of services
  - Philosophy of care
  - Gestational age of pregnancy
  - Maternal medical factors
  - Financial considerations
- Potential options
  - Adoption outside the family
  - Adoption within the family
  - Keeping and caring for the baby
  - Voluntary termination of pregnancy
    - Medical
    - Surgical
- Clear information should be provided regarding
  - All available services
  - The termination procedure(s)

- Medical
  - Avoids invasive procedure
  - No anesthesia
  - High success rate (≥ 95%)
  - Requires careful follow-up
  - May take up to 14 days to complete
  - Requires client participation
- Surgical
  - Invasive procedure
  - Sedation or anesthesia
  - One visit
  - High success rate (99%)
  - May not require follow-up
  - Coverage options should surgical services be required or desired
- Potential side effects of medical abortion
  - Nausea and vomiting
  - Diarrhea
  - Malaise
  - Necessary follow-up for medical abortion
    - 36–48 hours, and
    - 7–10 days
- Warning signs and symptoms post-procedure
  - Saturating sanitary pads in 30 minutes x 4
  - Heavy flow x 24 hours
  - Severe pain
  - Fever and chills lasting > 24 hours

Follow-up Care:
Follow-up Measures to Consider

- Following options counseling
  - Schedule prenatal care at client preference
  - Schedule termination following verification of dates
- Medical abortion
  - Return visit at 36–48 hours

- Provide misoprostol
- Observe for passage of products of conception
- Send to pathology for verification of tissue
- Provide RhIG if indicated (Varney et al., 2004)
  - Sign or symptoms of
    - Complications
    - Incomplete abortion
  - Return for care 7–10 days
    - Check β-HCG levels
      - Should be 50% of previous levels
      - Should drop continuously
      - May take up to 90 days to return to nonpregnant range
  - Follow-up ultrasound prn
    - If no FHR, can wait up to 36 days post-mifepristone before surgical intervention is necessary
  - Surgical interruption scheduled if full POC not passed by 2 weeks after initial dose
- For post-termination exam 2–4 weeks
    - Pelvic exam to verify complete abortion
    - Post-abortion counseling
    - Contraceptive management

Collaborative Practice:
Criteria to Consider for Consultation or Referral

- OB/GYN or women's health service
  - If midwife cannot provide objective care based on client preference for termination
  - For genetic counseling if anomaly or genetic disorder noted in fetus
  - To obtain surgical coverage for clients undergoing medical abortion when service is provided by the midwife
- Social service
  - Parenting resources

- ○ Adoption resources
- Mental health services
  - ○ Support groups
- For diagnosis or treatment outside the midwife's scope of practice

Caring for Women as They Age

The changes that occur as women age cannot be quantified simply by where she is on the chart of reproductive-life stages, but must include a broad view of how she sees herself and how the challenges of aging affect her. Many midwives provide comprehensive woman-centered care across the life span. Caring for women as they age requires a broad knowledge of the changes that occur and the ability to listen to women as they explore the many possibilities available to them through traditional and alternative health care.

During this time of transition women may have families that range from young children to adult children, grandchildren, and may include aging parents. The dream of retirement or financial security may be receding with the demands of providing care for aged parents or a diminished ability to work. Health problems may become more prevalent and use up a significant proportion of energy that was previously directed to home, family, or livelihood.

The hormonal changes that occur with aging may impact a woman's emotional responses to her life situation, her ability to rest well or sleep, her strength and stamina, and her self-image. Compassionate midwifery care offers women an opportunity to create a new view of themselves and the aging process, and provides a gateway to necessary services when problems develop.

Perimenopause

Key Clinical Information

Evaluation of the woman who stands on the threshold of menopause offers an opportunity to assess health attitudes and practices, while screening for common health problems that may occur following the change of life. This time of transition may last 1 day, the day when it has been 12 months since the last menstrual period, or it may last several years during which there are multiple signs and symptoms signaling the impending change. Each woman responds differently to the precursors of menopause—one may sigh with relief that her time of menstruation is nearly done, while another may be dismayed by the passing of her fertility.

Client History: Components of the History to Consider

- Age
- Reproductive and sexual history
  - ○ G, P
  - ○ Pap history
  - ○ STIs
  - ○ Presence or absence of cervix, uterus, ovaries
  - ○ Menstrual status
    - Frequency, duration, flow
    - Changes in menses
      - Pattern of bleeding
      - Intermenstrual bleeding
      - Prolonged
      - Excessive or scanty flow
  - ○ Vasomotor symptoms
    - Hot flashes
    - Night sweats
    - Flushing
  - ○ Urogenital symptoms
    - Vaginal dryness
    - Urinary symptoms
    - Decreased libido
  - ○ Other symptoms
    - Insomnia or sleep pattern changes
    - Emotional changes

- Lability
- Depression
- Diminished coping ability
  ○ Sexual activity and practices
- Medical/surgical history
  ○ Allergies
  ○ Medications
  ○ Chronic illnesses
  ○ Surgeries
- Family History
  ○ Osteoporosis
  ○ Female reproductive cancers
  ○ Colon or GI malignancy
  ○ Heart disease
  ○ Diabetes
- Social history
  ○ Drug/ETOC and tobacco use
  ○ Family support systems
  ○ Social activities
  ○ Ability to care for self
    ▪ Food, shelter
    ▪ Activities of daily living
    ▪ Ability to seek assistance prn
- Physical activity
- Nutritional assessment
- Review of systems
  ○ Integumentary
    ▪ Skin changes
    ▪ Lesions
  ○ HEENT
    ▪ Hearing loss
    ▪ Visual changes
  ○ Cardiopulmonary
    ▪ SOB
    ▪ Palpitations
    ▪ Edema
  ○ Gastrointestinal
    ▪ Bowel changes
    ▪ Rectal bleeding
  ○ Genitourinary
    ▪ Urinary frequency
    ▪ Dysparunia
  ○ Endocrine
    ▪ Fatigue
    ▪ Intolerance to cold/heat
  ○ Neurologic
    ▪ Confusion
    ▪ Headaches
  ○ Musculoskeletal
    ▪ Pain
    ▪ Range of motion

Physical Examination: Components of the Physical Exam to Consider

- Vital signs, including BP
- Height, weight
  ○ BMI
  ○ Changes in height or weight
- HEENT
  ○ Skin turgor
  ○ Hearing
  ○ Vision
  ○ Thyroid
- Back
  ○ CVA tenderness
  ○ Evaluate for kyphosis
  ○ Respiratory exam
  ○ Cardiac exam
    ▪ Rate and rhythm
    ▪ Murmurs

- Pulses
- Peripheral edema
- Breast exam
  - Masses
  - Discharge
  - Axilla
- Abdomen
  - Bowel sounds
  - Liver margins
- Extremities
  - Edema
  - Varicosities
  - Range of motion
- Genital exam
  - Genital atrophy
  - Lesions
  - Pap
  - Bimanual exam
    - Uterine
      - Size
      - Consistency
      - Contour
      - Mobility
    - Adnexa
      - Size
      - Consistency
      - Mobility
  - Rectal exam
    - Palpate for lesions/masses
    - Stool for occult bleeding

Clinical Impression:
Differential Diagnoses to Consider

- Well-woman exam
  - Perimenopausal

- Postmenopausal woman
- Risk factors or presence of conditions
  - Osteoporosis
  - Heart disease
  - Diabetes
  - Hypothyroid
  - Elevated BMI
  - Mood disorder
  - Colon cancer

Diagnostic Testing:
Diagnostic Tests and Procedures to Consider (ACOG, 1995)

- Pap smear
- Endometrial biopsy
- Mammogram
- Thyroid testing
- Liver function tests
- Fasting blood sugar
- Bone density testing
- Lipid profile or cholesterol
- ECG
- Stool for occult blood
- Colonoscopy
- TB testing

Providing Treatment:
Therapeutic Measures to Consider

- Immunization update
  - Tetanus-diphtheria
  - Influenza
  - Pneumococcal
- Birth control
- Hormone therapy (see Hormone Therapy)
  - Estrogen replacement therapy

- ◦ Combination hormone replacement therapy
- ◦ Estrogen/androgen therapy
- Treatment for medical conditions
  - ◦ Hypertension
  - ◦ Diabetes
  - ◦ Hypothyroid

Providing Treatment:
Alternative Measures to Consider

- Dietary changes
  - ◦ Decrease fat, caffeine, sugar, alcohol
  - ◦ Increase soy, whole grains, dietary fiber
  - ◦ Vitamin E, vitamin D, calcium, and magnesium
- Maintain regular weight-bearing exercise
  - ◦ Walking, jogging
  - ◦ Weight training
  - ◦ Aerobics
- Nonweight bearing exercise for joint mobility
- Sleep aids
  - ◦ Valarian root
  - ◦ Chamomile
  - ◦ Melatonin
- Utilize creative outlets
  - ◦ Journal writing
  - ◦ Dance, meditation, or singing
  - ◦ Prayer
- Community involvement, groups
  - ◦ Schools, childcare
  - ◦ Church
  - ◦ Libraries
  - ◦ Nature preserves
  - ◦ Homeless shelters
  - ◦ Soup kitchens
  - ◦ Nonprofit organizations
- Sexual comfort

- ◦ Vaginal lubricants
- ◦ Alternative sexual practices

Providing Support:
Education and Support Measures to Consider

- Review signs and symptoms of
  - ◦ Perimenopausal period
  - ◦ Thyroid dysfunction
  - ◦ Diabetes
- Screening recommendations
  - ◦ Benefits and drawbacks to testing
  - ◦ Prep for testing, prn
  - ◦ Interpretation of test results
- Discuss medical therapies for symptoms
  - ◦ Risks
  - ◦ Benefits
  - ◦ Alternatives
- Discuss alternative therapies for symptoms
  - ◦ Risks
    - ▪ May stimulate similar to estrogens
    - ▪ Difficult to quantify dose
  - ◦ Benefits
    - ▪ Natural
    - ▪ Client regulated
    - ▪ May relieve symptoms
  - ◦ Options
    - ▪ Soy
    - ▪ Plant estrogens
- Encourage regular physical activity
- Teach warning signs of female reproductive cancers
  - ◦ Bleeding
    - ▪ Irregular
    - ▪ Postmenopausal
  - ◦ Pain
  - ◦ Masses

○ Lesions

Follow-up Care:
Follow-up Measures to Consider

- Document
- Return for continued care
  ○ Annually
  ○ As indicated by test results
  ○ With onset of problem or symptoms

Collaborative Practice:
Criteria to Consider for Consultation or Referral

- OB/GYN service
  ○ For abnormal reproductive findings or test results
- Medical service
  ○ For continued care of medical problems
- Support services
  ○ Smoking cessation
  ○ Drug or alcohol rehab
  ○ Support groups
    - Diabetes
    - Domestic violence
    - Hypertension
    - Substance abuse
- For diagnosis or treatment outside the midwife's scope of practice

Hormone Replacement Therapy

Key Clinical Information

Hormone replacement therapy (HRT), like many other treatments, is a double-edged sword. It offers significant benefits to a carefully selected group of women, while for other women it holds significant risks. One major criticism of HRT is the way it was previously "mandated" for every woman after menopause as if it were the panacea for all the ills of women as they age. Obviously, no therapy should be used globally without evaluating the risks and benefits for the individual and offering information so that the client herself can be an active participant in her care. HRT may offer profound relief of vasomotor symptoms for women with severe effects of hormone depletion at menopause or during the perimenopausal period.

Unopposed estrogen (ERT) has been demonstrated to increase the risk of endometrial cancer for women with an intact uterus when compared to women who used estrogen in combination therapy or women who declined ERT. All women who have a uterus and use supplemental estrogen from *any* source should have it balanced with progesterone. Women who use long term HRT have a slight increase in their risk of heart disease and breast cancer over women who decline HRT. In women with severe symptoms and who are planning short-term therapy (< 5 yrs) to help them through menopause, this risk is considered low when there is no other significant risk of breast cancer or heart disease.

Client History:
Components of the History to Consider

- Age
- Reproductive history
  ○ LMP or age at
    - Menopause
    - Hysterectomy
- Current pattern of bleeding
  ○ Frequency
  ○ Duration
  ○ Amount of flow
- Presence or absence of vasomotor symptoms
  ○ Hot flashes
  ○ Night sweats

- ○ Vaginal atrophy and dryness
- Symptoms related to estrogen decline
  - ○ Urinary problems
  - ○ Mood disturbance
  - ○ Facial hair increase
- Reproductive cancers and disorders (e.g., leiomyomata)
- Most recent
  - ○ Exam
  - ○ Pap
  - ○ Mammogram
  - ○ Bone density testing
- Medical/surgical history
  - ○ Allergies
  - ○ Medications
  - ○ Heart disease
    - ■ Coronary artery disease
    - ■ Hypertension
  - ○ Hx of thromboembolus or thrombosis
  - ○ Risk factors for osteoporosis
    - ■ Recent fractures
    - ■ History of anorexia nervosa
    - ■ Long-term Depo-Provera use (especially immediately prior to menopause)
  - ○ Depression
  - ○ Gallbladder disease
  - ○ Liver disease
- Family history
  - ○ Osteoporosis
  - ○ Heart disease
  - ○ Alzheimer's disease
  - ○ Colon cancer
  - ○ Breast cancer
- Social history
  - ○ Tobacco and alcohol use

- ○ Physical activity patterns
- ○ Nutritional status
- ○ Domestic violence or abuse
- Contraindications for HRT
  - ○ History of estrogen sensitive tumors
    - ■ Breast cancer
    - ■ Endometrial hyperplasia
    - ■ Endometrial cancer
  - ○ Undiagnosed postmenopausal bleeding
  - ○ Impaired liver function
  - ○ Hx of thromboembolus or thrombosis
  - ○ Heart disease
- Review of systems (ROS)

Physical Examination: Components of the Physical Exam to Consider

- Vital signs, BP
- BMI
- Height, compare to previous
- Thyroid
  - ○ Palpation
  - ○ Size, contour
- Breast exam
  - ○ Presence of masses
  - ○ Documentation of contour
- Cardiopulmonary evaluation
- Pelvic exam
  - ○ Atrophy, pallor
  - ○ Presence of masses
- Bony integrity
  - ○ Range of motion
  - ○ Arthritis
  - ○ Kyphosis
- Rectal exam

Clinical Impression:
Differential Diagnoses to Consider

- HRT for the following indication(s)

  ○ Severe vasomotor symptoms

  ○ Osteoporosis (consider nonhormonal therapies first)

  ○ ASC-US Pap smear (local therapy preferred)

  ○ Mood disturbance related to hormone changes (consider other medications first)

- Contraindication to HRT in client with symptoms

Diagnostic Testing:
Diagnostic Tests and Procedures to Consider

- Pap smear

- Endometrial biopsy

- FSH/LH

- Blood lipid evaluation

- ECG

- Bone mineral density testing

- Mammogram

- Pelvic ultrasound

- Postmenopausal woman

  ○ Prior to initiation of HRT consider

    ▪ Endometrial biopsy

    ▪ Progestin challenge

      • Provera 5–10 mg daily x 10 days

      • Anticipate withdrawal bleed within 10 days of completion of medication

      • If little or no bleed consider continuous HRT therapy

      • If vigorous bleed consider cyclic HRT

Providing Treatment:
Therapeutic Measures to Consider

- Perimenopausal woman with moderate to severe vasomotor symptoms

  ○ Combination hormonal contraceptives

    ▪ 💣 Do not use in smokers > 35

  ○ Transdermal estrogen

    ▪ Estraderm 0.5 mg or 1.0 mg

    ▪ Progestin not required with regular monthly menses

    ▪ Add progestin when menses irregular

      • Provera 5–10 mg x 5–10 days

      • Prometrium 200 mg qhs x 12 days (Murphy, 2005)

- Postmenopausal woman

  ○ Continuous hormone replacement therapy (HRT)

  ○ Use for as brief a period as possible

  ○ Combination therapy

    ▪ CombiPatch (estradiol/norethindrone acetate transdermal system)

      • Apply patch at twice weekly interval

      • For more info: (877) 266-2448 or www.combipatch.com

    ▪ PremPro (oral conjugated estrogens/progestin)

- Use lowest effective dose

  ○ 0.3 mg/1.5 mg 1 po daily

  ○ 0.45 mg/1.5 mg 1 po daily

  ○ 0.625 mg /2.5 mg 1 po daily

  ○ 0.625/5 1 po daily

    ▪ Estrogen–daily

      • Conjugated estrogen 0.3-0.625 mg

      • Estropipate 0.625 mg

      • Esterified estrogen 0.3-0.625 mg

      • Micronized estradiol 0.5-1 mg

- Transdermal estrogen 0.05 mg
  - Progestin—daily
    - Provera 2.5 mg
- Cyclic hormone replacement therapy
  - Estrogen—days 1–25 of month or continuously
    - Dose range 0.3 mg–1.25 mg daily, varies with brand
    - 0.625 mg is lowest dose recommended to treat osteoporosis
    - Plant-based estrogens
      - Estrace
      - Cenestin
      - Gynodiol
      - EstraTab
      - Ogen
  - Progestin use with cyclic estrogen
    - Provera 5–10 mg x 5–10 days
    - Prometrium 200 mg qhs x 12 days
    - Use progestin days 11–25 to 16–25 of cycle month
- Estrogen–androgen therapy (Simon et al., 1999; Bachmann, 1993)
  - For decreased libido
  - Given cyclically (e.g., 3 weeks on, 1 week off)
  - Short-term therapy
  - Virilization may occur
  - Must use progestin in client with intact uterus
  - Products available
    - Esterified estrogen 0.625 mg/methyltesterone 1.25 mg
    - Esterified estrogen 1.25 mg/methyltesterone 2.5 mg
    - Conjugated estrogen 0.625 mg/methyltesterone 5 mg
    - Conjugated estrogen 1.25 mg/methyltesterone 10 mg

Providing Treatment: Alternative Measures to Consider

- See Vasomotor Symptoms
- Vitamin and mineral supplements
  - Calcium and magnesium supplementation
  - Vitamin E supplements 400 IU bid with meals

Providing Support: Education and Support Measures to Consider

- Provide information for informed choice
  - Indications for HRT
  - Limitations of HRT
  - Risks, benefits, and alternatives to HRT
  - Methods of HRT, dose, timing, side effects
  - Osteoporosis prevention and evaluation
- Provide medications instructions
  - Dose
  - Timing and method of use
  - Anticipated results
  - Warning signs and symptoms
- Reinforce need to return for evaluation for
  - Unscheduled vaginal bleeding
  - Symptoms of complications related to HRT
- Dietary recommendations
  - Limit caffeine, fat, white sugar, flour, and alcohol
  - Whole grains, dark leafy green vegetable, sea vegetables
  - Protein from legumes, nuts, and seeds
- Recommended lifestyle changes
  - Smoking cessation
  - Regular exercise, rest, and relaxation
  - Encourage participation in activities that support acceptance of the life changes

Follow-up Care:
Follow-up Measures to Consider

- Document
- Return for evaluation
  - Evaluate in 3 months after initiating HRT/ERT
    - Reduction in symptoms
    - Bleeding patterns
    - Satisfaction with treatment
    - Concerns or unexpected side effects
    - Weight, BP
  - Annually for well-woman exam
  - Unanticipated or unscheduled vaginal bleeding
  - Breast changes

Collaborative Practice:
Criteria to Consider for Consultation or Referral

- OB/GYN service
  - Symptoms that do not respond to standard HRT regimens
  - Unexplained or persistent vaginal bleeding
  - Breast mass or abnormal mammogram
  - Gynecological complications of HRT49p9
- Medical service
  - Diagnosis of osteoporosis (see Osteoporosis)
  - Signs or symptoms of heart disease
  - Medical complications of HRT
- For diagnosis or treatment outside the midwife's scope of practice

Screening for Osteoporosis
Key Clinical Information

Osteoporosis is defined as a disease that is characterized by a decrease in the level of bone mass itself, resulting in bones that are more porous. This leads to deterioration of the structural integrity of the remaining bone, and contributes to fragile bones that are more likely to fracture with minimal trauma. The diagnosis of osteoporosis and osteopenia (the onset of bone loss, but not yet to the degree that equals osteoporosis) are made using bone mineral density (BMD) evaluation. Osteoporosis is said to be present when the BMD is more than 2.5 standard deviations below the mean. Prevention measures include regular weight-bearing activities to both increase bone stress and maintain muscle mass to support the bone. Treatment is aimed at slowing the loss of bone and preferably building bone mass. Any woman with a history of a fracture after age 40 should consider BMD testing (WHO, 2003; ACOG, 2004).

Client History:
Components of the History to Consider

- Age
- Reproductive history
  - LMP, G, P
  - Age at menarche
  - Age at menopause
  - Length of time postmenopause
  - Use of hormonal
    - Contraceptives
    - Hormone replacement therapy
    - Herbs or plant extracts
  - Breastfeeding history
- Assess for risk factors for osteoporosis (Siris & Schussheim, 1998)
  - Small or thin frame or body size
  - Positive family history of osteoporosis
  - Prior fracture after minor trauma after age 40
  - Current history of cigarette smoking
  - Early/surgical menopause without estrogen replacement

- ○ Sedentary lifestyle
- ○ Low calcium intake
- ○ History of estrogen deficiency
  - ■ Surgical oopherectomy
  - ■ Premature menopause
  - ■ Endocrine disorders leading to amenorrhea
  - ■ Anorexia leading to amenorrhea
  - ■ Long-term breast-feeding
- ○ Long-term use of
  - ■ Corticosteroids ≥ 10 mg Prednisone/day
  - ■ Thyroxine ≥ 200 µg/day
  - ■ Heparin ≥ 12,000–15,000 U/day
  - ■ Alcohol (≥ 7 oz./week)
  - ■ Depo-Provera use during bone mass formation
- • Secondary causes of osteoporosis
  - ○ Cushing's disease
  - ○ Hyperthyroidism
  - ○ Hyperparathyroidism
  - ○ Diabetes
  - ○ Lymphoma
  - ○ Multiple myeloma
- • Assess for symptoms of osteoporosis
  - ○ Complaints of back pain
  - ○ Changes in posture/height
  - ○ Fractures after perimenopausal period
- • Current prevention measures
  - ○ Vitamin D intake/sun exposure
  - ○ Calcium intake
  - ○ Mineral supplementation
  - ○ Weight-bearing exercise
- • Health habits
  - ○ Daily physical activity
  - ○ Tobacco use
  - ○ Alcohol use

- ○ Safety measures to prevent falls

Physical Examination: Components of the Physical Exam to Consider

- • Vital signs
- • Height, compare to previous
- • Weight
- • Presence of kyphosis, "dowager's hump"
  - ○ Palpation of vertebrae for pain
- • Evidence of increased risk for falls
  - ○ Physical limitations
  - ○ Frailty
  - ○ Balance and coordination
  - ○ Eyesight
- • Other exam components as indicated by history

Clinical Impression: Differential Diagnoses to Consider

- • Osteopenia
- • Osteoporosis
- • At risk for fracture, secondary to
  - ○ Significant fall risk
  - ○ Calcium and vitamin D deficiency
  - ○ Diminished bone density

Diagnostic Testing: Diagnostic Tests and Procedures to Consider

- • Osteomark urine test
  - ○ Screens for bone collagen breakdown
  - ○ (800-99OSTEX)
- • Bone density testing
  - ○ Dual-energy X-ray absorptiometry (DXA)
  - ○ Low radiation dose
  - ○ T-score

- Bone mass in relation to young adult reference population
- T-score −1 = 1 SD decrease in bone mass
- > 1 SD = twofold risk in fracture
- T-score −2 = fourfold risk of fracture (ACOG, 2004; WHO, 2003)

Providing Treatment:
Therapeutic Measures to Consider

- For women with no contraindications to HRT
  - Single or combination hormone replacement therapy (see Hormone Replacement Therapy)
    - Short-term therapy (< 5 yrs)
    - Weigh risks vs. benefits
- Nonhormonal treatment (Murphy, 2004)
  - Raloxofene (Evista)
    - 60 mg po daily
  - Calcitonin-salmon (Miacalcin)
    - 200 units intranasally daily
  - Alendronate (Fosamax)
    - Must swallow whole
    - Not for use in clients with renal insufficiency
    - Osteopenia—5 mg po daily
    - Osteoporosis—10 mg po daily

Providing Treatment:
Alternative Measures to Consider

- Nutritional support
  - Calcium foods (see Calcium Foods List)
  - Vitamin and mineral supplements
    - Vitamin D 400-800 IU daily
    - Calcium 1000-1500 mg daily (ACOG, 2004)
- Weight-bearing exercise

- Sunlight exposure for vitamin D synthesis
  - Hands and face
  - 10 minutes daily

Providing Support:
Education and Support Measures to Consider

- Provide information regarding
  - Calcium sources and intake
  - Weight-bearing exercise
    - Walking
    - Weight training
    - Rowing
    - Sweeping, vacuuming
- Medication use
  - Side effects
  - Benefits
  - Risks (Ferris, 1998)
- Community preventive health programs
  - Smoking cessation
  - Alcoholics Anonymous
  - Exercise programs
- Encourage client to avoid or limit use of
  - Tobacco
  - Alcohol
  - Caffeine
  - Phosphorus-containing soft drinks

Follow-up Care:
Follow-up Measures to Consider

- Document
- Offer bone density testing at 1–2 year intervals
- Reevaluate behavioral modification for modifiable risk factors
  - Medication use
  - Smoking

- ○ Alcohol use
- ○ Physical activity patterns
- Review risk status annually with well-woman exam

Collaborative Practice:
Criteria to Consider for Consultation or Referral

- Physical therapy
  - ○ Assess for risk of falls
  - ○ Strengthening program
  - ○ Improve balance
  - ○ Ability to maintain activities of daily living
- OB/GYN or orthopedic service
  - ○ For initiation and management of treatment plan for diagnosis of osteoporosis
- For diagnosis or treatment outside the midwife's scope of practice

Evaluation and Treatment of Women with Perimenopausal Symptoms

Key Clinical Information

Many symptoms are common during both the perimenopausal period and early postmenopause. The symptoms result from a significant decline in estrogen and may considerably affect the quality of a woman's life. Many women believe that the changes that occur with menopause are natural and not a disease or illness that requires treatment with medication. For generations women have coped without hormone replacement therapy (HRT) and while some did very well, others suffered from severe symptoms. Women may opt to use, or decline, alternative therapies or HRT for treatment of menopausal symptoms after consideration of the associated risks, benefits, and costs (ACOG, 2001c).

Client History:
Components of the History to Consider

- Age

- Reproductive history
  - ○ G, P
  - ○ LMP or age at menopause
  - ○ Current menstrual status
  - ○ Sexual activity
  - ○ Sexual orientation
- Menopausal symptoms and perceived severity
  - ○ Vasomotor symptoms
    - Hot flashes or flushes
    - Night sweats
  - ○ Sleep disorders
    - Sleep habits
    - Insomnia
    - Wakefulness
    - Daytime sleepiness
  - ○ Urogenital symptoms
    - Vaginal atrophy and dryness
    - Urinary frequency or urgency
    - Dysparunia
    - Cervical changes
  - ○ Skin changes
    - Fine wrinkles
    - Increase in facial hair
  - ○ Decreased libido
  - ○ Mood disturbance and mental status changes
    - Mood swings
    - Depression
    - Irritability
    - Confusion
    - Memory loss (Varney et al., 2004)
- Effect of symptoms on
  - ○ Self-image
  - ○ Emotional well-being
  - ○ Relationships
  - ○ Stamina and physical well-being

- Medical/surgical history
  - Allergies
  - Medications
  - Conditions
    - Breast cancer
    - Gallbladder disease
    - Heart disease
    - Blood clots
    - Liver disease
    - Chronic illness
    - Depression
- Family history
  - Heart disease
  - Diabetes
  - Cancer
- Social history
  - ETOH/tobacco use
  - Coping ability
  - Domestic violence or abuse
  - Support systems
    - Partner
    - Friends
    - Social activities
  - Significant life stressors
  - Physical activity patterns
  - Diet assessment
- Review of systems (ROS)

Physical Examination:
Components of the Physical Exam to Consider

- Vital signs, BP
- Weight, height
- General physical exam with focus on
  - Thyroid palpation
  - Cardiopulmonary status

- Breast exam
- Pelvic exam
  - Observe for atrophy of tissues
    - Pale
    - Thin
    - Fragile
- Rectal exam

Clinical Impression:
Differential Diagnoses to Consider

- Symptoms related to menopause
  - Vasomotor
  - Affective
  - Physiologic
- Medical conditions with similar symptoms, such as
  - TB
  - Thyroid disorder
  - Adrenal disorder
  - Mood disorder
  - Sleep disorder

Diagnostic Testing:
Diagnostic Tests and Procedures to Consider

- Pap smear
- Endometrial biopsy
- FSH/LH
- Blood lipid evaluation
- Bone density testing
- Mammogram
- Pelvic ultrasound

Providing Treatment:
Therapeutic Measures to Consider

- Perimenopausal client

- Moderate to severe symptoms
  - Oral contraceptives
  - Transdermal estrogen
- Menopausal client
  - Consider HRT therapy (see Hormone Replacement Therapy)
- Abnormal Pap smear (ACUS)
  - Estrogen vaginal cream
- Antidepressants (see Mental Health)
- Sleep aids, short-term therapy
  - Use caution with
    - Depression suspected
    - ETOH use
    - Hepatic or renal disease
  - Reevaluate 2–3 weeks
  - Ambien 10 mg po hs
  - Dalmane 15–30 mg hs
  - Halcion 0.125–0.25 mg hs
  - Sonata 10 mg hs (Murphy, 2004)
- Vitamin and mineral supplements
  - Calcium 1200–1500 mg daily
  - Magnesium 400 mg daily
  - Vitamin E 400 IU bid with meals

Providing Treatment: Alternative Measures to Consider

- Natural hormones
  - Custom compounding of natural hormones
  - Professional compounding pharmacies
  - Hormone creams, absorbed via skin
- Nutritional support
  - Phytoestrogens may combat symptoms
    - May stimulate endometrial hyperplasia
    - Food sources include
      - Peanuts
      - Oats, corn

- Apples
- Soy (ACOG, 2001c)
- Flaxseed
  - Dietary recommendations
    - Whole grains
    - Dark leafy green vegetables
    - Sea vegetables
    - Protein from legumes, nuts, and seeds
    - Limited organic animal proteins and fats
- Vaginal dryness
  - Lubrication
    - Astroglide
    - Massage oil
    - Replens
- Mental acuity
  - Ginko biloba (Foster, 1996)
  - Puzzles, word games
  - Aerobic exercise
- Homeopathic and herbal remedies
  - Hot flashes
    - Belladonna
    - Lachesis
  - Herbal remedies (ACOG, 2001c)
    - St.-John's-wort (depression)
    - Black cohosh (vasomotor symptoms)
    - Soy and isoflavones (vasomotor symptoms)
    - Vitex or chasteberry (mood and headache)
  - Vaginal dryness
    - Bryonia
    - Natrum mur
- For additional herbal formulas see *The Roots of Healing* (Soule, 1996)
- Physical activity to release endorphins
  - Yoga

- ◦ Dance
- ◦ Aerobics

Providing Support:
Education and Support Measures to Consider

- Provide information about
  - ◦ Menopause and common symptoms
  - ◦ Recommendations for symptom relief
    - Skin care
    - Vaginal lubrication
    - Mental stimulation
  - ◦ Local support or women's groups
  - ◦ Other resources
- Informed choice regarding treatments
- Lifestyle recommendations
  - ◦ Regular daily exercise, rest, and relaxation
  - ◦ Limit intake of
    - Caffeine
    - Fat
    - Refined sugar and flour
    - Cigarettes and alcohol
    - Phosphorus-containing soft drinks
- Indications to return for evaluation
  - ◦ Unscheduled vaginal bleeding
  - ◦ Breast mass
  - ◦ Osteoporosis prevention and evaluation
  - ◦ Depression
  - ◦ Ineffective coping

Follow-up Care:
Follow-up Measures to Consider

- Document
- Return for continued care
  - ◦ As needed to provide ongoing support
  - ◦ Unscheduled vaginal bleeding for evaluation

- ◦ For worsening symptoms
  - Mood disorders
  - Mental status changes
  - Vasomotor symptoms
  - Physiologic symptoms
- ◦ For evaluation of treatment of side effects
- ◦ For annual evaluation

Collaborative Practice:
Criteria to Consider for Consultation or Referral

- OB/GYN service
  - ◦ Symptoms that do not respond, or worsen with
    - Alternative therapy
    - Standard HRT regimens
  - ◦ Unexplained or persistent vaginal bleeding
  - ◦ Breast mass
- Medical service
  - ◦ Osteoporosis
  - ◦ Abnormal liver or renal function test results
  - ◦ Symptoms of
    - Heart disease
    - Diabetes
- Mental health service
  - ◦ Depression
  - ◦ Psychosis
  - ◦ Ineffective coping
- Sleep specialist
  - ◦ Severe insomnia
- For diagnosis or treatment outside the midwife's scope of practice

References

American College of Obstetricians and Gynecologists [ACOG]. (1995). Health maintenance for peri-menopausal women. In *2002 compendium of selected publications* [Technical bulletin No. 210]. Washington, DC: Author.

ACOG. (2000). Use of hormonal contraception in women with co-existing medical conditions. In *2005 compendium of selected publications* [Practice Bulletin No. 18]. Washington, DC: Author.

ACOG. (2001a) Antibiotic prophylaxis for Gyn procedures. In *2005 compendium of selected publications* [Practice Bulletin No. 23]. Washington, DC: Author.

ACOG. (2001b). Emergency oral contraception. In *2005 compendium of selected publications* [Practice Bulletin No. 25]. Washington, DC: Author.

ACOG. (2001c). Use of botanicals for management of menopausal symptoms. In *2005 compendium of selected publications*. Washington, DC: Author.

ACOG. (2004). Osteoporosis. In *2005 compendium of selected publications* [Practice bulletin No. 50]. Washington, DC: Author.

Advocates for Youth. (n.d). Intrauterine device. Retrieved February 21, 2005, from http://www.advocatesfor youth.org/youth/health/contraceptives/iud.htm.

Bachmann, G. A. (1993). Estrogen-androgen therapy for sexual and emotional well-being. *The Female Patient, 18*, 15–24.

Centers for Disease Control and Protection [CDC]. (2002). *National Immunization Program.* Retrieved February 27, 2005, from http://www.cdc.gov/nip/recs/adult-schedule.htm.

deCosta, C. L., Younes, R. N., & Lorneco, M. T. (2002). Stopping smoking: A randomized double-blind study comparing nortriptyline to placebo. *Chest, 122*, 403–408.

Family Practice Notebook (2000). Xylocaine. Retrieved March 1, 2005 from http://www.fpnotebook.com/SUR84.htm.

Ferris, D., Brotzman, G., & Mayeaux, E. J. (1998). Improving compliance with estrogen therapy for osteoporosis. *The Female Patient, 23*(4), 29–45.

Foster, S. (1996). *Herbs for your health.* Loveland, CO: Interweave Press.

Hall, S. M., Humfleet, G. L., Rhus, V. I., Munoz, R. F., Hartz, D. T., & Maude-Griffin, R. (2002). Psychological intervention and antidepressant treatment in smoking cessation. *Archives General Psychiatry, 59*, 930–936.

Heatherton, T. F., Kozlowski, L. T., Frecker, R. C., & Fagerstrom, K.O. (1991). The Fagerstrom test for nicotine dependence: A revision of the Fagerstrom tolerance questionnaire. *British Journal of Addiction, 86*, 1119–1127.

Kass-Annese, B., & Danzer, H., (2003). *Natural birth control made simple.* Alameda, CA: Hunter House.

Mackenzie, S. J., & Yeo, S. (1997). Pregnancy interruption using Mifepristone (RU-487): A new choice for women in the USA. *Journal of Nurse-Midwifery, 42*, 86–98.

Murphy, J. L. (Ed.). (2004). *Nurse practitioner's prescribing reference.* New York: Prescribing Reference.

Program for Appropriate Technology in Health. (1997). *Emergency contraception: A resource manual for providers.* Seattle, WA: Author.

Rieder, J., & Coupey, S. M. (2000). Contraceptive compliance. *The Female Patient,* (Suppl.), 12–19.

Ringel, M. (1998). HRT: Is it for you? *The Female Patient, 11*(S), 13–17.

Scherger, J. E. (1993). *Preconception care: A neglected element of prenatal services. The Female Patient, 18*, 78–83.

Simon, J., Klaiber, E., Wiita, B., Bowen, A., Yang, H. M., (1999). Differential effects of estrogen-androgen and estrogen-only therapy on vasomotor symptoms, gonadotropin secretion, and endogenous androgen bioavailability in postmenopausal women. *Menopause, 6*, 138–146.

Singer, K. (2004). *The garden of fertility.* New York: Avery.

Siris, E. S., & Schussheim, D. H. (1998). Osteoporosis: Assessing your patient's risk. *Women's Health in Primary Care, 1*(1), 99–106.

Smith, T. (1984). *A woman's guide to homeopathic medicine.* New York: Thorsons.

Soule, D. (1996). *The roots of healing.* Secaucus, NJ: Citadel Press.

Sweet, B. R. (Ed.). (1999). *Mayes' midwifery* (12th ed.). London: Bailliere Tindall.

Trapani, F. J. (1984). *Contraception naturally.* Coopersburg, PA: CJ Frompovich.

Varney, H., Kriebs, J. M., & Gegor, C. L. (2004). *Varney's midwifery* (4th ed.). Sudbury, MA: Jones and Bartlett.

Weed, S. (1985). *Wise woman herbal for the childbearing year.* Woodstock, NY: Ashtree.

Weinstein, M. (1994). *Your fertility signals.* St. Louis, MO: Smooth Stone Press.

World Health Organization [WHO]. (2003). *Prevention and management of osteoporosis* [WHO Technical Report No. 921]. Geneva: Author.

Wyeth Pharmaceuticals. (2003). Norplant system package insert. Retrieved February 21, 2005, from http://www.norplantinfo.com.

Bibliography

Barger, M. K. (Ed.). (1988). *Protocols for gynecologic and obstetric health care.* Philadelphia: W. B. Saunders.

Frye, A. (1998). Holistic midwifery. Portland, OR: Labrys Press.

Foster, S. (1996). *Herbs for your health.* Loveland, CO: Interweave Press.

Gardner, J. (1986). A difficult decision: A compassionate book about abortion. Berkeley, CA: Crossing Press.

Gordon, J. D., Rydfors, J. T., et al. (1995) *Obstetrics, gynecology & infertility* (4th ed.). Glen Cove, NY: Scrub Hill Press.

Murphy, J. L. (Ed.). (2004). *Nurse practitioner's prescribing reference.* New York: Prescribing Reference.

Scott, J. R., DiSaia, P. J., Hammond, C. B., Gordon J. D., & Spellacy W. N. (1996). *Danforth's handbook of obstetrics and gynecology.* Philadelphia, PA: Lippincott-Raven.

Starr, D. S., (2000). The legal advisor: Missing a smoking gun. *The Clinical Advisor,* March 25, 2000, 105–106.

Varney, H., Kriebs, J. M., & Gegor, C. L. (2004). *Varney's midwifery* (4th ed.). Sudbury, MA: Jones and Bartlett.

Weed, S. (1985). *Wise woman herbal for the childbearing year.* Woodstock, NY: Ashtree.

Care of the Woman with Reproductive Health Needs: Reproductive Health Problems

Midwifery care includes the care of select women's health problems and variations from normal.

The ability to discern the difference between which conditions or findings represent the wide spectrum of "normal" and which may be subtle presentations of the abnormal is a skill that midwives must work to develop. Skill as a diagnostician is necessary for midwifery practice, and it is an essential part of comprehensive care of women's reproductive health needs. Many women rely on their midwife for their reproductive health needs outside of pregnancy.

There is a wide range of resources available to the midwife to help her develop, maintain, and improve her competence in the diagnosis and treatment of commonly encountered women's health problems. A problem-oriented, directed history is essential to accurate diagnosis and the validation of the woman's concerns. The exam should focus on pertinent body systems and the organs that influence them. The resulting clinical impression, or list of potential differential diagnoses, should guide the midwife as to what diagnostic studies are appropriate or whether prompt consultation or referral is indicated. The midwifery plan of care should clearly include anticipatory thinking and planned follow-up both with and without resolution of symptoms.

Abnormal Mammogram

Key Clinical Information

Women with an abnormal mammogram are understandably anxious, as most assume that an abnormal mammogram is an indication of breast cancer. Mammography is one method of identifying and evaluating solid breast lesions that may be benign or malignant. An abnormal mammogram may indicate the need for scheduled reevaluation or biopsy for tissue diagnosis to determine whether additional treatment is indicated. Prompt treatment of early breast cancer provides the best chance for long-term survival. Women who have negative lymph nodes at time of biopsy have a 70% chance for 5-year survival without recurrence (Simpson et al., 2000). Many communities have breast centers where specialty care of breast abnormalities is available.

Client History:
Components of the History to Consider

- OB/GYN history
  - Current menstrual status
  - G, P
  - Age at first birth
  - Infant feeding method(s)
  - Breast history
    - Mastitis
    - Prior breast masses
    - Previous breast surgery
    - Previous treatment for breast disease
- Current symptoms, if any
  - Onset
  - Duration
  - Severity
- Family history
  - Breast cancer
  - Ovarian cancer
  - Benign breast disease
- Screening for risk factors for breast cancer (ACOG, 2003)
  - Most breast cancer is random, not risk associated
  - Older age
  - Early menarche
  - Alcohol use
  - Hormone replacement therapy
  - 🌐 Eastern European Jewish heritage
  - Nulliparous status

- Never having breast fed
- Strong family history
- Personal history of breast cancer

Physical Examination:
Components of the Physical Exam to Consider

- Complete breast exam
  - Positioning
    - Sitting, arms at sides
    - Sitting, arms raised
    - Sitting, leaning forward
    - Supine
  - Evaluate for
    - Mass
    - Dimpling
    - Nipple retraction
    - Nipple discharge
    - Redness
    - Induration
    - Axillary lymphadenopathy
    - Breast or axillary tenderness

Clinical Impression:
Differential Diagnoses to Consider

- Breast cancer
  - In situ
  - Focal
  - Disseminated
- Benign breast mass
  - Fibroadenoma
  - Fibrocystic breast
- Enlarged lymph nodes
- Other benign lesions

Diagnostic Testing:
Diagnostic Tests and Procedures to Consider

- Ultrasound (ACOG, 2003)
  - Benign process suspected
  - Differentiates solid from cystic mass
- Follow-up mammogram
  - Based on radiologist recommendations
    - Magnification views
    - 3–6 months follow-up
- Biopsy
  - Based on
    - Clinical findings
    - Radiologist recommendations
    - Client preference
  - Biopsy methods
    - Fine-needle aspiration
    - Core-needle biopsy
    - Stereotactic biopsy
    - Excisional biopsy
- Genetic testing

Providing Treatment:
Therapeutic Measures to Consider

- Excisional biopsy
  - Definitive treatment for benign masses
  - Treatment for small malignancies, combined with
    - Chemotherapy
    - Radiation treatment
- Cancer treatments
  - Surgery
    - Lumpectomy
    - Mastectomy
      - Partial
      - Simple

- Modified radical
- Radical
  - Axillary node evaluation
    - Sentinel node(s)
    - Axillary node dissection
- Medical therapy
  - Treatment
    - Radiation treatment
    - Chemotherapy
  - Prevention
    - Tamoxifen

Providing Treatment:
Alternative Measures to Consider

- 🔔 Alternative therapies should not take the place of diagnostic measures
- Herbal and homeopathic remedies
  - May interact with medications
  - Immune support
    - Echinacea—use with caution (Foster, 1996; Soule, 1995)
  - Emotional support
    - Rescue remedy
    - Bach flower essences
    - Saint-John's-wort
    - Lemon balm tea (Foster, 1996)
- Love and laughter have been shown to fight cancer
  - Rent comedy videos
  - Enjoy time with friends
  - Enjoy each day as a gift

Providing Support:
Education and Support Measures to Consider

- Advise client of abnormal screening test results
- Provide information

- ○ Abnormal mammograms
- ○ Options for diagnostic testing
- ○ Tissue sample (biopsy) is diagnostic test
- ○ Options for treatments
- ○ Written information helpful
- Allow time for client to express concerns
  - ○ Validate concerns
  - ○ Address fears
  - ○ Provide information
- With cancer diagnosis, information on
  - ○ Community resources
  - ○ Reach to Recovery
  - ○ American Cancer Society
  - ○ Cancer support groups

Follow-up Care:
Follow-up Measures to Consider

- Document
- Coordinate referral, prn
  - ○ Provide client with
    - ▪ Appointment time and date
    - ▪ Directions
    - ▪ Anticipated sequence of events
- Return for care
  - ○ To review findings
  - ○ Provide client education
  - ○ For support and counseling
  - ○ For well-woman care

Collaborative Practice:
Criteria to Consider for Consultation or Referral

- Surgery or breast care service
  - ○ Suspicious mammogram result
  - ○ Evaluation of lesion
  - ○ Solid mass
  - ○ Second opinion

- Community resources
  - ○ Social service
  - ○ Transportation
  - ○ Counseling
  - ○ Support groups
- For diagnosis or treatment outside the midwife's scope of practice

Abnormal Pap Smear
Key Clinical Information

Triage of the woman with an abnormal smear can be confusing. The American Society for Colposcopy & Cervical Pathology (ASCCP) has developed algorithms for this process. The algorithms may be purchased from ASCCP, or viewed online at www.asccp.org. Pap smear slides remain the most effective and cost-efficient means of screening a large population of women. However, liquid-based cytology offers the opportunity to perform "reflex" HPV testing should an atypical result be returned. HPV testing is useful for determining which clients require more aggressive follow-up, but it is of limited value with an abnormal result other than "abnormal cells of unknown significance" (ACUS). Atypical glandular cells of unknown significance (AGUS), high grade squamous intraepithelial lesions (HSIL), or cancer findings should prompt immediate evaluation by a skilled colposcopist. When in doubt about the interpretation of any Pap result, discussion with the cytology lab is recommended.

Client History:
Components of the History to Consider

- LMP, G, P
- Special circumstances
  - ○ Pregnant client
  - ○ Adolescent client
  - ○ Postmenopausal client
- History of prior

- ◦ Abnormal Pap smears
- ◦ Diagnostic testing
- ◦ Treatment
- • Sexual history
  - ◦ Age at onset of sexual activity
  - ◦ Number of sexual partners
  - ◦ Condom use
  - ◦ History of STIs
    - ▪ HPV
    - ▪ HIV
- • Social history
  - ◦ Smoking
  - ◦ Drug and alcohol use
- • Family history
  - ◦ Cervical disease
  - ◦ DES exposure in utero
- • Medical history
- • Risk factors for abnormal Pap
  - ◦ More than three sexual partners
  - ◦ History of STIs, especially HPV and HIV
  - ◦ Prior abnormal Pap smears
  - ◦ Lack of self-care, noncompliance
  - ◦ Cigarette smoking
  - ◦ Presence of CIN (cervical intraepithelial neoplasia)
    - ▪ Persistent CIN I
    - ▪ Progressive CIN
    - ▪ Any CIN II or greater lesion
- • 🩺 Symptoms consistent with cervical cancer
  - ◦ Persistent watery discharge
  - ◦ Intermenstrual bleeding

Physical Examination:
Components of the Physical Exam to Consider

- • Examination of the external genitalia for HPV lesions (Saslow, et al., 2003)

- ◦ Visible HPV is considered low-risk for CIN
- ◦ External HPV may contribute to
  - ▪ Vulvar intraepithelial neoplasia (VIN)
  - ▪ Vaginal intraepithelial neoplasia (VaIN)
- • Visualization of the cervix and vaginal vault
  - ◦ Presence of gross lesions
  - ◦ Signs of genital atrophy
  - ◦ Colposcopic exam, if indicated
    - ▪ Squamocolumnar junction
    - ▪ Presence of acetowhite lesions
      - • Punctation
      - • Mosaicism
      - • Abnormal vessels
      - • Lesion borders
      - • Abnormal Lugol's uptake

Clinical Impression:
Differential Diagnoses to Consider

- • Genital infection
  - ◦ Cervicitis
  - ◦ Vaginitis
  - ◦ STI
- • Trauma
- • Abnormal cervical cytology
  - ◦ DES exposure
  - ◦ Atypical squamous cells of unknown significance (ACUS)
  - ◦ Atypical glandular cells of unknown significance (AGUS)
  - ◦ Atypical endometrial cells of unknown significance (AEUS)
  - ◦ Low-grade squamous intraepithelial lesion (LSIL)
  - ◦ High-grade squamous intraepithelial lesion (HSIL)
  - ◦ Suspicious for invasive cervical cancer
    - ▪ Adenocarcinoma

- Squamous cell carcinoma

Diagnostic Testing:
Diagnostic Tests and Procedures to Consider

- Atypical cells of unknown significance (ACUS) (Wright, et al., 2002)
  - Evaluation
    - HPV hybrid capture testing, *or*
    - Repeat Pap smear in 3–4 months, *or*
    - Colposcopic evaluation
    - If evaluation is within normal limits (WNL), repeat Pap smear at next annual
    - Liquid cytology preferred
    - HPV on Pap specimen for ACUS result
  - Colposcopy indicated
    - Abnormal repeat Pap smear after ACUS
    - Presence of high-risk HPV
    - 💣 AGUS
    - Colposcopic evaluation
      - Biopsy of lesions
      - Endocervical curettage
      - Endometrial biopsy AGUS
- LSIL (Wright, et al., 2002)
  - Colposcopic evaluation
    - Identification of lesions
    - Directed biopsy
    - Endocervical curettage
- 💣 HSIL (Wright, et al., 2002)
  - Colposcopic evaluation
    - Identification of lesion
    - Directed punch biopsy
    - Loop electrical excision procedure (LEEP) biopsy
    - Endocervical curettage
- High-risk patient (Wright, et al., 2002)
  - Inflammation

- Treat underlying condition
- Repeat Pap smear
- Follow Pap smear with acetic acid wash to look for gross lesions
  - Biopsy lesions
- If repeat normal
  - Repeat in 3 months
  - Liquid medium preferred
- Inflammation persists
  - Acetic acid wash for gross lesions
  - Biopsy if lesions present
- If repeat is abnormal → colposcopy

- Hyperkeratosis/parakeratosis (Wright, et al., 2002)
  - Common post-LEEP
    - Indicates scarring
    - May mask HSIL lesion
  - Repeat Pap smear in 3 months
  - Acetic acid wash for gross lesions
  - Biopsy if lesions present
  - If the repeat Pap smear is normal
    - Follow-up in 9 months
  - If repeat Pap smear shows persistent HK/PK
    - Evaluate with acetic acid wash for gross lesions
    - Biopsy if lesions present
  - If repeat Pap is abnormal, colposcopy indicated

Providing Treatment:
Therapeutic Measures to Consider

- Dietary support (Soule, 1995)
  - Beta-carotene—50,000 IU bid with meals
  - Vitamin C—1000-2000 mg tid
  - Vitamin E—400 IU daily
  - Folic acid—2 mg daily x 3 months then 0.4 mg daily

- ○ Selenium—200 mg daily
- ○ Zinc—30 mg daily
- Conservative management
  - ○ Appropriate for adolescents (Wright, et al., 2002)
    - ▪ Follow with Pap smear and colposcopy
    - ▪ Rebiopsy as indicated
    - ▪ 📞 Triage to treatment with progression
  - ○ Menopausal clients
    - ▪ Vaginal estrogen x 3 months
    - ▪ Repeat Pap smear
- Ablation therapies
  - ○ Cryotherapy
  - ○ Laser
- Excisional therapies
  - ○ LEEP procedure
  - ○ Cold knife cone

Providing Treatment:
Alternative Measures to Consider

- 🖐 Alternative therapies are not a substitute for evaluation and treatment
- Herbs to support the immune and reproductive systems
  - ○ Echinacea (Foster, 1996)
  - ○ Red raspberry leaf (Soule, 1995)
  - ○ Vitex (Foster, 1996; Soule, 1995)
- Visualization of healing

Providing Support:
Education and Support Measures to Consider

- Provide information regarding cervical disease
  - ○ Written information preferred
  - ○ Meaning of abnormal Pap result
  - ○ Information about diagnostic testing options
  - ○ Potential treatment measures
  - ○ Importance of, and schedule for, follow-up

- ○ Smoking cessation, prn
- ○ Recommended vitamin and mineral supplements
- ○ Safe sexual practices

Follow-up Care:
Follow-up Measures to Consider

- Document
- Repeat screening as recommended by ASCCP
- CIN I—confirmed with biopsy
  - ○ Follow with Pap smears (compliant clients)
    - ▪ q 4 months x 12 months then q 6 months x 12 months
    - ▪ Repeat biopsy for persistent lesion
    - ▪ Treat according to biopsy results
  - ○ 📞 Arrange for treatment
    - ▪ Large lesion
    - ▪ Noncompliant client
  - ○ Posttreatment
    - ▪ Pap q 4 months x 12 months then q 6 months x 12 months
    - ▪ Repeat biopsy for persistent lesion
    - ▪ Treat according to biopsy results
- CIN II or greater
  - ○ 📞 Arrange for treatment
  - ○ Posttreatment
  - ○ Pap q 4 months x 12 months then q 6 months x 12 months
  - ○ Repeat biopsy for persistent lesion
  - ○ Treat according to biopsy results

Collaborative Practice:
Criteria to Consider for Consultation or Referral

- OB/GYN service
  - ○ Unusual cervical configuration or appearance

- Visually
- By palpation
- By colposcopy
  - Colposcopy for HSIL lesions
  - Evaluation of AGUS lesions
  - Treatment
    - CIN lesions
    - Malignancy
- For diagnosis or treatment outside the midwife's scope of practice

Amenorrhea

Key Clinical Information

Primary amenorrhea is defined as an absence of menses in a young woman who by age 14 has not begun developing secondary sex characteristics, or who by age 16 or older has developed secondary sex characteristics (Varney et al., 2004). Up to 10% of young women with primary amenorrhea will have a constitutional delay of menarche. Secondary amenorrhea is defined as the absence of menses for 3–6 months in a woman who has previously menstruated, and is not pregnant or menopausal. There is crossover between potential causes of primary and secondary amenorrhea, and all differential diagnoses should be considered when evaluating the woman with amenorrhea.

Client History:
Components of the History to Consider

- Age
- BMI
- Presence of secondary sex characteristics
- Menstrual history
  - Age at menarche
  - Previous menstrual pattern
  - Onset and duration of amenorrhea
- Presence of other symptoms

  - Galactorrhea
  - Hirsutism
- Medical and surgical history
  - Thyroid disorders
  - Weight loss
  - Systemic illness
  - Medications
  - GYN and uterine surgery
- Sexual history
  - Sexual activity
  - Sexual abuse
  - Contraceptive history
    - Injectable contraceptives
    - Hormonal IUD
- Pregnancy and breast-feeding history
  - Pregnancy terminations
  - Length of breastfeeding
- Psychosocial assessment
  - Nutrition patterns
    - Adequacy
    - Eating disorders
  - Physical activity level
  - Effects of amenorrhea on self-image
- Review of systems

Physical Examination:
Components of the Physical Exam to Consider

- Weight, vital signs
- Hair distribution
  - Mons and genital area
  - Axilla
- Thyroid exam
  - Enlargement
  - Nodularity
  - Physical findings consistent with thyroid disorders

- Breast exam
  - Development
  - Nipple discharge
- Pelvic exam
  - Presence of secondary sex characteristics
  - Examination for congenital anomalies
    - Absence of vagina, cervix, or uterus
    - Ambiguous genitalia

Clinical Impression:
Differential Diagnoses to Consider

- Amenorrhea, due to
  - Pregnancy
  - Hormonal contraception use
  - Perimenopause
  - Constitutional rate of maturation
  - Anorexia, causing hypothalamic dysfunction
  - Hormonal imbalance or insufficiency
    - Premature ovarian failure
    - Polycystic ovary syndrome
    - Androgen-producing tumors
    - Hyperprolactinemia
    - Hypothyroidism
    - Pituitary disease
  - Congenital anomalies
    - Congenital absence of uterus/ovaries
    - Congenital adrenal hyperplasia
  - Genetic factors (Varney et al., 2004)

Diagnostic Testing:
Diagnostic Tests and Procedures to Consider

- Secondary amenorrhea
  - Serum HCG
  - If HCG negative
    - TSH (elevated TSH = hypothyroidism)

- Prolactin (< 100 ng/ml normal)
- Consider progesterone trial
- Normal secondary sex characteristics
  - Uterus present
    - Serum HCG
    - Serum T4, TSH
    - Prolactin level
- Elevated prolactin level, get CT scan
- Normal prolactin level, evaluate for vaginal and cervical patency
  - Uterus absent
    - Evaluate testosterone level, and/or
    - Karyotype
- No secondary sex characteristics
  - FSH/LH levels
    - FSH 5–30 IU/L
    - LH 5–20 IU/L
    - Elevated FSH/LH ⇒ Karyotype
    - Normal or low FSH/LH ⇒ 📞 Refer for trial with gonadotropin releasing hormone (Varney et al., 2004)

Providing Treatment:
Therapeutic Measures to Consider

- Progesterone trial
  - Medication options
    - Provera 10 mg x 10 days *or*
    - Prometrium 400 mg qhs x 10 days or
    - Crinone 4%, progesterone gel 45 mg per vagina qid x 6 doses
  - Expect withdrawal bleeding within 10 days following medication
  - 📞 No withdrawal bleed refer
- 📞 Refer for treatment based on working diagnosis
  - Gynecological

○ Endocrine

○ Congenital

Providing Treatment: Alternative Measures to Consider

- Herbal remedies that support menstruation (Soule, 1995)
  ○ Red raspberry leaf tea
  ○ Dong quai tea (not to be used while nursing)
  ○ Wild yam root tea or tincture
  ○ Blue cohosh root tea or tincture
  ○ Use for 3 months, even after cycle resumes
- Acupuncture

Providing Support: Education and Support Measures to Consider

- Provide age appropriate information
  ○ Menstrual cycle and function
  ○ Potential causes
    ▪ Breast-feeding and amenorrhea
    ▪ Exercise and amenorrhea
    ▪ Endocrine disorders
  ○ Plan for testing and results
  ○ Expectation for treatment
  ○ Amenorrhea is associated with
    ▪ Infertility
    ▪ Endometrial hyperplasia
    ▪ Osteopenia and osteoporosis (Sinclair, 2004)

Follow-up Care: Follow-up Measures to Consider

- Document
- Office follow-up
  ○ As indicated by results and diagnosis
  ○ Results of progestin challenge

▪ Positive withdrawal bleed with normal prolactin and TSH = anovulation

▪ Negative withdrawal bleed requires further workup

○ For support during GYN workup

○ As indicated for routine care

Collaborative Practice: Criteria to Consider for Consultation or Referral

- OB/GYN service or GYN endocrinologist
  ○ Primary amenorrhea
  ○ Presence of anomalies
  ○ Abnormal lab results
    ▪ Reproductive
    ▪ Endocrine
    ▪ Genetic
  ○ Secondary amenorrhea
    ▪ Primary evaluation
    ▪ Following progestin challenge
      • If no withdrawal bleed
      • Following a withdrawal bleed
- Mental health service
  ○ Presence of eating disorder
- Social service
  ○ Evidence of malnutrition
- For diagnosis or treatment outside the midwife's scope of practice

Bacterial Vaginosis

Key Clinical Information

Bacterial vaginosis is a commonly occurring problem. Controversy exists as to whether bacterial vaginosis (BV) contributes to the onset of preterm labor. BV has been linked to background mycoplasma infection. BV may contribute to endometritis and postoperative wound infections following gynecological procedures. Many women consider all vaginal infections as yeast infections and may self-treat with over-the-counter medications before coming for evaluation. Cultural practices related to genital hygiene may impact development of BV.

Client History:
Components of the History to Consider

- Age
- G, P, LMP
- Onset and duration of symptoms
  - Vulvovaginal irritation or burning
  - Presence of discharge
    - Copious
    - Smooth
    - Thin or thick
    - Grayish white
  - Odor
    - Described as foul or "fishy"
    - Stronger after menses and intercourse
  - Treatments used and results
- OB/GYN history
  - BV associated with
    - Early pregnancy losses
    - Preterm labor (ACOG, 2001)
    - Endometritis
  - STI
    - Testing
    - Treatment
  - Sexual practices
    - Oral-genital contact
    - Vaginal contact following anal penetration
    - Multiple partners for self or partner
  - Use of
    - Condom
    - Spermicide
    - Lubricants
    - Douches
  - Birth control method
- Medical history
  - Allergies
  - Medications
    - Antibiotics
    - Hormones
  - Systemic illness
    - Diabetes

Physical Examination:
Components of the Physical Exam to Consider

- Genital examination for
  - Redness
  - Erythema
  - Lesions
  - Discharge
  - Retained tampon or foreign body
  - Presence of odor
- Collection of specimens
  - Wet prep
  - STI testing as indicated by history

Clinical Impression:
Differential Diagnoses to Consider

- Bacterial vaginosis
- Candida vaginosis
- Chronic cervicitis
- Cervical cancer
- Foreign body
- Chlamydia
- Gonorrhea
- Mycoplasma

Diagnostic Testing:
Diagnostic Tests and Procedures to Consider

- Wet prep
  - Positive KOH whiff test
  - Positive clue cells
  - Negative mycelia or branching hyphae
  - Rare lactobacilli
  - Occasional white blood cells
  - Vaginal pH > 4.5
- Gram stain (CDC, 2002)

Providing Treatment:
Therapeutic Measures to Consider

- Metronidazole (CDC, 2002)
  - Pregnancy category B
    - Use in second or third trimester preferred
  - MetroGel-Vaginal
    - 1 applicator per vagina
      - bid x 5 days, *or*
      - qhs x 5 days
  - Flagyl ER (extended release)
    - 750 mg po qid x 7 days
  - 500 mg po bid x 7 days, or
  - 2 gm po as single dose, or
  - 250 po tid x 7 days
- Cleocin (clindamycin)
  - Pregnancy category B
  - Vaginal cream
    - 5 gm intravaginally qhs x 7 days
    - Avoid use in pregnancy (CDC, 2004)
  - 300 mg po bid x 7 days
    - May use in pregnancy (CDC, 2002)
- Ampicillin
  - 500 mg po qid x 7 days
  - Pregnancy category B

- Amoxicillin
  - 500 mg po tid x 7 days
  - Pregnancy category B

Providing Treatment:
Alternative Measures to Consider

- Boric acid capsules (Soule, 1996)
  - Boric acid powder
  - Slippery elm powder
  - 1 per vagina qhs x 5
  - Follow with
    - Lactobacillus capsules
      - 1 per vagina qhs x 5, or
      - Yogurt douche
        - 1 cup live culture yogurt
        - 1 quart warm water
- Garlic vaginal suppository
  - 1 clove garlic, peeled
  - Attach 6″ length of dental floss
  - Use nightly x 5 nights
- Herbal douche
  - Tincture of
    - Calendula—2 parts
    - Echinacea root—2 parts
    - Myrrh—2 parts
  - Place 50 gtts in 1 cup warm calendula tea
  - Douche x 6 nights
- Homeopathic remedies (Smith, 1984)
  - Graphites—discharge is thin and watery and causes burning
  - Sepia—discharge is offensive and may be yellowish

Providing Support:
Education and Support Measures to Consider

- Review genital hygiene

- ○ Limit alkaline soaps (Soule, 1996)
- ○ Wipe front to back
- ○ Urinate after sexual relations
- ○ Cotton panties or liners
- ○ Avoid close-fitting clothing
- Provide information about BV
  - ○ Treatment instructions
    - ▪ Avoid sexual relations during treatment
  - ○ Return for care for persistent symptoms
    - ▪ Additional testing may be needed
    - ▪ Partner may need treatment
  - ○ Diagnosis during pregnancy
    - ▪ Warning signs of preterm labor

Follow-up Care:
Follow-up Measures to Consider

- Document
- If symptoms recur or persist
  - ○ Consider testing for chlamydia and/or mycoplasma
  - ○ Treat partner and retreat patient
- Diagnosis during pregnancy
  - ○ Reevaluate at 28–35 weeks
  - ○ Assess for signs of
    - ▪ Preterm labor
    - ▪ Postpartum endometritis
    - ▪ Post-op wound infection

Collaborative Practice:
Criteria to Consider for Consultation or Referral

- OB/GYN service
  - ○ For persistent or unresponsive vaginitis
  - ○ For preterm labor
- For diagnosis or treatment outside the midwife's scope of practice

Breast Mass
Key Clinical Information

Every breast mass must be considered suspicious for breast cancer until shown to be otherwise. Breast cancer is second only to lung cancer as a cause of mortality in women, and it is the leading cause of cancer-related deaths in women aged 35–54. Up to 80% of women who develop breast cancer have no risk factors for breast cancer. Pregnancy does not exclude breast cancer from the differential diagnosis as 2% of all breast cancers are diagnosed during pregnancy (Simpson et al., 2000; Varney et al., 2004).

Client History:
Components of the History to Consider

- Age
- G, P
- LMP and menstrual status
- Location and onset of symptoms
  - ○ When first noted
  - ○ Relation to menstrual cycle
  - ○ Characteristics of mass
    - ▪ Location
    - ▪ Consistency
    - ▪ Mobility
    - ▪ Pain
  - ○ Associated breast changes
    - ▪ Nipple discharge
    - ▪ Dimpling
    - ▪ Skin changes
    - ▪ Axillary masses
- Previous mammography
- Risk factors (ACOG, 2003)
  - ○ Positive family history
  - ○ Loss of ovarian function before age 35

- Age at menopause (> 40 menstrual years increases risk 2–5 times)
- Obesity, diabetes, high-fat diet
- Nulliparous, or first child born after age 35
- Use and duration of HRT
- Previous or current breast conditions
  - Lactation
  - Benign disorders, such as
    - Fibrocystic breasts
    - Mastitis
    - Breast abscess
  - Biopsies
- Self-breast exam habits and techniques

Physical Examination: Components of the Physical Exam to Consider

- Complete breast exam, sitting and supine
- Visual findings
  - Scarring
  - Dimpling and retraction
  - Skin changes
    - Peau d'orange
    - Paget's
  - Asymmetry
  - Nipple retraction
  - Redness
- Palpable findings of mass(es)
  - Single or multiple
  - Location(s)
    - Upper outer quadrant most common for cancer
    - Diffuse distribution more common with cystic breasts
  - Contour
    - Smooth
    - Stellate

- Size
  - Describe in cm
  - Round, oval, or irregular
- Mobility
  - Mobile
  - Fixed
- Consistency
  - Firm
  - Hard
  - Soft
- Heat
- Spontaneous nipple discharge
- Evaluation for palpable axillary nodes

Clinical Impression: Differential Diagnoses to Consider

- Benign breast mass(es)
  - Fibroadenoma
  - Fibrocystic breasts
  - Traumatic hematoma
  - Breast infection
    - Enlarged lymph node(s)
    - Breast abscess
    - Blocked duct
    - Mastitis
- Breast cancer

Diagnostic Testing: Diagnostic Tests and Procedures to Consider

- Mammogram
  - Difficult to interpret with
    - Young women
    - During lactation
- Ultrasound
  - Cyst or abscess suspected

- May support or oppose physical findings
- Shows fluid-filled soft-tissue changes best
- Biopsy
  - Definitive diagnosis with tissue specimen
  - Each technique has limitations
    - Needle aspiration biopsy
    - Stereotactic biopsy
    - Excisional biopsy
- Genetic screening
  - Controversial
  - Negative screen does not exclude risk (ACOG, 2003)

Providing Treatment: Therapeutic Measures to Consider

- Cystic mass
  - Observation
  - Aspiration
  - Excision
- Abscess
  - Treat with oral antibiotics (see Mastitis)
  - May require incision and drainage
- Solid mass with
  - Sharp margins
  - Uniform shape
  - No characteristics of malignancy
  - Observation and reevaluation within 3 months
  - Needle or stereotactic biopsy
  - Excision of mass
- Characteristics of malignant or premalignant lesions
  - Needle or stereotactic biopsy
  - Excisional biopsy

Providing Treatment: Alternative Measures to Consider

- Alternative measures are not a substitute for prompt evaluation and treatment
- Decrease or eliminate
  - Caffeine
  - Chocolate
  - Alcohol
  - Carbonated beverages
  - Fat intake
  - Products from hormone-fed animals
    - Meat
    - Poultry
    - Milk
    - Cheese
- Increase vitamin intake
  - Vitamin C
  - Beta-carotene
  - Vitamin E
  - B complex
- Dietary recommendations
  - Organically raised food
  - Deep green vegetables
  - Grains
  - Legumes
  - Sea vegetables
  - Fruit
- Homeopathic treatment for fibrocystic breast discomfort (Smith, 1984)
  - Belladonna for tenderness and sensitivity
  - Conium for premenstrual tenderness
  - Lapis albis for a painful nodule with burning
- Homeopathic remedies for cysts
  - Use only after malignancy has been ruled out
  - Calcarea for single cyst without tenderness or pain

  ○ Conium for right-sided, hard, mobile cyst
- Breast cancer
  ○ Healthy diet to promote healing
  ○ Homeopathic arnica to promote healing
  ○ Rescue Remedy for emotional distress

Providing Support:
Education and Support Measures to Consider

- Teach self-breast exam techniques
  ○ Daily vs. monthly
  ○ Familiarity with breast changes through cycle
  ○ No reminder needed monthly
- Provide information related to
  ○ Working diagnosis
  ○ Informed choice
    ▪ Evaluation modalities
    ▪ Testing recommendations
    ▪ Treatments
  ○ Support services and options

Follow-up Care:
Follow-up Measures to Consider

- Document
- Assess emotional state
  ○ Understanding of information
  ○ Ability to proceed with recommendations
  ○ Need for counseling/support
- Return for care
  ○ Cystic mass
    ▪ 1–3 months
    ▪ Following menses if menstruating
    ▪ Immediately if enlargement occurs
  ○ Solid masses, not referred for biopsy
    ▪ Must appear benign by
      • Clinical findings, and

  • Mammogram and/or ultrasound
    ▪ 1 month rechecks
      • Following menses (if cycling)
      • No growth or regression
  ○ 🔔 Remember a benign breast mass may mask a malignancy

Collaborative Practice:
Criteria to Consider for Consultation or Referral

- Breast center or surgery service
  ○ Breast mass that is suspicious for cancer
  ○ Diagnostic evaluation
    ▪ Abnormal mammogram
    ▪ Abnormal ultrasound
    ▪ Persistent mass
- For excision if cyst recurs after aspiration
- Client preference for definitive therapy (e.g., excisional biopsy)
- For diagnosis or treatment outside the midwife's scope of practice

Chlamydia

Key Clinical Information

Chlamydia remains the most common sexually transmitted infection in the U.S. Women with chlamydial infection may present with symptoms that range from asymptomatic to fulminant PID. Chlamydia infection may cause or contribute to blocked tubes, infertility, persistent pelvic pain, ectopic pregnancy, preterm labor or rupture of membranes and neonatal conjunctivitis and/or trachoma. Chlamydia and gonorrhea or other sexually transmitted infections frequently coexist (CDC, 2002).

Client History:
Components of the History to Consider

- G, P

- LMP
  - Onset, duration
  - Symptoms of pregnancy
  - Ectopic pregnancy may mimic chlamydia
  - Gestational age if pregnant
- Onset, duration, and type of symptoms
  - Pain
    - Location
    - Severity
    - Precipitating factors
  - Discharge
    - Amount
    - Color
    - Consistency
  - Other associated symptoms (Burst, 1998)
    - Urethritis
    - Conjunctivitis
    - Arthritis
- Sexual history
  - Previous diagnosis of STIs
  - New sexual partner for self or partner
  - Multiple sexual partners
  - Method of birth control, e.g., IUD
  - Consistency of condom use
  - Sexual practices
- Medical/surgical history
  - Allergies
  - Medications
  - Chronic health problems
- Social history
  - Alcohol or drug use
- ROS

Physical Examination:
Components of the Physical Exam to Consider

- Vital signs
- Abdominal palpation for
  - Rebound tenderness
  - Guarding
- Pelvic exam
  - External genitalia
  - Speculum exam
    - Vaginal discharge
    - Appearance of cervix
      - Presence of mucopurulent cervical discharge
      - Edema, erythema of cervix
  - Bimanual exam
    - Cervical motion tenderness
    - Uterine enlargement or tenderness
    - Painful adnexal mass

Clinical Impression:
Differential Diagnoses to Consider

- Chlamydia
- Gonorrhea
- PID
- Vaginitis
- Cervicitis
- Cervical cancer
- Ectopic pregnancy
- Round ligament pain
- Ovarian cyst
- Appendicitis

Diagnostic Testing:
Diagnostic Tests and Procedures to Consider

- Cervical swab for chlamydia and gonorrhea

- Vaginal wet mount
- Serum/urine pregnancy testing
- Serum testing for
  - HIV
  - Hepatitis B
  - Syphilis

Providing Treatment: Therapeutic Measures to Consider

- Remove IUD if present
  - Provide alternate method of birth control
- Medications—nonpregnant client (CDC, 2002)
  - Azithromycin 1 g po in a single dose—pregnancy category B
  - Doxycycline 100 mg po bid x 7 days—pregnancy category D
  - Ofloxacin 300 mg po bid x 7 days—pregnancy category C
  - Levofloxacin 500 mg po qid x 7 days
  - Sulfisoxazole (Gantrisin) 500 mg po qid x 10 days—pregnancy category C
- Medications—pregnant client (CDC, 2002)
  - Erythromycin base 500 mg po qid x 7 days—pregnancy category B
  - Erythromycin ethylsuccinate 800 mg po qid x 7 days—pregnancy category B
  - Amoxicillin 500 mg tid x 7 days—pregnancy category B

Providing Treatment: Alternative Measures to Consider

- Alternative measures are not a substitute for antibiotic therapy
- Balanced diet
- Herbal/homeopathic remedies to boost immune response
  - Echinacea
  - Homeopathic merc. sol.

- Acidophilus to offset effects of antibiotics on gut
  - Capsules
  - Yogurt
  - Probiotics

Providing Support: Education and Support Measures to Consider

- Provide information regarding
  - Infection cause and transmission
  - Effects on reproductive organs and future fertility
  - Treatment plan
  - Prevention measures
  - Risk behaviors
  - Safe sexual practices
  - Need to evaluate and/or treat partner(s)
- Medication instructions
  - Avoid intercourse until
    - Partner has been tested and treated
    - 7 days after medication is completed
      - Self and partner

Follow-up Care: Follow-up Measures to Consider

- Document
- Return to office or clinic
  - 3-4 weeks posttreatment for test of cure
    - Pregnancy
    - Noncompliant client
    - High-risk behaviors (CDC, 2002)
  - For continued symptoms
    - For persistent pain
    - New partner for self or partner
    - Client preference for testing
  - Re-screen within 4-12 months
  - With new diagnosis of pregnancy

- Test all clients
- Early ultrasound following PID
- Assess postpartum and newborn clients
  - Endometritis
  - Salpingitis
  - Newborn ophthalmic infection
  - Newborn respiratory infection (CDC, 2002)

Collaborative Practice:
Criteria to Consider for Consultation or Referral

- OB/GYN service
  - For complicated infection, such as with
    - Persistent symptoms
    - Pelvic infection
    - Unresponsive infection
    - Positive HIV or Hep B status
  - Persistent pelvic pain
  - Ectopic pregnancy
- Pediatric service
  - Imminent delivery with
    - Chlamydia infection or symptoms
    - Preterm labor
    - Newborn with signs of chlamydia
      - Ophthalmia neonatorum
      - Pneumonia
- For diagnosis or treatment outside the midwife's scope of practice

Colposcopy

Key Clinical Information

Colposcopy is the "gold standard" for the evaluation of abnormal Pap smear results. It involves using a colposcope to look at the cervix under magnification while applying one or more solutions that help delineate or highlight abnormal lesions. Biopsies are then taken from the most abnormal area(s). Many midwives perform col-

poscopy on women who have low-grade lesions that often do not require treatment. There is a significant education and training process that is required in order to become a skilled colposcopist. For information contact the American Society for Colposcopy and Cervical Pathology at (800) 787-7227 or www.asccp.org.

Client History:
Components of the History to Consider

- Age
- G, P
- LMP
- Method of birth control
- Indication for colposcopy
  - Abnormal squamous cells of unknown significance (ASCUS)
  - Low-grade squamous intraepithelial neoplasia (LGSIL)
  - Genital lesions
- GYN history
  - History of STIs
  - Prior abnormal Pap smears
    - HPV testing
    - Diagnostic procedures
    - Treatment
  - Intermenstrual or postcoital bleeding
  - Maternal DES use
- Medical history
  - HIV infection
  - Decreased immune response
- Family history
  - Maternal or sibling history
    - Abnormal Pap smears
    - Cervical cancer
- Social history
  - Smoking

- ◦ Factors that contribute to risk
  - Multiple sexual partners
  - Unprotected sex
  - Limited access to health care
  - Immunocompromised state
  - Smoking (Nyirjesy, et.al., 1998)
- • Verify client preparation for procedure
  - ◦ Premedication (see below)
  - ◦ Informed consent
  - ◦ Questions and concerns

Physical Examination: Components of the Physical Exam to Consider

- • Vulvar examination
  - ◦ Apply 5% acetic acid soaked 4 x 4 pads
  - ◦ Examine for evidence of potential vulvar intraepithelial lesion (VIN)
    - Pigmented or acetowhite lesions
    - Visible warts
    - Discharge
- • Vaginal examination
  - ◦ Apply 5% acetic acid wash
  - ◦ Examine for evidence of vaginal intraepithelial lesion (VaIN)
    - Acetowhite lesions
    - Warts or other signs of HPV
    - Punctation and/or mosaicism
  - ◦ Visible lesion present
    - Gentle biopsy
    - 📞 Refer for biopsy
    - 🕐 Vagina is very thin
- • Cervical examination
  - ◦ Obtain specimens if indicated
    - Pap smear
    - HPV testing
  - ◦ Apply 5% acetic acid wash

- ◦ Examine without magnification
- ◦ Examine colposcopically
  - No filter
  - Green filter
- ◦ Transformation zone
- ◦ Squamocolumnar junction
- ◦ Evaluate lesion(s)
  - Size
  - Location
  - Clarity of margins
  - Thickness of edge
  - Brightness of acetowhite tissue
  - Presence of punctation and/or mosaicism
  - Intercapillary distance
  - Fine versus coarse changes
  - Abnormal vessels (Wright & Lickrish, 1989)
- ◦ Apply Lugol's solution if needed to clarify presence of lesion or borders
- ◦ Obtain biopsies as indicates
- ◦ Following biopsies of lesion(s)
  - Ensure hemostasis
    - • Pressure
    - • Monsel's paste
      - ◦ Ferric subsulfate solution
      - ◦ Leave open to thicken to paste
    - • Silver nitrite application
      - ◦ Insert 1–3 sticks into biopsy wound
      - ◦ Apply gentle steady pressure
      - ◦ Release pressure
      - ◦ Do not pull on sticks
      - ◦ Tap gently until sticks spontaneously release

Clinical Impression:
Differential Diagnoses to Consider

- Colposcopy for
  - Evaluation of abnormal Pap smear
  - Follow-up after diagnosis and/or treatment of cervical intraepithelial lesion (CIN)
  - Persistent vaginal discharge with negative testing
  - Visible cervical lesion on gross exam
  - Perinatal DES exposure

Diagnostic Testing:
Diagnostic Tests and Procedures to Consider

- Pap smear—if > 6 weeks since abnormal pap
- HPV DNA testing (Wright, et al., 2002)
  - ASC-US Pap smear
- Biopsies as indicated by colposcopic exam
  - Directed cervical biopsies
  - Endocervical curettage
    - If unsatisfactory exam *or*
    - All clients
- STI testing per client history

Providing Treatment:
Therapeutic Measures to Consider

- Treatment options
  - Cryotherapy (ablative therapy)
  - LEEP (excisional therapy)
  - Laser (ablative therapy)
  - Cold knife cone (excisional therapy)
- Treatment triage (Wright, et al., 2002)
- Client with consistent results
  - No high-risk HPV, no lesion, AS-US Pap
  - No treatment indicated
  - Observation with close follow-up x 2 years
  - High-risk HPV, ASC-US/LSIL

- Pap, lesion and biopsy consistent with CIN I
- Conservative mgmt: no treatment
- Treatment if lesion is persistent or progressive
- Treatment if client is likely to be noncompliant with follow-up
  - High-risk HPV, ASC-US/LSIL
    - Lesion and biopsy consistent with CIN II/III
    - ☎ Treatment indicated
- Client with ASC-US, LSIL and inconsistent results
  - ☎ Consult with pathologist, review
    - Cytology
    - HPV result
    - Histology
    - Clinical presentation
  - Close follow-up, *or*
    - ☎ Further evaluation with expert colposcopist

Providing Treatment:
Alternative Measures to Consider

- Increase folic acid intake
- Whole foods diet
- Support immune system
  - Echinacea
  - Visualization
  - Vitamin C and E
- Herbal support formula see Soule's *The Roots of Healing* (1996, pp. 176–178)

Providing Support:
Education and Support Measures to Consider

- Provide information
  - Indication for colposcopy

- Colposcopic procedure
  - Premed with NSAID
  - In stirrups with speculum
  - Takes 5–20 minutes
  - May cause cramping
  - Occasional vagal response (syncope)
- Postcolposcopy instructions
  - Brownish discharge common
  - Vaginal rest x 7 days
  - Call with bright bleeding
- Postcolposcopy information
  - Working diagnosis
  - Anticipated treatment and/or follow-up
- Provide written information
  - Abnormal Pap smears
  - HPV
  - Anticipated 2-year follow-up

Follow-up Care:
Follow-up Measures to Consider

- Document
  - Indication for colposcopy
  - Findings: pictorial and descriptive
  - Anticipated biopsy result(s)
  - Actual biopsy result(s)
- Correlate results to formulate plan
  - Pap
  - HPV
  - Clinical picture
  - Biopsy results
- Close follow-up for 2 years
  - Interval based on results and correlation
  - Pap *or* HPV DNA testing
  - HPV DNA testing indications (Wright, et al., 2002)
    - 12 month postnegative colposcopy

- ASC-H
- LSIL
- HPV DNA positive ASC-US
- Positive → Colposcopy
  - Biopsy confirmed CIN I
    - HPV testing in 12 months for surveillance
      - Positive → Colposcopy
      - Negative → Annual Pap smear
  - CIN II, III posttreatment
    - HPV DNA 6+ months posttreatment
      - Positive → Colposcopy
      - Negative → Annual Pap smear
- Pap at 6 and 12 months
- Reevaluate with biopsy
  - Persistent lesion on colposcopy
  - Progressive Pap smear result
  - Positive high risk HPV DNA

Collaborative Practice:
Criteria to Consider for Consultation or Referral

- OB/GYN or colposcopy service
  - Colposcopy not within midwife's scope of practice
  - High-grade lesions
  - Lesions CIN II or greater for treatment
  - Clients with demonstrated progression
  - Noncompliant clients for treatment
  - For management plan for woman in whom results are not consistent
- For diagnosis or treatment outside the midwife's scope of practice

Dysfunctional Uterine Bleeding
Key Clinical Information

Dysfunctional uterine bleeding has many causes. Many of them may be a physiologic process that is age related, or it may be secondary to a pathologic process. Differentiation of the causes of irregular or intermenstrual bleeding is essential to developing a plan of care that is acceptable to the woman and appropriate to treat the problem. A common cause of noncyclic bleeding in adolescents and peri-menopausal women is anovulation. In the woman of childbearing age, causes such as thyroid disease or pelvic infection are more common (ACOG, 2000a).

Client History:
Components of the History to Consider

- Age
- G, P, LMP, menarche
- Medical history
  - Allergies
  - Prescription medications
    - Hormones
    - Anticoagulants
  - Herbal or OTC remedies
    - Aspirin and NSAIDs
    - Blue or black cohosh
- GYN history
  - Current method of contraception
    - IUD
    - Hormonal methods
  - History of and risk for STIs
  - Pap smears
    - Results of prior Pap smears
    - Date of last Pap smear and exam
  - Onset, frequency, and duration of bleeding
    - Onset, frequency, and duration of bleeding
    - Usual flow
    - Changes in menses
    - Association of bleeding with
      - Menstrual cycle
      - Intercourse
      - Pain

  - Other associated symptoms
    - Hypotension
    - Hypovolemia
    - Fatigue, breathlessness
    - Changes in metabolism
    - Hirsutism
    - Eating disorder
    - Pain with intercourse
    - Urinary frequency
    - Abdominal bloating

Physical Examination:
Components of the Physical Exam to Consider

- Vital signs
- Weight: note changes
- Thyroid
- Speculum exam
  - Cervix and vagina
    - Erosion
    - Lesions
    - Friability
    - Discharge
    - Presence of polyps
- Bimanual exam
  - Uterine, cervical, and adnexal
    - Position
    - Size
    - Contour
    - Consistency
    - Masses
    - Pain
    - Cervical motion tenderness

Clinical Impression:
Differential Diagnoses to Consider

- Functional DUB (primary ovarian dysfunction)

- Endocrine disorder
  - Thyroid dysfunction
  - Premature ovarian failure
  - Diabetes
  - Adrenal disorders
- Pregnancy disorders
  - Ectopic
  - Placenta previa
  - Septic abortions
  - Threatened abortion
- Uterine disorders
  - Fibroids
  - Endometrial hyperplasia
  - Endometrial cancer
  - Endometriosis
  - Endometritis
- Cervical disorders
  - Cervicitis
  - Malignant lesions
  - Polyps
- Vaginal disorders
  - Foreign body
  - Malignancy
  - Congenital anomalies
- Systemic disease
  - Coagulation disorders
  - Aplastic anemia
  - Coagulation factor deficiencies
  - Blood dyscrasias
  - Leukemia
  - Thrombocytopenia
  - Von Willebrand's disease (ACOG, 2000a)

Diagnostic Testing:
Diagnostic Tests and Procedures to Consider

- Pregnancy testing
- Pap smear
- Chlamydia and/or gonorrhea testing
- Thyroid testing: TSH, T3, T4
- Hormonal evaluation
  - FSH and LH
  - Prolactin (ACOG, 2000a)
  - Estradiol
  - Testosterone
- CBC with differential
- H & H
- Bleeding time, PT, PTT (Varney et al., 2004)
- Pelvic ultrasound to evaluate for
  - Placenta previa
  - Uterine fibroids
  - Thickness of endometrial stripe
  - Intrauterine polyps
  - Ovarian or adnexal masses (Varney et al., 2004)
- CT scan: abdomen and pelvis
- Endometrial biopsy

Providing Treatment:
Therapeutic Measures to Consider

- Consider differential diagnoses
- Functional DUB (primary ovarian dysfunction)
  - Trial of treatment with
    - Combination hormonal contraceptives
    - Cyclical progestins
      - Begin 14 days before next anticipated menses
      - Provera 10 mg x 10 days
      - Prometrium 400 mg x 10–12 days
- 📞 Refer for treatment as indicated by differential diagnosis

Providing Treatment:
Alternative Measures to Consider

- Reduce stress
  - Counseling for emotional issues
  - Adequate rest
  - Regular planned physical activity
  - Balanced nutrition
- Herbal remedies
  - Red raspberry
  - Black cohosh
  - Dong quai
  - Vitex (Soule, 1995)
- Iron foods to treat anemia (see Iron Foods)

Providing Support:
Education and Support Measures to Consider

- Provide information
  - Normal menstrual functioning
  - Workup related to working diagnosis
  - Results and diagnosis
  - Informed choice regarding treatment options
- Follow-up plan
  - Maintain menstrual calendar
  - Medication instructions
  - Consultation and/or referral criteria
  - When to call for problems

Follow-up Care:
Follow-up Measures to Consider

- Document
- Return for continued care
  - As indicated by diagnosis
  - For persistent or worsening symptoms
  - For support during evaluation and/or treatment
  - For well-woman care following treatment

Collaborative Practice:
Criteria to Consider for Consultation or Referral

- OB/GYN service
  - Diagnosis of cancer or precancerous condition
  - DUB
    - In presence of
      - Fibroids
      - Pregnancy
      - Congenital anomaly
    - Persistent and progressive
    - Unresponsive to herbal or hormone therapy
    - Endocrine or systemic cause
    - Unknown cause
- For diagnosis or treatment outside the midwife's scope of practice

Dysmenorrhea

Key Clinical Information

Painful periods may be functional or may be caused by endometriosis, infection, or enlarging fibroids. When dysmenorrhea does not respond to treatment, evaluation for endometriosis should be considered. The pain of endometriosis frequently begins prior to the onset of menses unlike physiologic pain, which is caused by uterine contractions expelling the menstrual flow (ACOG, 1999a). Pain with menstruation is often accompanied by heavy flow, headache, diarrhea, or other symptoms, and may cause women lost days from work or limit their ability to care for themselves or their family. Careful investigation into this common problem may provide options for relief or a decrease in symptoms.

Client History:
Components of the History to Consider

- Age

- ○ Common in women < 20 (Varney et al., 2004)
- OB/GYN history
  - ○ G, P
    - ▪ Common in nulliparous women
  - ○ Menstrual history
    - ▪ Age of menarche
    - ▪ Usual menstrual patterns
    - ▪ Age of onset of dysmenorrhea
    - ▪ Characteristics of discomfort
      - • Location
      - • Duration
      - • Severity
      - • Timing in cycle at onset
      - • Association with other body functions
      - • Bowel and bladder changes with pain
      - • Other associated symptoms
    - ▪ Relief measures used and results
    - ▪ Impact on lifestyle and daily functioning
  - ○ Current method of birth control
    - ▪ Hormonal contraceptive use
    - ▪ IUD use, type
  - ○ PID/STIs
  - ○ Endometriosis
    - ▪ Symptoms
    - ▪ Diagnosis
  - ○ Previous pelvic surgery
  - ○ Congenital pelvic anomaly
- Medical/surgical history
  - ○ Medications
  - ○ Allergies
  - ○ Health conditions
- Family history
  - ○ Dysmenorrhea
  - ○ Endometriosis
- Social history
- Review of systems

Physical Examination: Components of the Physical Exam to Consider

- Vital signs
- BMI
- Abdominal palpation
  - ○ Lower abdominal tenderness
  - ○ CVA tenderness
- Pelvic exam
  - ○ Speculum exam
    - ▪ Appearance of cervix
    - ▪ Appearance of vagina
    - ▪ Specimen collection prn
  - ○ Bimanual exam
    - ▪ Uterine size, position, and contour
    - ▪ Uterine or cervical motion tenderness
  - ○ Uterine and adnexal mobility
  - ○ Adnexal tenderness
  - ○ Pelvic masses
  - ○ Cystocele or rectocele
- Rectal exam

Clinical Impression: Differential Diagnoses to Consider

- Functional dysmenorrhea
- Endometriosis
- PID
- Pelvic anomaly
- Pelvic tumor, e.g., fibroids
- Pelvic prolapse
- PMS
- Urinary tract dysfunction or infection
- Bowel disorder or disease

Diagnostic Testing: Diagnostic Tests and Procedures to Consider

- Pap

- Chlamydia/gonorrhea testing
- Urinalysis
- Stool for occult blood following rectal exam
- Pelvic ultrasound based on pelvic exam findings

Providing Treatment:
Therapeutic Measures to Consider

- Functional dysmenorrhea
  - Ibuprofen 300–600 mg tid
  - Naproxen 275–500 mg bid
  - Begin 24 hours before menses expected
- Hormonal control
  - Combination hormonal birth control
  - Mirena IUD
- Suspected endometriosis
  - Low-dose birth control pills
    - Regulate menses
    - Diminish symptoms
  - Consider definitive diagnosis and treatment
  - Laparoscopy is used for evaluation and treatment
- 📞 Other diagnoses, evaluate and treat as appropriate

Providing Treatment:
Alternative Measures to Consider

- Heat to abdomen
- Balanced diet
  - Vitamin E
  - Decrease salt intake
  - Natural diuretics
    - Tea, coffee
    - Asparagus
  - Plenty of fiber
- Vigorous exercise for endorphin release
- Herbal remedies

- Dandelion root tea or tincture (Soule, 1996, p. 78)
  - 3–5 x daily 5 days/week
  - Continue 1–6 months
  - Safe for use in pregnant and nursing women
- Evening primrose oil, 3–6 capsules/day
- Dong quai tea (not to be used while pregnant or nursing, or if menses are excessive)
- Crampbark tea or tincture, may combine with valerian root

Providing Support:
Education and Support Measures to Consider

- Provide age-appropriate information
  - Reproductive anatomy and physiology
    - Symptoms may improve following pregnancy
    - Teach fertility awareness
      - Foster awareness of cycle
      - NSAID use before onset of menses
  - Working diagnosis
    - Evaluation options
    - Testing and treatment recommendations
    - Self-help measures
    - When to return for care
  - Indications for consult or referral
- Validate client concerns

Follow-up Care:
Follow-up Measures to Consider

- Document
- Return for care
  - After treatment to evaluate effectiveness
  - As indicated by test results
  - For worsening symptoms

Collaborative Practice:
Criteria to Consider for Consultation or Referral

- OB/GYN service
  - For evaluation and treatment of suspected endometriosis
  - For symptoms that do not improve with treatment
  - For abnormal ultrasound, prolapse, or occult bleeding
- For diagnosis or treatment outside the midwife's scope of practice

Endometrial Biopsy

Key Clinical Information

Endometrial biopsy is performed for a wide variety of indications. The most common indication is peri- or postmenopausal bleeding. Persistent dysfunctional uterine bleeding may also be evaluated with endometrial biopsy (ACOG, 1999a). Evaluation of atypical glandular cells (AG-US) on a Pap smear is another indication for endometrial biopsy; however, endometrial biopsy is best performed in conjunction with colposcopy performed by an expert colposcopist because of the possibility of highly aggressive disease associated with AG-US (Wright, et al., 2002). Gentle technique minimizes discomfort during the procedure and aids in avoiding complications.

Client History:
Components of the History to Consider

- Age
- G, P
- Interval history related to indication for endometrial biopsy
  - Postmenopausal bleeding
  - Dysfunctional uterine bleeding (DUB)
  - Thickened endometrium on ultrasound
  - Infertility investigation
  - AG-US (Grube & McCool, 2004)
- LMP or menstrual status
  - Luteal phase for infertility investigation
  - Potential for pregnancy
  - Method of birth control if applicable
- Last Pap smear and results
- Medical conditions (Grube & McCool, 2004)
  - Allergies
  - Medications, such as
    - HRT
    - Hormonal contraception
    - Aspirin
  - Bleeding or clotting disorders
  - Heart valve replacement
  - Current undiagnosed fever
  - Coronary artery disease
- Contraindications for endometrial biopsy
  - Genital tract infection
  - Positive HCG or suspected pregnancy
  - Cervical cancer
- Verify client preparation
  - Questions or concerns
  - Informed consent
  - Premedication, prn
  - Nutritional intake
  - Support person available

Physical Examination:
Components of the Physical Exam to Consider

- Vital signs pre- and postprocedure
- Evaluate for
  - Presence of reproductive tract infection
  - Size and position of uterus

Clinical Impression:
Differential Diagnoses to Consider

- Endometrial biopsy for evaluation of
  - Postmenopausal bleeding
  - Postmenopausal HRT
  - Endometrial hyperplasia on ultrasound
  - Persistent DUB
  - Infertility (Grube & McCool, 2004)
  - AG-US (Saslow, et al., 2003)

Diagnostic Testing:
Diagnostic Tests and Procedures to Consider

- Urine or serum HCG
- Pelvic ultrasound
- Endometrial biopsy procedure
- With speculum in place
  - Examine cervix and vagina for signs of infection
  - If present do not proceed
  - Cleanse cervix with prep solution
- Using careful aseptic technique
  - Apply tenaculum to straighten uterus
    - Slow application decreases cramping
    - Upper lip of cervix for anteverted/anteflexed uterus
    - Posterior lip of cervix for retroverted/retroflexed uterus
    - Avoid 3 and 9 o'clock positions
  - Apply gentle, steady traction to tenaculum
  - Sound uterus
    - Helps to dilate cervix
    - Determines depth of
      - Endometrial cavity
      - Biopsy collection device insertion
    - *Gently* insert sound in direction of uterine curvature

- Apply gentle pressure at os to relax os
- When resistance lets go
  - Gently advance sound to fundus
  - ⏱ Do not force sound
  - ⏱ If perforation occurs, remove sound and *do not proceed*
- Remove sound
- Note centimeter marking on sound
  - Insert endometrial biopsy collection device to fundus
    - Determine depth by sound measurement
    - Apply suction according to manufacturer's instructions
    - Rotate 360° while gently moving along length of uterus several times
    - Suction lost when tip removed from uterus
  - Deposit specimen into formalin
    - Cut end of collection device (into formalin)
    - Label formalin container
- Allow client to rest supine
  - Vasovagal response may be prevented
  - Obtain postprocedure vital signs (Grube & McCool, 2004)

Providing Treatment:
Therapeutic Measures to Consider

- Preprocedure medication
  - Ibuprofen 600–800 mg po
  - 1–2 hours before procedure
- Vasovagal syncope
  - Atropine sulfate indicated for heart rate under 40
  - Preferred route is IV, but may be given IM
  - Dose: 0.4 mg
  - ⏱ Be prepared for CPR

Providing Treatment:
Alternative Measures to Consider

- ☕ Alternative measures are not a substitute for evaluation of abnormal uterine bleeding
- Herbal support
  - Red raspberry leaf
  - Yarrow
  - Ginko (Foster, 1996, pp. 46)
  - Dong quai (Foster, 1996, p. 28)
  - Black cohosh
- Homeopathic support
  - Lachesis
  - Natrum mur.
  - Sepia

Providing Support:
Education and Support Measures to Consider

- Provide information
  - Potential side effects
    - Cramping
    - Light bleeding
    - Vasovagal syncope
  - Potential complications
    - Cervical stenosis preventing adequate biopsy
    - Uterine perforation
    - Postprocedure infection
  - Plan for continued care
    - Obtaining results
    - Warning signs of complications
    - Indications for consultation or referral
    - When to return for care

Follow-up Care:
Follow-up Measures to Consider

- Document

- Return for continued care
  - As indicated by biopsy results
  - Treatment based on diagnosis
  - With bleeding, pain, or fever
  - Recurrent or unresolved symptoms

Collaborative Practice:
Criteria to Consider for Consultation or Referral

- OB/GYN service
  - Treatment recommendations
    - Postprocedure infection
    - Uterine perforation
  - Cervical stenosis
  - Pathology result diagnostic of
    - Endometrial cancer
    - Endometrial atypia
    - Endometrial hyperplasia
- Medical service
  - Clearance for clients with
    - Valve replacement
      - Antibiotic prophylaxis recommendations
    - Coronary artery disease
  - Follow-up of clients with CAD and significant vagal response
- For diagnosis or treatment outside the midwife's scope of practice

Evaluation of Postmenopausal Bleeding
Key Clinical Information

Postmenopausal bleeding requires prompt evaluation for endometrial cancer. Endometrial cancer is a highly treatable malignancy of the uterine lining. It commonly goes undetected until abnormal bleeding occurs. Use of combination hormone replacement therapy decreases risk of endometrial cancer when compared to both nonhormone users and those women with a uterus who take only estrogen. Women who use natural estrogen-containing products for the treatment of menopause should be advised to report any unexpected or unusual bleeding and may want to consider the cyclic use of a progestin to diminish the growth of the endometrium.

Client History: Components of the History to Consider

- Age
- OB/GYN history
  - G, P
  - LMP or age of menopause
  - Presenting symptoms
    - Onset, duration, and severity of bleeding
    - Bleeding intervals
    - Amount, consistency, and color of bleeding
    - Other accompanying symptoms
      - Pain and cramping
      - Diarrhea
      - Backache
      - Respiratory symptoms
- Medical history
  - Diabetes
  - Hypertension
  - Heart disease
  - Biliary disease
  - Medication use
    - Tamoxifen therapy
    - Estrogen replacement therapy
    - Hormone replacement therapy
    - Aspirin or anticoagulant use
- Contributing factors
  - Early menarche
  - Late menopause
  - Nulliparous
  - Infertility
  - Polycystic ovary syndrome
  - Estrogen-producing tumors
  - Estrogen from natural sources
  - Diabetes
  - Previous or current breast cancer (ACS, 2005)
  - Family history
    - Northern European or North American
- Review of systems (ROS)

Physical Examination: Components of the Physical Exam to Consider

- Vital signs
- Speculum exam
  - Blood in vaginal vault
  - Appearance of cervix
  - Presence of lesions or masses
- Bimanual exam
  - Uterine size and contour
  - Cervical contour
  - Adnexal masses
  - Firmness and mobility of reproductive organs
- Inguinal lymph nodes
- Rectal exam
  - Confirm pelvic exam
  - Evaluate posterior pelvis
    - Masses
    - Mobility of tissues
    - Rectal involvement

Clinical Impression: Differential Diagnoses to Consider

- Abnormal vaginal bleeding

- ○ Pre- or postmenopausal
- ○ Consistent with endometrial abnormality

Diagnostic Testing:
Diagnostic Tests and Procedures to Consider

- Pelvic ultrasound
  - ○ Abdominal
  - ○ Transvaginal
  - ○ Evaluation of endometrial stripe
    - ■ 4–6 mm is within normal limits
- Endometrial biopsy
- 🌀 Endometrial curettage (D & C)
- 🌀 Hysteroscopy
- 🌀 Sonohysterography

Providing Treatment:
Therapeutic Measures to Consider

- 🌀 Refer for treatment
  - ○ Surgical treatment (ACS, 2005)
    - ■ Hysterectomy
    - ■ Oopherectomy
    - ■ Pelvic lymph nodes for staging
    - ■ Additional surgery may be required
  - ○ Radiation therapy
  - ○ Chemotherapy

Providing Treatment:
Alternative Measures to Consider

- 🌀 Alternative therapies should not delay evaluation and treatment
- Alternative therapies should be aimed at supporting healing
  - ○ Nutritional support
    - ■ Vitamin C and E
    - ■ Antioxidant foods
    - ■ Avoid hormone-containing

- • Meat
- • Poultry
- • Dairy products
  - ■ Balanced diet
- ○ Visualization
- ○ Prayer
- Avoid herbs prior to surgery (Murphy, 1999)
  - ○ May decrease clotting ability
  - ○ Stop use 7–14 days before procedure
    - ■ Feverfew
    - ■ Garlic
    - ■ Ginger
    - ■ Ginseng
    - ■ Ginko

Providing Support:
Education and Support Measures to Consider

- Discussion regarding
  - ○ Significance of symptoms
  - ○ Need for diagnostic workup
  - ○ Results of
    - ■ Physical exam
    - ■ Diagnostic testing
  - ○ Plan for referral and ongoing care
  - ○ Options for support services
- Active listening
  - ○ Client fears and concerns
  - ○ Questions
  - ○ Preferences for care

Follow-up Care:
Follow-up Measures to Consider

- Document
- Offer continued support, as appropriate
  - ○ Assess for

- Depression
- Altered self-image
- Barriers to healing
  - Encourage
    - Positive attitude
    - Return for care, prn

Collaborative Practice:
Criteria to Consider for Consultation or Referral

- OB/GYN service
  - Evaluation of postmenopausal bleeding
  - Diagnosis of
    - Endometrial atypia
    - Endometrial hyperplasia
    - Endometrial cancer
- Support services, such as
  - Social services
  - Nutritionist
  - Support groups

Endometriosis

Key Clinical Information

Endometriosis is found in 5–20% of women of reproductive age during pelvic laparoscopy. As many as one third of these women have endometriosis-related fertility issues. Pain is the primary presenting complaint in women who are diagnosed with endometriosis. Pelvic laparoscopy may be used to both diagnose and treat endometriosis. Endometriosis implants may affect the reproductive organs, the bowel, the bladder, and the pelvic sidewalls (ACOG, 1999b).

Client History:
Components of the History to Consider

- Age
- OB/GYN history
  - G, P
  - Menstrual history
    - Age at menarche
    - LMP
    - Usual menstrual patterns
  - Sexual activity
  - Contraception
    - Hormonal contraceptives
    - IUD
  - STIs
- Onset, duration, and frequency of symptoms
  - Age at onset of symptoms
  - Presence of symptoms related to endometriosis (ACOG, 1999b)
    - Significant cyclic pre- and perimenstrual pain
    - Dysparunia
    - Infertility
    - Dysfunctional uterine bleeding
    - Urinary urgency or frequency
    - Effect on bowel and bladder function
    - Other symptoms
  - Relief measures used and their effect
- Medical/surgical history
  - Cystitis
  - Pelvic surgery
  - Diverticular disease
  - Appendicitis
- Family history
  - Dysmenorrhea
  - Infertility
  - Endometriosis
  - Bowel disorders
- Social history
  - Risk factors for
    - PID

- Ectopic
- Review of systems (ROS)

Physical Examination:
Components of the Physical Exam to Consider

- Vital signs
- Abdominal exam
  - Tenderness
  - Rebound
  - Guarding
  - Masses
- Speculum exam
- Bimanual exam
  - Uterine position, size, and consistency
  - Cervical motion tenderness
  - Adnexal size, location, and tenderness
  - Findings suggestive of endometriosis
    - Fixed, retroverted uterus
    - Adnexal thickening, nodularity, or irregularity
    - Limited mobility of
      - Uterus
      - Adnexa

Clinical Impression:
Differential Diagnoses to Consider

- Pelvic pain consistent with
  - Endometriosis
  - Fibroid uterus
  - Chronic salpingitis
  - Pelvic infection
  - Ectopic pregnancy
  - Interstitial cystitis
  - Appendicitis
  - Adhesions secondary to

- PID
- Pelvic surgery
- Peritonitis
- Diverticular disease

Diagnostic Testing:
Diagnostic Tests and Procedures to Consider

- STI testing
- CBC
- Pelvic ultrasound
  - May be suggestive of endometriosis
  - Used to rule out other differential diagnoses
- Laparoscopy to confirm diagnosis (ACOG, 1999b)
  - Visualization of pelvis
  - Tissue sample for histology

Providing Treatment:
Therapeutic Measures to Consider

- Symptomatic treatment while awaiting diagnosis
  - Anti-inflammatory medication
    - Naproxen sodium
    - Ponstel
  - Initiation of hormonal birth control
- Laparoscopy for diagnosis and preliminary treatment
  - Ablation of endometrial implants
- Medications for treatment of persistent symptoms (ACOG, 1999b)
  - Danazol
  - Progestins
  - Oral/hormonal contraceptives
  - GnRH agonist
- Surgical treatment
  - Retreat with ablative therapy

○ Hysterectomy with oopherectomy

Providing Treatment:
Alternative Measures to Consider

- Symptomatic treatment (see also Dysmenorrhea)
  - ○ Local heat
    - ■ Castor oil packs
    - ■ Heating pad
  - ○ Yoga
  - ○ Massage
  - ○ Acupuncture
  - ○ Meditation
  - ○ Pregnancy

Providing Support:
Education and Support Measures to Consider

- Active listening
  - ○ Encourage participation in evaluation and treatment process
  - ○ Women may opt to live with symptoms
- Provide information
  - ○ Endometriosis
  - ○ Fertility awareness
  - ○ Evaluation process
  - ○ Potential modes of treatment

Follow-up Care:
Follow-up Measures to Consider

- Document
- Return for care
  - ○ PRN during diagnosis and/or treatment
  - ○ For well-woman care
  - ○ With pregnancy

Collaborative Practice:
Criteria to Consider for Consultation or Referral

- OB/GYN service
  - ○ Suspected endometriosis
  - ○ Persistent pelvic pain
  - ○ Pain accompanied by bowel or bladder involvement
  - ○ Pain accompanied by fever or elevated WBC
- Endometriosis Association: (800) 992-3636 or http://www.endometriosisassn.org
- For diagnosis or treatment outside the midwife's scope of practice

Fibroid Uterus

Key Clinical Information

Fibroids are a common benign tumor of the uterus. Fibroids may enlarge continuously in the pre-menopausal woman, but generally regress during menopause. While fibroids are most often benign, there is a small chance of malignancy developing or being masked by fibroids. In addition, blood supply to fibroids may become occluded resulting in degeneration of fibroids. Most fibroids simply represent an overdevelopment of the muscle cells of the uterus. They may occur anywhere in the uterus: the fundus, the wall of the uterus, inside the uterus, or the cervix. Treatment is based primarily on relieving symptoms: pain, bleeding, and abdominal enlargement (ACOG, 1999b).

Client History:
Components of the History to Consider

- Age, G, P
- Symptoms
  - ○ Onset, duration, severity
  - ○ Symptoms of uterine fibroids
    - ■ Pelvic pressure
    - ■ Abdominal enlargement

- Changes in bowel or bladder function
- Menstrual changes
- OB/GYN history
  - LMP and menstrual status
  - Menstrual history
    - Duration, frequency, and length
    - Amount of flow
    - Dysmenorrhea
    - Intermenstrual bleeding
- Previous clinical findings
  - Uterine size and contour
  - Previous pelvic ultrasounds
  - Previous GYN problems
- Social history
  - Fibroids more common in African-American women
- Review of systems (ROS)

Physical Examination:
Components of the Physical Exam to Consider

- Vital signs, including BP and weight
- Abdominal exam
  - Fundal height
  - Abdominal girth
- Bimanual exam
  - Uterine size and position
  - Uterine contour
  - Uterine consistency
  - Presence of adnexal masses
  - Tenderness
  - Signs of other processes
    - Discharge
    - Pain on cervical motion
- Rectal or rectovaginal exam
  - Palpate posterior uterus

Clinical Impression:
Differential Diagnoses to Consider

- Enlarged uterus secondary to
  - Uterine fibroids
  - Pregnancy
  - Malignancy
    - Uterine
    - Cervical
    - Ovarian
- Anemia secondary to
  - Menorrhagia
  - Occult GI bleeding

Diagnostic Testing:
Diagnostic Tests and Procedures to Consider

- Pelvic ultrasound
- Hemoglobin and hematocrit
- Stool for occult bleeding
- Endometrial biopsy

Providing Treatment:
Therapeutic Measures to Consider

- Hormonal regulation of menses
- Iron supplementation as indicated (Murphy, 2004)
  - Ferrosequels 1–2 po daily
  - Niferex 150 1–2 po daily
  - Ferrous gluconate 1–2 po daily
- Lupron Depot (Murphy, 2004; NIH, 2004)
  - Short-term treatment
  - Indicated to decrease uterine size prior to surgery
  - Dosing
    - 3.75 mg IM monthly x 3 month, *or*
    - 11.25 mg IM x 1 (lasts 3 months)

- ○ 💣 Do not use for undiagnosed uterine bleeding
- ○ Exclude pregnancy prior to use
- ○ May cause vasomotor symptoms
- Uterine artery embolization (NIH, 2004)
- Myomectomy (ACOG, 1999b)
  - ○ Excision of fibroid(s)
  - ○ Retains fertility
  - ○ Uterine scarring may require Cesarean birth
- Hysterectomy (ACOG, 1999b)
  - ○ Grossly enlarged uterus
  - ○ Degenerative fibroids
  - ○ Potential malignancy
  - ○ Severe menorrhagia
  - ○ Client preference

Providing Treatment:
Alternative Measures to Consider

- Dietary sources of iron replacement (see Iron Foods)
- Floradix iron supplement
- Avoid phytoestrogens
- Homeopathic remedies (Smith, 1984)
  - ○ Aurum mur.
  - ○ Belladonna
  - ○ Calc. iod.
  - ○ Tarentula hisp.

Providing Support:
Education and Support Measures to Consider

- Discussion regarding
  - ○ Clinical findings
  - ○ Recommended testing
  - ○ Planned follow-up
  - ○ Medications recommended

- ■ Indications
- ■ Side effects
- ■ Anticipated results
  - ○ Warning signs
    - ■ Excessive bleeding
    - ■ Pain
    - ■ Change in bowel or bladder function
- Provide information and support if surgery indicated
  - ○ Preoperative testing
  - ○ Anticipated hospital stay
  - ○ Self-care following discharge
  - ○ Active listening to elicit
    - ■ Concerns
    - ■ Family/personal support
    - ■ Coping mechanisms
  - ○ Allow grieving
    - ■ Loss of fertility/body part
    - ■ Body image changes with surgery
    - ■ Potential perceived loss of femininity

Follow-up Care:
Follow-up Measures to Consider

- Document
- Return for care
  - ○ Reevaluation of uterine size
    - ■ Annual or semiannual
    - ■ Serial ultrasound sizing
  - ○ With significant change in bleeding pattern
  - ○ Progression of symptoms
  - ○ Preop history and physical, prn
- Informed consent as indicated for
  - ○ Lupron Depot
  - ○ Operative procedures

Collaborative Practice:
Criteria to Consider for Consultation or Referral

- OB/GYN service
  - Grossly enlarged uterus
  - Client preference
  - Progression of symptoms
  - Evidence or suspicion of pathologic process
  - Surgical and/or anesthesia consultation
- Social service support, prn
- For diagnosis or treatment outside the midwife's scope of practice

Gonorrhea

Key Clinical Information

Gonorrhea is often accompanied by chlamydia or trichomonas, and may infect eyes, mouth, and joints as well as the reproductive tract. Significant effects of gonococcal infections include infertility, premature rupture of membranes, preterm labor, and infection of the newborn's eyes resulting in blindness if left untreated. Gonorrhea, like other STIs, may increase the transmission risk of those exposed to HIV infection. More information may be obtained from the CDC at www.cdc.gov. Additionally, the treatment guidelines may be downloaded to a handheld device from the Web site (CDC, 2002).

Client History:
Components of the History to Consider

- Age
- G, P LMP
- GYN history
  - Review previous history
    - Pap smear
    - STI testing
    - STI treatments
  - Sexual history

- Sexual practices
  - Monogamous
  - Multiple partners for self or partner(s)
  - Vaginal, oral, anal intercourse
- Condom use
  - Male condom
  - Female condom
- Birth control method
- Problem history
  - Onset, duration, and severity of symptoms
  - Last unprotected intercourse
  - Symptom profile for gonorrhea
    - May be asymptomatic
    - Urinary frequency and dysuria
    - Urethritis
    - Vaginal or anal discharge
    - Sore throat
    - PID
      - Pain with intercourse
      - Genital pain and discharge
      - Fever
      - Lower abdominal pain
      - Intermenstrual bleeding
      - Painful bowel movements
- Medical/surgical history
  - Allergies
  - Medications
  - Chronic health conditions
- Social history
  - Behavioral risk factors
    - ETOH/drug use
    - Exposure to more than five sexual partners
    - Male partner who is bisexual
    - Travel to or residence in fluoroquinolone-resistant GC areas (CDC, 2004a)
      - Asia

- Pacific Islands
- California
  - ○ Social support
  - ○ Access to health care

Physical Examination:
Components of the Physical Exam to Consider

- Vital signs including temperature
  - ○ Temp > 38°C suspicious for PID
- Pelvic exam (Varney et al., 2004)
  - ○ Bartholin's, urethra, and Skene's for evidence of
    - ■ Discharge
    - ■ Inflammation
  - ○ Vaginal, cervical, or anal discharge
    - ■ Yellow or mucopurulent
  - ○ Evidence of PID
    - ■ Pain on cervical motion
    - ■ Adnexal or uterine tenderness
    - ■ Lower abdominal pain
    - ■ Presence of inflammatory mass on pelvic exam

Clinical Impression:
Differential Diagnoses to Consider

- Chlamydia
- Gonorrhea
- PID
- Cervicitis
- Cervical cancer
- Ectopic pregnancy
- Ovarian cyst
- Ovarian torsion
- Appendicitis

Diagnostic Testing:
Diagnostic Tests and Procedures to Consider

- Gonorrhea testing (Payne, 2003)
  - ○ Gram stain
    - ■ Positive Gram stain
    - ■ Gram negative intracellular diplococci
    - ■ > 10 WBC/hpf
  - ○ Culture
  - ○ DNA probe
  - ○ Elisa test (antigen specific)
  - ○ Nucleic acid amplification tests (NAAT)
- Chlamydia testing
- Wet mount
- Pelvic ultrasound
  - ○ Presence of inflammatory mass
- WBC with sedimentation rate
  - ○ Sed. rate > 15 mm/hour suspicious
- HIV counseling and testing

Providing Treatment:
Therapeutic Measures to Consider

- Begin treatment based on symptoms
- One time dosing
  - ○ May be provided on site
- Compliance assured by direct observation
- CDC recommendations for uncomplicated gonorrhea (CDC, 2002)
- Single-dose regimens
  - ○ Cefixime 400 mg po (pregnancy category B)
  - ○ Ceftriaxone 125mg IM (pregnancy category B)
    - ■ 1% lidocaine may be used as diluent to reduce pain of injection
    - ■ Indicated for use when fluoroquinolone-resistant GC suspected or confirmed (CDC, 2004a)

- Ciprofloxin 500 mg po (pregnancy category C)
- Ofloxacin 400 mg po (pregnancy category C), *plus*
  - Azithromycin 1 gm po (pregnancy category B)
- Levofloxin 250 mg po
- Plus, if chlamydia has not been ruled out
  - Azithromycin 1 g po
  - Doxycycline 100 mg po (🚫 pregnancy category D) bid x 7 days
- Alternate medications
  - Spectinomycin 2 gm IM (pregnancy category B)
    - Indications
      - Pregnant women
      - Those who cannot tolerate cephalosporins or quinolones
  - Ceftizoxime 500 mg IM
  - Cefoxitin 2 g IM with probenecid 1 g po
  - Cefotaxime 500 mg IM
- Pharyngeal infection
  - Ceftriaxone 125 mg IM (pregnancy category B); 1% lidocaine may be used as diluent to reduce pain of injection
  - Ciprofloxin 500 mg po (pregnancy category C) as one time dose, *or*
  - Plus, if chlamydia has not been ruled out
    - Azithromycin 1 g po one time dose
    - Doxycycline 100 mg po (🚫 pregnancy category D) bid x 7 days

Providing Treatment: Alternative Measures to Consider

- 🚫 Alternative therapies are not a substitute for medical treatment
- Supportive measures to promote healing

- Adequate rest
- Sitz baths with comfrey leaf tea or Epsom salts
- Nutritional support
  - Balanced diet
  - Live culture yogurt
  - Blue-green algae
  - Vitamins C and E
- Herbal support formulas (Soule, 1995)
  - Adjunct to medical therapy
  - Use 2–3 times daily
  - Prepare as tea or tincture
    - Red clover—2 parts
    - Calendula—2 parts
    - Yarrow—1 part
    - Dandelion root—1 part
- Homeopathic remedies
  - Adjunct to medical therapy
  - Use 30x grains three times daily
  - Arnica montana (promotes soft tissue healing)
  - Merc. sol (to offset side effects of antibiotic treatment)
- Acidophilus capsules per vagina to prevent yeast overgrowth

Providing Support: Education and Support Measures to Consider

- Information regarding
  - Gonorrhea
    - Diagnosis
    - Prevention
    - Potential sequelae
  - Client notification of results
  - Treatment recommendations
  - Partner
    - Notification
    - Evaluation

- ▪ Treatment
  - ◦ State reporting requirements
  - ◦ Symptoms of acute PID
  - ◦ When and how to access care
- Medication instructions
  - ◦ Avoid sexual relations
    - ▪ Until treatment is completed
    - ▪ Symptoms have resolved
- Educate regarding STI transmission and prevention

Follow-up Care:
Follow-up Measures to Consider

- Document
- Indications to return for care
  - ◦ Symptoms of acute PID
  - ◦ Persistent symptoms
    - ▪ May represent reinfection
    - ▪ Consider testing for drug resistance
- Repeat testing
  - ◦ Persistent symptoms
  - ◦ New partner for self or partner
- Offer HIV and other STI counseling and testing

Collaborative Practice:
Criteria to Consider for Consultation or Referral

- OB/GYN service or STI clinic
  - ◦ Signs and symptoms of PID
  - ◦ Client requiring hospitalization
  - ◦ Gonorrhea infection with
    - ▪ Symptoms of meningitis
    - ▪ Disseminated infection
- Social services
  - ◦ Support services as indicated
- For diagnosis or treatment outside the midwife's scope of practice

Human Immunodeficiency Virus
Key Clinical Information

HIV infection in women is increasing. HIV may be transmitted to women by infected male or female partners during insertive intercourse, oral/genital, or digital/genital contact. Virus transmission is affected by the viral load of the infected partner. Transmission is enhanced when the HIV-exposed woman is menstruating or has nonintact skin or mucous membrane such as occurs with ulcerative STIs or trauma. Not all exposed women contract HIV; genetic and/or immunologic factors may protect against HIV infection (Greenblatt & Hessel, 2001). Infection is diagnosed by HIV testing. The stage of illness is determined by CD4 counts and clinical presentation (CDC, 2002). A client's *partner* means any sexual *or* needle-sharing partner. HIV prevention vaccines (for use in HIV-negative clients) and therapeutic HIV vaccines (to improve the immune system of HIV-positive individuals) are currently undergoing clinical trials. No vaccines are available at this time.

Client History:
Components of the History to Consider

- Age
- OB/GYN and sexual history
  - ◦ HIV risk assessment (CDC, 2002; Varney et al., 2004)
    - ▪ Knowledge and understanding of HIV transmission
    - ▪ Current HIV prevention behaviors
    - ▪ Transmission risk since last visit, such as
      - • IV drug use
      - • Unprotected sex
      - • Sex with incarcerated male
      - • Sexual abuse or assault
  - ◦ Sexual orientation for self and partner(s)
    - ▪ Sexual practices

- Contraception
  - Previous HIV/STI testing
    - Previous diagnosis of STIs or abnormal Pap smear
    - Treatment of previous STI or abnormal Pap smear
- Medical/surgical history
  - Allergies
  - Medications
  - Chronic diseases or disorders
- Social history (Varney et al., 2004)
  - IV drug use
  - Living situation
    - Economic factors
    - Mental health issues
    - Substance abuse
    - Support systems
  - Access to services
- Review of systems (ROS)
- Risk factors for HIV-1 infection
  - Client or partner with more than five partners
  - Diagnosis or symptoms of any STI
  - IV drug use, self or partner
  - Exposure to blood or body fluids
- Risk factors for HIV-2 infection
  - 🌐 Travel or residence in HIV-2 endemic areas
    - West Africa
    - Angola
    - France
    - Mozambique
    - Portugal
  - Clinical evidence of HIV infection with negative HIV-1 test

- Signs & symptoms of acute retroviral syndrome (Niu, Stein, & Schnittman, 1993; CDC, 2002)
  - Fever
  - Lymphadenopathy
  - Pharyngitis
  - Rash
    - Maculopapular lesions
    - Mucocutaneous ulceration
  - Myalgia or arthralgia
- Signs and symptoms of active HIV infection
  - Abnormal pap: CIN II or III
  - PID
  - Constitutional symptoms > 1 month
    - Fever
    - Weight loss
    - Diarrhea
  - Herpes zoster
  - Oral hairy leukoplakia
  - Candidiasis
    - Oral
    - Persistent vaginal
  - Idiopathic thrombocytopenic puerpera
  - Listerosis
  - Peripheral neuropathy

Physical Examination: Components of the Physical Exam to Consider

- Vital signs, including temp
- Weight—compare to previous
- HEENT
  - Cervical lymph nodes
  - Oral candidiasis or ulcerative lesions
  - Throat for redness
- Chest
  - Cardiac assessment
  - Lung sounds

- Presence of cough
- Skin
  - Rash
    - Erythematous maculopapular rash
    - Mucocutaneous ulceration
  - Lesions
    - Herpes zoster
- Abdomen
  - Enlargement of liver or spleen
  - Bowel sounds
- Extremities
  - Range of motion
  - Joint tenderness or swelling
  - Femoral lymph nodes
- Pelvic exam
  - Lesions
    - Mucocutaneous ulceration of genitals
  - Discharge
    - Mucopurulent cervicitis
    - Bacterial vaginosis
  - Cervical lesions
    - Cervicitis
    - Friability
    - Masses
  - Uterine motion tenderness
  - Adnexal mass or pain
- Neurologic exam
  - Peripheral neuropathy
  - Facial palsy
  - Cognitive impairment (Niu, Stein, & Schnittman, 1993)

Clinical Impression: Differential Diagnoses to Consider

- Acute retroviral syndrome
- HIV infection

- AIDS
- Malignancy
- IV drug abuse/addiction
- TB
- Cervical cancer
- STIs
- Hepatitis

Diagnostic Testing: Diagnostic Tests and Procedures to Consider

- HIV-1 antibody testing
  - Antibody screen is positive > 2–14 weeks postinfection
  - Collection: venous sample in tiger-top tube
- Other labs
  - GC and chlamydia
  - Pap smear
  - Wet mount
  - Hepatitis A, B, and C serology
  - Syphilis serology
- HIV infection strongly suspected
  - Toxoplasmosis antibody test
  - TB testing
    - Skin test
    - Chest X-ray
  - CD4 cell count
  - CBC
  - Chemistry profile
  - Bun and creatinine

Providing Treatment: Therapeutic Measures to Consider

- Acute retroviral syndrome
  - Occurs in first weeks after infection prior to positive antibody test
  - Immediate initiation of antiretroviral therapy

- May delay onset of HIV-related complications
- ☏ Antiretroviral therapy following current recommendations (DHHS, 2004)
  - Most recent updates available at http://atAIDSinfo.nih.gov
- Drug classes
  - Nucleoside reverse transcriptase inhibitors
  - Nonnucleotide reverse transcriptase inhibitors
  - Protease inhibitors
  - Fusion inhibitors
- Problem specific treatments as indicated

Providing Treatment: Alternative Measures to Consider

- ⬙ Avoid echinacea and other immunostimulants with HIV
- General measures to support immune function
  - Adequate rest
  - Balanced diet
  - Stress reduction
- HIV immune support herbal formulas
  - Improve bone marrow function
  - See *The Roots of Healing* (Soule, 1996, pp. 254–255)

Providing Support: Education and Support Measures to Consider

- HIV-1 antibody testing
  - Antibody screen is positive > 2–14 weeks postinfection
  - Perform pretest counseling to obtain informed consent
    - Routes of transmission
    - Prevention measures
    - Information regarding testing

- Venipuncture
- Confidentiality
- Test interpretation
- Timing and return visit for results
- Availability of anonymous testing
  - Client must return for results and posttest counseling
  - Partner notification
- Client Resources
  - CDC Division of HIV/AIDS Prevention: www.cdc.gov/hiv/dhap.htm
  - AMA HIV/AIDS Patient Info: www.ama-assn.org
  - HIV/AIDS Treatment Information Center: www.aidsinfo.nih.gov
  - National AIDS Hotline
    - English (800) 342-AIDS
    - Spanish (800) 344-7432
- Encourage creative and supportive measures, such as
  - Meditation or spiritual practices
  - Art therapy
  - Dance
  - Support groups
  - Religious involvement
  - Community involvement
  - Participation in HIV prevention programs
- HIV risk-reduction practices
  - Abstaining from intercourse
  - Selecting low-risk partners
  - Negotiating partner monogamy
  - Condom use

Follow-up Care: Follow-up Measures to Consider

- Document

- Provide posttest counseling
- HIV positive client
  - ◦ 📞 Arrange case management
  - ◦ Provide ongoing reproductive health care as appropriate
- HIV-negative client (Wang & Celum, 2001)
  - ◦ Provide HIV prevention education
  - ◦ Perform HIV risk assessment at return visits
    - ▪ Risk may come from male partner

Collaborative Practice: Criteria to Consider for Consultation or Referral

- HIV/AIDS expert
  - ◦ HIV-positive clients for
    - ▪ Medical evaluation
    - ▪ Treatment plan
    - ▪ Coordination of case management
- Clients with new HIV diagnosis
  - ◦ Behavioral services
    - ▪ Risk reduction
    - ▪ Prevention management
  - ◦ Case management and medical care
    - ▪ Substance abuse services
    - ▪ Reproductive health counseling
    - ▪ Psychosocial services
      - • Mental health
      - • Crisis counseling
      - • Housing and financial support services
  - ◦ Medical evaluation and treatment
    - ▪ Detailed medical history
    - ▪ Physical exam including pelvic
    - ▪ Comprehensive lab work
    - ▪ TB testing
    - ▪ Chest X-ray
    - ▪ Psychosocial evaluation
    - ▪ Monitoring of medical status

- HIV-negative women with HIV behavioral risk factors
  - ◦ Behavioral services
    - ▪ Risk reduction
    - ▪ Prevention management
  - ◦ Psychosocial services
  - ◦ Drug rehab services
- For diagnosis or treatment outside the midwife's scope of practice

Hepatitis

Key Clinical Information

Hepatitis is defined as inflammation of the liver (Dorland's, 2002). It includes a number of liver diseases that may be broken down, based on viral characteristics, into the categories of hepatitis A, hepatitis B, hepatitis C, hepatitis D, and hepatitis E. Hepatitis B and C are the forms of hepatitis that are most frequently seen by the midwife. Hepatitis B is 100 times more infectious that HIV. Risk of developing chronic infection is age related. Only 10% of infected adults develop chronic HBV infections. Hepatitis may also be caused by an autoimmune disorder, alcohol abuse, or drug-related behavior, particularly with acetaminophen use, and may result in permanent liver damage, liver failure, or liver cancer.

Client History: Components of the History to Consider

- Age
- Medical/surgical history
  - ◦ Allergies
  - ◦ Medications
    - ▪ Acetaminophen-based products
  - ◦ Chronic illnesses
    - ▪ Organ transplant
    - ▪ Anemia

- HIV/AIDS
- Social history
  - Drug & alcohol use
  - ⊛ Emigration, travel, or adoption from endemic areas
    - Asia
    - Africa
    - Pacific Islands (including Hawaii)
    - South or Central America
- Presence, onset, duration, and severity of symptoms
  - May be asymptomatic
  - Malaise and lethargy
  - Fever and chills
  - Right upper quadrant pain
  - Jaundice
  - Nausea and vomiting
  - Dark urine
  - Pale colored stools (Mercksource, 2003)
- Review of systems (ROS)
- Potential for exposure to hepatitis
  - Health care professional
  - IV drug use, shared needles
  - Sexual contacts
  - Presence of tattoos
  - Ingestion of raw shellfish
  - Hemodialysis patients
  - Blood or organ recipient prior to 1992
- Indications for hepatitis B vaccine (CDC, in press)
  - Adolescents before sexual activity
  - Diagnosis of STI
  - Travel to hepatitis B endemic areas
  - Multiple sexual partners
  - IV drug use
- Contraindications to hepatitis B vaccine

  - Allergy to yeast

Physical Examination:
Components of the Physical Exam to Consider

- VS, including weight
- Examine for evidence of jaundice
  - Skin
  - Mucous membranes
  - Sclera
- Palpate and percuss for
  - Liver margins
  - Splenomegaly
  - RUQ pain
  - Abdominal ascites

Clinical Impression:
Differential Diagnoses to Consider

- Hepatitis B immunization
- Jaundice secondary to
  - Hepatitis
  - Biliary disease
  - Obstructive cholelithiasis
  - Other liver disorders
- Asymptomatic HBV infection found via
  - STI testing
  - Blood donation

Diagnostic Testing:
Diagnostic Tests and Procedures to Consider

- Hepatitis panel
- Hepatitis B
  - HBsAg (hepatitis B surface antigen)
    - Detected 1–12 weeks postinfection
- Positive result indicates infection with HBV
- Negative result indicates susceptibility to HBV

- HBsAb or anti-HBs (hepatitis B surface antibody)
  - Positive result indicates immunity
  - Negative result indicates infection
- HBcAb or anti-HBc (hepatitis core antibody)
  - Indicates past or present infection
  - May be present in those chronically infected
  - False positive is possible
  - With HBsAb indicates recovery
  - With HbsAg indicates chronic infection
- Liver function testing (LFTs)
  - SGOT (AST), SGPT (ALT), LDH, bilirubin
  - ↑ during acute phase
- Ultrasound, RUQ
  - Gallbladder

Providing Treatment:
Therapeutic Measures to Consider

- Hepatitis B vaccines (CDC, 2002)
  - Recombinant vaccines
  - Age-related doses by manufacturer
  - Series of immunizations (3 doses)
  - Given with HBIG immediately postexposure
- HB immune globulin (HBIG)
  - Given ASAP postexposure (up to 7 days)
  - 1 or 2 doses
- Active infection
  - Must run its course
  - ☏ Acute illness refer for treatment

Providing Treatment:
Alternative Measures to Consider

- Supportive care

- Whole foods diet with minimum of toxins
- Adequate rest
- Herbal support
  - Milk thistle tea (Soule, 1996)
  - Silymarin 140–560 mg tid x 6 weeks (Hepatitis C Technical Advisory Group, 2005; Ferenci, Dragosics, Dittrich, et al., 1989)
  - Licorice root tincture

Providing Support:
Education and Support Measures to Consider

- Provide information about hepatitis
  - Types
  - Route(s) of transmission
    - Fecal-oral
    - Blood transfusion
    - Sexual contacts
  - Prevention measures (Mercksource.com, 2003)
    - Avoid contact with blood or body fluids
    - Wash hands before eating and following toileting
    - Safe sexual practices
    - Avoid undercooked food in endemic areas
    - Avoid shared needles or razors
    - Acetaminophen use
      - Abstain from alcohol when taking
      - Do not exceed recommended dose
      - OTC meds may contain acetaminophen
- Discussion regarding
  - Immunization
  - Options for treatment and supportive care, prn
    - Potential effects of illness
    - Medications
    - Parameters for referral

- Client resources
  - Hepatitis Foundation International: http://www.hepfi.org/
  - The Hepatitis Information Network: http://www.hepnet.com/
  - CDC Viral Hepatitis: http://www.cdc.gov/ncidod/diseases/hepatitis/
  - Hepatitis B Foundation: http://www.hepb.org
  - Hepatitis C Information Center: http://hepatitis-central.com/

Follow-up Care:
Follow-up Measures to Consider

- Document
- Testing
  - Screening
  - Postimmunization
  - With symptoms
    - Incubation lasts 1–4 months
    - It may take up to 6 months to
      - Determine if a client has recovered, *or*
      - Remains chronically infected
- Return for care
  - Weekly during acute phase of infection
  - Periodic LFTs
  - STI testing, prn
  - Reproductive health care

Collaborative Practice:
Criteria to Consider for Consultation or Referral

- Medical service
  - Diagnosis of hepatitis for detailed evaluation and treatment
  - Evidence of
    - Liver failure
    - Ascites

- Acetaminophen overdose
- For diagnosis or treatment outside the midwife's scope of practice

Human Papillomavirus
Key Clinical Information

There are more than 20 types of HPV that can affect the genital tract, but only a few that are considered high-risk types. Types 16, 18, 31, 33, and 35 are associated with cervical dysplasia, and may contribute to the development of anal cancer as well as cervical cancer. Women may be infected with more than one type of HPV. Current screening tests indicate the presence or absence of one or more high-risk types of HPV and may be used to guide clinical management of women infected with HPV (CDC, 2002; Saslow, et al., 2003).

Client History:
Components of the History to Consider

- Age
- Reproductive history
  - LMP, chance of pregnancy
  - Current method of birth control
    - Previous
- HPV testing
- Pap smear results
  - Sexual practices
    - Condom use
    - Number of sexual partners
    - Anal sex
- Medical/surgical history
  - Allergies
  - Medications
  - Chronic illnesses
- Social history
  - Tobacco use (increases risk of progression)

- ○ Drug and/or ETOH use
- Onset, duration, and severity of current symptoms
  - ○ Location of lesions
  - ○ Other associated symptoms
  - ○ Risk factors for HPV infection
    - Previous or current STIs
    - Diminished immune response
    - Unprotected sexual activity
    - Multiple sexual partners for self or partner(s)
    - Previous abnormal Pap smear
- Review of systems (ROS)

Physical Examination:
Components of the Physical Exam to Consider

- Pelvic exam
  - ○ Careful evaluation
    - Internal and external genitalia
      - Genital warts
      - Friable lesions
    - Consider application of
      - 5% acetic acid (white vinegar)
        - ○ HPV lesions turn acetowhite
      - Lugol's solution (strong iodine)
        - ○ Normal squamous cells stain mahogany brown
        - ○ HPV lesions and columnar cells remain unstained
    - Consider colposcopy of
      - External genitalia
      - Vagina
      - Cervix
- Bimanual exam
  - ○ Palpate for abnormality of cervix or vagina
    - Contour
    - Consistency
    - Mass

Clinical Impression:
Differential Diagnoses to Consider

- Condyloma
  - ○ Genital warts
  - ○ Microscopic HPV
    - Vulvar
    - Vaginal
    - Cervical
    - Anal
  - ○ Syphylitic condyloma
- Musculosum contagiosum
- Other genital lesions

Diagnostic Testing:
Diagnostic Tests and Procedures to Consider

- HPV testing
  - ○ Cervicovaginal
  - ○ Anal
- Other STI testing as indicated
  - ○ GC/CT
  - ○ RPR
  - ○ HIV counseling and testing
- Pap smear
  - ○ Slide (most cost effective for screening)
  - ○ Liquid-based cytology
    - Allows for reflex HPV testing
- HCG as indicated, before treatment
- Stool for occult blood

Providing Treatment:
Therapeutic Measures to Consider

- Vitamin therapy

- ○ Vitamin E 400 IU daily
- ○ Vitamin C 500–1000 mg daily
- Client-applied therapy (CDC, 2002)
  - ○ Imiquimod cream 5%
    - ▪ Apply q hs 3 x week until clear
    - ▪ Wash off after 6–10 hours
    - ▪ More info: (800) 428-6397 or www.3M.com/ALDARA
  - ○ Podofilox 0.5% solution or gel
    - ▪ Apply bid x 3 days
    - ▪ No treatment x 4 days
    - ▪ Repeat up to 4 cycles
- Provider applied therapy (CDC, 2002)
  - ○ Podophyllin resin
    - ▪ Apply weekly to lesions
    - ▪ Wash off in 6–8 hours
  - ○ Trichloracetic (TCA) or bichloracetic acid (BCA)
    - ▪ Apply weekly to lesions
    - ▪ Protect normal tissue with petrolatum

Providing Treatment:
Alternative Measures to Consider

- Balanced whole foods diet
- Antioxidant foods
  - ○ Blueberries
  - ○ Red peppers
  - ○ Plums
  - ○ Pumpkin
  - ○ Tomatoes
- Herbal remedies
  - ○ Echinacea tea or tincture daily to boost immune response
  - ○ Rub broken end of fresh green bean over visible lesions

- ○ See *The Roots of Healing* (Soule, 1996) for additional herbal formulas
- Stress reduction
- Visualization of area healed and whole

Providing Support:
Education and Support Measures to Consider

- Information
  - ○ Male and female condoms provide limited protection
    - ▪ Uncovered areas not protected
  - ○ Wart virus is not curable, but may become dormant
    - ▪ Regression most likely in adolescents
    - ▪ May spread virus with no visible warts
    - ▪ Oral, pharyngeal, or anal warts may occur with exposure
- Discuss treatment recommendations
  - ○ Medication/remedy use
  - ○ Anticipated response to treatment
  - ○ Signs or symptoms indicating need to return for care
- Encourage smoking cessation
- Emphasize need for annual Pap smears
  - ○ Increased risk of abnormal Pap results
    - ▪ Smoking increases risk of progression
    - ▪ Immune response affects regression or progression
- Suggest partner be evaluated and treated if visible lesions present
- For more information contact the American Social Health Association: www.ashastd.org

Follow-up Care:
Follow-up Measures to Consider

- Document
- Provide results and interpretation

- Return for care
  - As necessary for treatment chosen
  - Annually for Pap smear
  - As indicated by HPV test results

Collaborative Practice:
Criteria to Consider for Consultation or Referral

- OB/GYN service
  - Ablative therapy
    - Cryotherapy
    - Laser
  - Interferon injection of lesions
  - Extensive lesions
  - Anal lesions
- Behavior risk modification
  - Safe sex habits
  - Smoking cessation
- For diagnosis or treatment outside the midwife's scope of practice

Herpes Simplex Virus

Key Clinical Information

Herpes virus is caused by HSV-I or HSV-2. This common virus can be sexually transmitted and frequently causes significant discomfort to those with active lesions. The goal of therapy is to encourage the virus to become dormant and to support the immune system so that it stays dormant and the client remains asymptomatic. Herpes infection in the HIV-positive client increases the likelihood of transmission of HIV (CDC, 2004b). Unfortunately, it is possible to spread herpes infection without a noticeable lesion. Infants who are exposed to HSV may acquire systemic infection resulting in serious illness or death. For this reason, Cesarean birth may be offered to pregnant women with a history of recurrent HSV outbreaks during pregnancy.

Client History:
Components of the History to Consider

- Present symptoms
  - Onset, duration, and severity
  - Presence and location of lesions
    - Vesicular lesions
    - Ulcerative lesions
  - Pain, tingling, dysuria
  - Other associated symptoms
  - Precipitating factors
    - Stress
    - Fever or infection
    - Menses
    - Sun exposure
- Reproductive history
  - LMP, chance of pregnancy
  - Current method of birth control
  - Partner with oral or genital HSV
  - Previous history of genital or oral lesions
  - Sexual orientation
  - Sexual practices
    - Oral-genital sex
    - Anal sex
    - Safe sex practices
  - Last exam and testing results
    - HSV and other STI testing
    - HIV status
    - Pap smear results
- Medical/surgical history
  - Allergies
  - Medications
  - Chronic illnesses
    - HIV/AIDS
    - Immunosuppression
      - Cancer

- Burns
- Organ transplant
- Steroid use
- Review of systems
    - Primary HSV infection may be associated with
        - Fever
        - Headache
        - Malaise
        - Local lesions at site of infection
        - Lymphadenopathy
        - Herpes meningitis (CDC, 2004)
- Psychosocial assessment
    - Impact of symptoms
    - ⊛ African-Americans more likely to test positive for HSV
    - ⊛ Caucasians more likely to have active symptoms
    - ⊛ Caucasian teens fastest growing HSV-positive population (CDC, 2000)

Physical Examination:
Components of the Physical Exam to Consider

- Vital signs
- Pelvic exam
    - Palpate inguinal lymph nodes
    - Examine for characteristic lesions
        - Vesicles
        - Shallow ulcers
    - Lesions may occur on
        - Vulva
        - Urethra
        - Vagina
        - Cervix
        - Thighs
        - Anus
        - Buttocks
    - Examine for presence of other STI symptoms
        - Cervical discharge
        - Cervical or uterine motion tenderness
- Neurologic exam
    - Neck tenderness
    - Light sensitivity

Clinical Impression:
Differential Diagnoses to Consider

- Primary herpes infection
    - Local
    - Systemic
- Recurrent herpes outbreak
- Non-HSV lesions
    - Trauma
    - Chancre
- Bacterial meningitis

Diagnostic Testing:
Diagnostic Tests and Procedures to Consider

- Culture lesions for
    - HSV (CDC, 2002)
- Serum testing for HSV-1 or -2 antibody titer (CDC, 2002)
    - Documents primary infection
    - Important in early pregnancy
    - Repeat 7–10 days
    - Four-fold increase documents primary infection
- Additional STI testing as indicated

Providing Treatment:
Therapeutic Measures to Consider

- Valtrex (valacyclovir hydrochloride) (CDC, 2002)

- ○ Pregnancy category B
- ○ Pregnancy registry: (800) 722-9292, ext. 39437
- ○ Dose: 1000 mg bid x 7–10 days for initial outbreak
- ○ Dose: 500 mg bid x 3–5 days, or 1000 mg bid x 5 days for recurrent outbreak
- ○ Begin medication within 24 hours of first symptom
- Famvir (famciclovir)
  - ○ Pregnancy category B
  - ○ Dose 250 mg tid x 7–10 days for initial outbreak
  - ○ Dose: 125 mg bid x 5 days for recurrent outbreak
  - ○ Begin medication within 6 hours of first symptom
- Zovirax (Acyclovir)
  - ○ Pregnancy category C
  - ○ Pregnancy registry: (800) 722-9292, ext. 58465
  - ○ Dosages
    - ■ Topical ointment 5% apply 3 x day x 7 days
    - ■ Initial outbreak: 200 mg po 5 x day or 400 mg tid x 10 days
    - ■ Recurrent outbreak: 200 mg po 5 x day, or 400 mg tid, or 800 mg bid x 5 days
    - ■ Suppression, severe recurrent outbreaks 400 mg po bid x 12 months
- Acetaminophen or ibuprofen for pain relief

Providing Treatment: Alternative Measures to Consider

- Nutritional supplements
  - ○ L-lysine
    - ■ 500 to 1000 mg qid for prevention
    - ■ 2,000 mg bid or qid for outbreak (Soule, 1995)
  - ○ Vitamin C 250–500 mg
    - ■ bid with outbreak
    - ■ Combine with acidophilus
      - • 1 cap with meals
  - ○ Zinc 30 mg daily (Sinclair, 2004)
  - ○ Vitamin A
    - • 200,000 IU po x 3 days, *or*
    - • 50,000 IU daily
    - ■ Decreases length and severity of symptoms
    - ■ Not for use during pregnancy or with liver disorders
  - ○ Selinium 0.25 mg (250 mcg) daily
- Echinacea
  - ○ Topical applied to lesions
  - ○ po as tea, tincture, tablets or capsules tid x 2 weeks
- Aloe vera ointment
- Sitz bath or salve made with
  - ○ Lemon balm (Foster, 1996)
  - ○ Calendula
  - ○ Comfrey
- Homeopathics (University of Maryland, n.d.)
  - ○ Graphites
    - ■ Large itchy lesions
    - ■ Overweight client
  - ○ Natrum muriaticum
    - ■ Outbreaks caused by emotional stress
    - ■ Symptoms that are worse in daytime
  - ○ Petroleum
    - ■ Lesions on anus and thighs
    - ■ Symptoms worse in winter
  - ○ Sepia
    - ■ Stubborn outbreaks
    - ■ Client with lack of energy and cold intolerant

Providing Support:
Education and Support Measures to Consider

- Diet
  - Avoid foods high in arginine: chocolate, cola, peanuts, cashews, pecans, almonds, sunflower and sesame seeds, peas, corn, coconut, and gelatin
  - Include foods high in lysine: brewer's yeast, potatoes, fish, chicken, eggs, dairy (Soule, 1996)
- Rest and comfort measures
- Discuss and provide written information about
  - Herpes management
    - Medications
    - Nutritional support
    - Lifestyle changes
      - Abstinence during outbreaks
      - Wash hands after lesion contact
      - Avoid handling infants during active lesion
  - Effects on
    - Sexuality
    - HIV susceptibility
    - Childbearing
    - Self-image
- Review warning signs and symptoms
  - Meningitis
  - Secondary infection
  - Depression
- Client resources
  - The American Social Health Association: www.ashastd.org
  - National Women's Health Network: www.womenshealthnetwork.org
  - Centers for Disease Control and Prevention: (800) 311-3435 www.cdc.gov

Follow-up Care:
Follow-up Measures to Consider

- Document
- Return for care
  - Symptoms persist > 10 days
  - Worsening symptoms
    - Stiff neck
    - Unremitting fever
    - Inability to urinate
  - Ineffective coping

Collaborative Practice:
Criteria to Consider for Consultation or Referral

- OB/GYN service
  - Symptoms of
    - Herpes meningitis
    - Systemic infection
    - Ocular herpes
  - Pregnancy
    - Initial outbreak during pregnancy
    - Cesarean birth during active genital outbreak
- For diagnosis or treatment outside the midwife's scope of practice

Genital Candidiasis

Key Clinical Information

Genital candidiasis is so common that many women assume that every form of vaginitis is a "yeast infection." Candidal vulvovaginitis has many different appearances, from a curdy white vaginal discharge to the excoriated skin creases common in undiagnosed diabetic women. Careful attention to the wet mount is necessary to determine the presence of yeast, and the absence of additional causes of vaginitis.

Client History:
Components of the History to Consider

- Age
- Reproductive health history
  - G, P, LMP
  - Current method of birth control
  - Douching
  - Sexual practices
    - Change in sexual partners/habits
    - Anal/vaginal intercourse
    - Sex toys
- Symptoms
  - Onset, location, and duration
  - Exacerbating factors
    - Menses
    - Intercourse
  - Common description (CDC, 2004c)
    - Intense itching
    - Curdy discharge
    - Moist, raw skin
  - Other associated symptoms
    - Burning with urination
    - Pain
  - Treatments tried and efficacy
- Medical/surgical history
  - Allergies
  - Medications
    - Antibiotic use
    - Steroid use
  - Acute illness
  - Chronic illness
    - Diabetes or gestational diabetes
    - Immunocompromised condition
      - HIV/AIDS
      - Cancer

- Social history
  - Use of tight or damp clothing
  - Stress

Physical Examination:
Components of the Physical Exam to Consider

- Pelvic exam
  - Presence of red, excoriated external genitalia
  - White, adherent, curdy discharge within vagina
  - Collect wet mount specimen
- Assess for signs of monilia
  - On skin folds
  - Cutaneous infection
  - Oral cavity
- Observe for signs or symptoms of STIs

Clinical Impression:
Differential Diagnoses to Consider

- Vulvovaginal candidiasis
- Oral candidiasis (Thrush)
- Intertriginous candidiasis
- Bacterial vaginitis
- Chlamydia
- Gonorrhea
- Chronic cervicitis
- Foreign body irritation
- Medical conditions
  - Diabetes mellitus
  - HIV
  - Candida secondary to antibiotic use
- Impetigo

Diagnostic Testing:
Diagnostic Tests and Procedures to Consider

- Wet mount for

- Budding yeast
- Mycelia
- Branching hyphae (Varney et al., 2004)
- Vaginal pH testing, prn
- Severe or recurrent infection
  - Fasting blood sugar
  - HIV testing (CDC, 2004c)
- Other STI testing as indicated by history

Providing Treatment:
Therapeutic Measures to Consider

- Diflucan 150 mg po x 1 or 2 doses
- Terazol (Terconazole) 3-day or 7-day therapy
- Monistat Derm for cutaneous symptoms (Murphy, 2004)
- Over-the-counter antifungals
  - Mystatin (Mycostatin)
  - Miconazole (Monistat)
  - Clotrimazole (Gyne-Lotrimin, Mycelex)
  - Butoconozole (Femstat)

Providing Treatment:
Alternative Measures to Consider

- Acidophilus capsules 1 per vagina qhs x 5–7 days
- Boric acid capsules 1 per vagina qhs x 5–7 days
  Poisonous if taken orally!
- Herbal douche 2 x week (use acidophilus capsules other nights)
  - 1 tbs ti tree oil
  - 2 tbs cider vinegar
  - 2 cups warm water

Providing Support:
Education and Support Measures to Consider

- Dry genital region thoroughly before dressing (use blow drier on warm setting)
- Wear cotton panties, loose clothing (boxer shorts are good)
- Wear no panties to allow maximum ventilation
- Avoid excessive sugar or alcohol in diet
- Tub bath with 1 cup vinegar in water
- Avoid intercourse while using medication

Follow-up Care:
Follow-up Measures to Consider

- Document
- Return for care
  - Symptoms not improved within 5 days
    - For additional testing
    - Consider vaginal culture
  - As indicated by other test results

Collaborative Practice:
Criteria to Consider for Consultation or Referral

- OB/GYN service
  - Recurrent or unresponsive infection
  - For fasting glucose over 126 gm/dl (diagnostic of diabetes)
- Medical service
  - Positive HIV titer
  - Evidence of immunocompromise
- For diagnosis or treatment outside the midwife's scope of practice

Nipple Discharge

Key Clinical Information

Nipple discharge in the absence of pregnancy and lactation must be evaluated. It may represent a physiologic variation from normal or be the presenting symptom of a pathologic process. In evaluating galactorrhea of > 6–12 months duration the possibility of a pituitary tumor must be considered. Fortunately, many such tumors are exceedingly slow growing and not malignant. Large untreated tumors may cause pressure on optic nerves resulting in permanent visual loss or blindness.

Client History:
Components of the History to Consider

- Onset and duration of symptoms
  - Nature of discharge
    - Bloody, greenish, or milky
    - Unilateral or bilateral
    - Volume of discharge
  - Recent breast changes
  - Associated symptoms
    - Breast pain, tenderness, masses
    - Fever
    - Decreased libido
    - Headache
    - Visual changes
    - Presence of menstrual dysfunction
      - Amenorrhea
      - Irregular or scanty menses
- Reproductive history
  - G, P, LMP
  - Usual menstrual patterns
  - Current method of birth control
  - Infertility
  - Breast history
    - Lactation, duration, and most recent dates
    - Self-breast exam practices
    - Mastitis
    - Breast abscess
    - Fibrocystic breast disorder

- Breast cancer
- Breast surgery
- Breast stimulation or trauma
- Medical/surgical history
  - Medications that may cause nipple discharge
    - Phenothiazine
    - Cimetidine
    - Methyldopa
    - Metoclopramide
    - Oral contraceptives
    - Reserpine
    - Tricyclic antidepressants
    - Verapamil (Thompson, 2004)
  - Health conditions
- Family history
  - Breast disease
  - Endocrine disorder
- Review of systems (ROS)

Physical Examination:
Components of the Physical Exam to Consider

- Breast examination
  - Breast asymmetry or retraction
  - Masses
  - Presence of spontaneous nipple discharge
  - Crusting of discharge on nipple
  - Skin changes; thickening, coarseness, edema, scaling, redness
  - Palpate axillary lymph nodes
- Observe for hirsutism
- Thyroid palpation

Clinical Impression:
Differential Diagnoses to Consider

- Pregnancy

- Galactorrhea post breast-feeding
- Galactorrhea secondary to
  - Benign conditions
    - Infection
    - Pituitary adenoma
    - Intraductal papilloma (Thompson, 2004)
    - Ductal ectasia
    - Idiopathic galactorrhea
  - Breast cancer

Diagnostic Testing:
Diagnostic Tests and Procedures to Consider

- Pregnancy testing
- Infection suspected
  - Culture of discharge
  - Ultrasound for fluctuant mass
- Malignancy suspected
  - Cytology of discharge
  - Mammogram
  - 📞 Breast biopsy
    - Fine-needle aspiration cytology (Breast Cancer Care, 2003)
    - Core biopsy
- Endocrine disorder suspected
  - Thyroid testing, TSH
  - Prolactin
    - Nonpregnant < o–20 ng/ml
    - Pregnant 10–300 ng/ml
  - Head CT for prolactinoma
  - MRI for abnormalities of prolactin or sella turcica

Providing Treatment:
Therapeutic Measures to Consider

- Treatment is based on final diagnosis
  - Breast infection (see Mastitis)

- Ductal ectasia
  - Observation
  - 📞 Surgical repair of duct
- Intraductal papilloma
  - Observation
  - 📞 Surgical removal
- Pituitary tumor
  - 📞 Refer for evaluation and treatment
  - Bromocriptine used to return prolactin levels to normal
  - Large or bromocriptine-resistant tumors
- Surgical removal
- Stereotactic radiosurgery
  - Breast cancer
    - 📞 Refer for evaluation and treatment

Providing Treatment:
Alternative Measures to Consider

- Provide emotional support
- Bach flower remedies to balance emotional state
- Comfort measures
  - Warm castor oil packs
  - Immune support formulas

Providing Support:
Education and Support Measures to Consider

- Provide information related to
  - Diagnosis
  - Recommendations for evaluation
  - Treatment options
- Teach or review self-breast exam
- Offer active listening
  - Client fears and concerns

Follow-up Care:
Follow-up Measures to Consider

- Document
- By diagnosis
  - Pregnancy: options counseling as indicated
  - Galactorrhea, simple
    - Periodic prolactin levels to confirm stability
  - Galactorrhea, pathologic
    - Return for care following evaluation, and medical or surgical treatment
    - Assess for
      - Symptom recurrence
      - Prolactinoma tumor regrowth
      - Contralateral breast disease
  - For routine well-woman care

Collaborative Practice:
Criteria to Consider for Consultation or Referral

- OB/GYN or breast care service
  - Pituitary adenoma
  - Treatment of persistent galactorrhea
    - Ductal ectasia
    - Intraductal papilloma
  - Breast cancer
- Social service
  - Community support groups or organizations
- For diagnosis or treatment outside the midwife's scope of practice

Pediculosis

Key Clinical Information

Lice and scabies can be a particularly challenging problem in midwifery practice. An infestation of lice can be hard to eradicate, and since they are mobile, may affect the office environment and housekeeping practices after a client has been diagnosed. Lice and scabies live on human blood, and may contribute to the spread of impetigo. Head lice prefer the nape of the neck, while body lice inhabit seams of clothing or bedding and move onto the host to feed. Pubic or crab lice live in the genital region, but may be found on any hairy aspect of the body.

Client History:
Components of the History to Consider

- Symptoms
  - Onset, duration, location
  - Itching
  - Presence of nits (lice)
  - Presence of skin tracks (scabies)
  - Other associated symptoms
- Exposure to lice, nits, or scabies
  - Household contacts
  - Intimate contacts
  - Public contacts
  - International travel
- Medical/surgical history
  - Allergies
  - Medications
  - Health conditions
    - Asthma
- Reproductive history
  - LMP
  - Current method of birth control
  - Sexual partner with symptoms
- Social history
  - Environmental exposure
  - Shared personal items
  - Bathing habits
- Review of systems (ROS)

Physical Examination: Components of the Physical Exam to Consider

- Observe for signs of parasites (Emmons, 1997)
  - Anogenital region
  - Extremities
  - Nape of neck
  - Presence of
    - Lice (1 mm crablike organism)
    - Nits (small white orb attached to hair shaft)
    - Skin tracks from scabies burrows
  - Secondary signs due to itching
- Skin
  - Secondary infection
  - Rash
- Pelvic exam as indicated
  - STI symptoms
  - Lymph nodes for enlargement

Clinical Impression: Differential Diagnoses to Consider

- Pediculosis
- Scabies
- Impetigo
- Other parasitic infestation

Diagnostic Testing: Diagnostic Tests and Procedures to Consider

- Microscopic examination of parasites
- Evaluation of type of parasite
- Culture of skin lesions
- Wet mount
- STI testing
- Additional testing prn per H & P

Providing Treatment: Therapeutic Measures to Consider

- Avoid pyrethrum or permethrin with
  - Asthma
  - Ragweed allergy
- Avoid lindane with
  - Client weight under 110 lb
  - Nonintact skin
  - HIV/AIDS
  - History of seizures
- Scabies treatment
  - Permathrim cream 5%
  - Crotamiton cream
  - Malathion lotion 0.5% (Rx)
- Lice treatment
  - Use alternative therapies as first-line treatment
  - Pyrethrum 0.33% with butoxide
  - Pregnancy category C
- Lindane 1% lotion, cream or shampoo
  - Second-line treatment (FDA, 2003)
    - May cause severe neurotoxic reaction

Providing Treatment: Alternative Measures to Consider

- Lice R Gone Shampoo
  - Safe Solutions, Inc. (888) 443-8738 or www.safesolutionsinc.com
- Head or pubic lice
  - Coat affected area in olive oil
  - Comb with fine-toothed comb
  - Wash with soap or shampoo
  - Apply cream rinse
  - Comb again
  - Apply vinegar rinse
    - Use caution as may cause burning of

- Eyes
- Genitals
  - Blot dry
- Salt scrub to affected area
  - Mix coarse salt with oil
  - Follow with soap wash
- Sauna
- Wash of Painted Daisy
  - Source of pyrethrins
  - Use wash to affected area tid
- Shave affected area

Providing Support:
Education and Support Measures to Consider

- Provide written medication instructions
- Recommend treatment for all contacts
- Avoid sexual contact until treatment complete
- Review transmission mechanisms
  - Cleanse bedding and clothing
  - Hot water wash with bleach
  - Hot dryer
  - Vacuum living quarters
  - Wash throw rugs

Follow-up Care:
Follow-up Measures to Consider

- Document
- Return for care
  - 1 week if symptoms not eliminated
  - Symptoms of
    - Reinfestation
    - Secondary infection
    - Medication side effects

Collaborative Practice:
Criteria to Consider for Consultation or Referral

- Laboratory
  - Identification of unusual parasite
- Emergency department or medical service
  - Symptoms of neurotoxicity
- For diagnosis or treatment outside the midwife's scope of practice

Pelvic Pain, Acute
Key Clinical Information

Pelvic pain may have many potential causes, both GYN and non-GYN related. Acute pelvic pain requires prompt diagnosis in order to institute corrective action. The ability to differentiate between acute and nonacute pain is essential so that appropriate emergency care can be obtained when indicated.

Client History:
Components of the History to Consider

- Age
- Symptoms
  - Location: local or radiating
  - Onset: sudden, gradual, or cyclic
  - Duration of pain
  - Severity of symptoms
  - Precipitating or exacerbating factors
  - Associated symptoms
    - Fever and chills
    - Nausea and vomiting
    - Diarrhea
    - Constipation or obstipation
    - Vaginal discharge
      - Bleeding
      - Mucopurulent
- Reproductive history
  - LMP, G, P

- ○ Potential for pregnancy
- ○ Method of birth control
- ○ Last exam, Pap smear, and STI testing
- ○ History of
  - STIs/PID
  - Endometriosis
  - Ectopic pregnancy
- ○ Change in sexual partner for self or partner
- Medical/surgical history
  - ○ Medications
  - ○ Allergies
  - ○ Health conditions
    - Diverticular disease
    - Appendicitis
  - ○ Previous abdominal surgery
- Psychosocial history and status
  - ○ Physical or sexual violence
  - ○ Drug/ETOH use
  - ○ Living situation
  - ○ Mental health status
  - ○ Client affect and presentation
- Review of systems (ROS)

Physical Examination:
Components of the Physical Exam to Consider

- Vital signs
- Abdominal exam
  - ○ Distention
  - ○ Mass
  - ○ Rebound tenderness
  - ○ Guarding
  - ○ Presence or absence of bowel sounds
- Pelvic exam
  - ○ Speculum exam
    - Presence of cervical discharge

- Bimanual exam
  - ○ Cervical motion tenderness
  - ○ Uterine enlargement or tenderness
  - ○ Palpation of
    - Adnexa
    - Fornices
    - Rectum

Clinical Impression:
Differential Diagnoses to Consider

- Reproductive system
  - ○ Mucopurulent cervicitis
  - ○ PID
  - ○ Ectopic pregnancy
  - ○ Septic abortion
  - ○ Spontaneous abortion or miscarriage
  - ○ Ovarian cyst
  - ○ Torsion of ovary
  - ○ Endometriosis
  - ○ Degenerating fibroids
- Urinary system
  - ○ Renal calculi
  - ○ Acute cystitis
- Gastrointestinal system
  - ○ Acute appendicitis
  - ○ Diverticulitis
  - ○ Ulcerative colitis
  - ○ Bowel obstruction
- Incarcerated inguinal hernia
- Lower abdominal trauma

Diagnostic Testing:
Diagnostic Tests and Procedures to Consider

- Urinalysis
- Serum or urine HCG

- STI testing
- Pelvic ultrasound
- CBC with differential
- ESR
- 📞 Diagnostic laparoscopy

Providing Treatment:
Therapeutic Measures to Consider

- 🩺 Medical care is indicated for acute abdominal or pelvic pain
- Acetaminophen or ibuprofen for fever or pain
  - Take medication with sips of water
- Avoid eating or drinking until definitive diagnosis

Providing Treatment:
Alternative Measures to Consider

- Symptomatic treatment while test results pending
  - Rest
  - Local heat
  - Positioning

Providing Support:
Education and Support Measures to Consider

- Provide information regarding
  - Working diagnosis
  - Recommendations for evaluation
  - How to access care if condition worsens
  - Indications for consultation and/or referral

Follow-up Care:
Follow-up Measures to Consider

- Document
- Return for care
  - Nonacute presentation
    - 24–48 hours

- Reevaluation
- Phone or face to face
  - ASAP for
    - Worsening symptoms
    - Persistent symptoms
    - As indicated by testing

Collaborative Practice:
Criteria to Consider for Consultation or Referral

- OB/GYN service
  - Suspected or confirmed OB/GYN cause such as
    - Pelvic abscess
    - Ectopic pregnancy
    - Septic abortion
- Medical/surgical or emergency service
  - Non-GYN surgical emergency
  - Uncertain diagnosis
  - Temp 102°F with rebound tenderness or guarding
  - Clients with no improvement in 24–48 hours with treatment
- For diagnosis or treatment outside the midwife's scope of practice

Pelvic Pain, Chronic
Key Clinical Information

Chronic pelvic pain is a common finding in women's health and may be related to reproductive functioning, the bladder or bowels, or residual effects from previous infection or surgery of the abdomen or pelvis. Low-grade pelvic pain is not uncommon in women who have been subject to sexual assault or molestation. Ovarian cancer may present with vague pelvic symptoms. Client involvement and support during investigation of chronic pelvic pain is essential. Validation of the client's discomfort and concerns are needed as much as a skilled history, review of systems, and thorough physical examination.

Client History:
Components of the History to Consider

- Age
- Symptom profile
  - Location: radiating or fixed
  - Onset
    - Intermittent or constant
    - Relation to events
      - Pelvic infection
      - Sexual violence
      - Abortion
  - Duration and severity of symptoms
    - Precipitating factors
    - Relation to menses
  - Character of symptoms, such as
    - Crampy
    - Aching
    - Knifelike
  - Presence of associated symptoms
    - Fever and chills
    - Nausea and vomiting
    - Vaginal discharge
    - Change in bowel or bladder function
    - Weight loss
    - Dysparunia
- Relief measures used and client response
- Reproductive history
  - LMP
  - Number of births—vaginal and/or Cesarean
  - Last exam, Pap smear, and STI testing
  - History of
    - PID
    - Endometriosis
    - Ectopic pregnancy
  - New sexual partner for self or partner
- Medical/surgical history
  - Medications
  - Allergies
  - Health conditions
    - Diverticular disease
    - Renal calculi
  - Abdominal surgery
- Family history
  - Endometriosis
  - Dysmenorrhea
  - Ovarian cancer
  - Diverticular disease
  - Colon cancer
- Psychosocial history and status
  - Physical or sexual violence
  - Drug/ETOH use
  - Living situation
  - Mental health status
  - Affect and presentation
- Review of systems (ROS)

Physical Examination:
Components of the Physical Exam to Consider

- Vital signs
- Abdominal exam
  - Palpate for masses and/or pain
  - Note guarding or rebound tenderness
  - Auscultate bowel sounds
- Pelvic exam
- Speculum exam
  - Vaginal discharge
  - Bleeding
  - Cervical discharge or lesions

- Bimanual exam
  - Urethra
  - Cervical motion tenderness
  - Uterus: contour, position, or pain
  - Adnexa: size, mass, or pain
  - Fornices and posterior pelvis: mass or pain
  - Rectovaginal exam
  - Assess for
    - Cystocele
    - Rectocele
    - Enterocele
    - Uterine prolapse
- Rectal exam

Clinical Impression:
Differential Diagnoses to Consider

- Physiologic
  - Midcycle pain
  - Pelvic relaxation
- Infection
  - Chlamydia
  - Gonorrhea
  - Low-grade PID
  - Urinary tract infection
- Pelvic disorder
  - Endometriosis
  - Uterine fibroids
  - Chronic pelvic pain post-PID
  - Ovarian mass or cancer
  - Ectopic pregnancy
- Non-GYN pelvic disorder
  - Peritoneal adhesions
  - Hernia
  - Gastrointestinal cause
- Psychogenic pain

Diagnostic Testing:
Diagnostic Tests and Procedures to Consider

- Urinalysis
- Stool for occult blood
- Pregnancy testing
- Pap smear
- STI testing
- CBC, with differential
- CA 125 (postmenopausal clients)
  - Nonspecific
  - > 35 u/ml suspicious
  - May be elevated in premenopausal women
- Pelvic ultrasound

Providing Treatment:
Therapeutic Measures to Consider

- Symptom relief
  - Anti-inflammatory medications (NSAIDs)
    - Ibuprofen 600 mg tid x 5–7 days
    - Naproxen sodium 500 mg bid x 7–10 days
- Other treatments based on diagnosis

Providing Treatment:
Alternative Measures to Consider

- Local symptomatic relief measures
  - Heat
  - Positioning
  - Physical activity
- Dietary support
  - Well-balanced diet
  - Limit fatty foods, caffeine, and alcohol
  - Adequate fluid intake

Providing Support:
Education and Support Measures to Consider

- Discuss
  - Differential diagnosis
  - Recommendations for evaluation
  - Treatment options
- Encourage client to keep symptom and menstrual record
- Review danger signs, e.g., fever, acute pain, syncope
- Encourage client participation in evaluation process
  - Provide reassurance, comfort, active listening
  - Provide coping skills for living with chronic pain
- Provide information about community resources
  - Acupuncture
  - Expressive therapy
  - Support groups

Follow-up Care:
Follow-up Measures to Consider

- Document
- Return for continued care
  - At frequent intervals until pathology ruled in/out
  - 📞 Consider laparoscopic evaluation for diagnosis, prn
  - For support, prn if no pathology found

Collaborative Practice:
Criteria to Consider for Consultation or Referral

- OB/GYN service
  - Suspected endometriosis
  - Pain of suspected or documented pathologic origin

- Persistent low-grade pelvic pain unresponsive to therapy
- For signs of pelvic prolapse
- Mental health service
  - Pain with apparent psychogenic basis
- For diagnosis or treatment outside the midwife's scope of practice

Pelvic Inflammatory Disease

Key Clinical Information

Pelvic inflammatory disease (PID) is one of the most common and serious complications of STIs. PID is caused by bacteria that ascend from the vagina into the upper genital tract. The most common causative bacteria are gonorrhea and chlamydia; however, the normal flora of the genital tract may also cause PID. It is essential that the sexual partner(s) of women with suspected PID are treated before resumption of sexual activity. PID may cause significant scarring in the fallopian tubes as well as in the pelvis. Scarring may contribute to infertility, chronic pelvic pain, and other related disorders. Women with HIV are more likely to require hospitalization with PID (CDC, 2002).

Client History:
Components of the History to Consider

- Location, onset, duration, severity of symptoms
  - Common symptoms
    - Lower abdominal pain
    - Abnormal vaginal discharge
    - Dysparunia
  - Associated symptoms
    - Fever
    - Referred pain
    - Nausea and vomiting
    - Diarrhea
    - Malaise

- Reproductive history
  - LMP, G, P
  - Most recent Pap smear and STI testing
  - History of STIs
  - Current method of birth control
  - Sexual orientation and practices
  - New sexual partner for self or partner
  - Recent procedure, delivery, or termination of pregnancy
- Medical/surgical history
  - Allergies
  - Medications
  - Chronic illnesses
  - Previous surgery
- Social history
  - Drug or alcohol use
  - Living situation
- Review of systems (ROS)
- Risk factors for PID
  - Active infection with chlamydia or gonorrhea
  - Previous infection with STI
  - Sexually active adolescent
  - Intrauterine device (IUD)
  - Multiple sexual partners
  - Douching

Physical Examination:
Components of the Physical Exam to Consider

- Vital signs
- Abdominal exam
  - Lower abdominal tenderness
  - Guarding
  - Distention
  - Rebound tenderness
  - Presence or absence of bowel sounds
- Pelvic exam

- Speculum exam
  - Mucopurulent cervical discharge
  - Collection of cervical cultures
- Bimanual exam
  - Cervical motion tenderness
  - Uterine enlargement or tenderness
  - Adnexal mass or tenderness

Clinical Impression:
Differential Diagnoses to Consider

- Diagnostic criteria for PID (CDC, 2002)
  - Fever > 101°F, 38.3°C
  - Mucopurulent cervical or vaginal discharge
  - WBCs on wet mount of vaginal secretions
  - Elevated ESR
  - Elevated CRP
  - Positive testing for *N. gonorrhoeae* or *C. trachomatis*
- Genitourinary tract disorders
  - PID
  - Ectopic pregnancy
  - Ovarian cyst
  - Septic abortion
  - Endometriosis
  - Degenerating fibroids
  - Acute cystitis
- GI tract disorders
  - Acute appendicitis
  - Diverticulitis
  - Ulcerative colitis
  - Bowel obstruction

Diagnostic Testing:
Diagnostic Tests and Procedures to Consider

- Urinalysis
- Serum or urine HCG

- STI testing, including HIV
- CBC with differential
- Erythrocyte sedimentation rate (ESR)
- C-reactive protein (CRP)
- Gram stain and culture of cervical discharge
  - Presence of gram negative intracellular diplococci
  - > 10 WBC/hpf
- Pelvic ultrasound or MRI
  - Thickened fluid-filled tubes
  - Free fluid in pelvis
  - Tubo-ovarian complex
- 📞 Diagnostic laparoscopy

Providing Treatment:
Therapeutic Measures to Consider

- Choice and location of treatment varies with
  - Severity of illness
  - Anticipated client compliance
- Minimum treatment indications (CDC, 2002)
  - Uterine/adnexal tenderness
  - Cervical motion tenderness
- Outpatient treatment for PID (CDC, 2002)
  - Regimen A
    - Ofloxacin 400 mg po bid x 14 days, *or*
    - Levofloxin 500 mg po qid x 14 days, *with or without*
    - Metronidazole 500 mg po bid x 14 days
  - Regimen B
    - Cefoxitin 2 gm IM, *plus* probenicid 1G po, *or*
    - Ceftriaxone 250 mg IM, *PLUS*
    - Doxycycline 100 mg po bid x 14 days, *with or without*
    - Metronidazole 500 mg po bid x 14 days
- Hospital-based treatment (CDC, 2002)

- Treatment is continued until 24 hours after client improves clinically
- Oral antibiotics are given to provide 14 days of coverage
- Regimen A
  - Cefoxitin 2 gm IV q 6 hours, *or*
  - Cefotetan 2 gm IV q 12 hours, *plus*
  - Doxycycline 100 mg po or IV q 12 hours
    - po route preferred
- Regimen B
  - Clindamycin 900 mg IV q 8 hours, *plus*
  - Gentamycin
    - Loading dose (2mg/kg) IV or IM
    - Maintenance dose 1.5 mg/kg IV or IM q 8 hours

Providing Treatment:
Alternative Measures to Consider

- 💧 Alternative therapies are not a substitute for prompt medical care
- Comfort measures
  - Warm heat to abdomen
  - Adequate rest
- Remedies for healing and immune support
  - Balanced nutrition
  - Echinacea
  - Rescue Remedy
  - Visualization

Providing Support:
Education and Support Measures to Consider

- Provide information related to
  - Diagnosis
  - Treatment recommendations
    - Compete all medication
    - Avoid intercourse until

- Meds completed + 7 days
- Partner treated + 7 days
  - Test of cure as indicated
  ○ Mandatory STI reporting
  ○ Need to evaluate and/or treat partner(s)
- Provide written information
  ○ Medication instructions
  ○ Transmission of infection
  ○ Prevention of recurrence
    - Abstinence
    - Condom use
    - Mutual monogamy
    - Regular STI screening
  ○ Potential complications
    - Pelvic abscess
    - Infertility
    - Ectopic pregnancy
    - Chronic pelvic pain
  ○ Warning signs
  ○ When to return for care

Follow-up Care:
Follow-up Measures to Consider

- Document
- Outpatient therapy
  ○ Client contact within 24–48 hours
  ○ Hospitalization if limited improvement by 72 hours (CDC, 2002)
- For test of cure 4–6 weeks with diagnosis of
  ○ Chlamydia
  ○ Gonorrhea
- HIV testing if not done with initial workup

Collaborative Practice:
Criteria to Consider for Consultation or Referral

- OB/GYN service
  ○ Acutely ill women requiring hospitalization
  ○ Pregnant women with PID
  ○ Clients who do not improve within 24–72 hours of treatment
- For diagnosis or treatment outside the midwife's scope of practice

Premenstrual Syndrome

Key Clinical Information

Premenstrual syndrome or PMS is a common cyclical hormonal disorder that may manifest with physical or emotional signs and symptoms. Women who suffer from PMS frequently feel that they are not in control of their moods or actions. Treatment is aimed at finding relief measures that are acceptable to the individual woman and supporting her within the context of her life. Attention to lifestyle, diet, home life, and other life choices is an integral part of the assessment and treatment for PMS.

Client History:
Components of the History to Consider

- Age
  ○ Age 30–45 may have most severe symptoms
- Reproductive history
  ○ LMP, G, P
  ○ Review of last exam, Pap results, etc.
  ○ Menstrual history
    - Age at menarche
    - Years of menstruation
    - Timing of PMS in cycle
  ○ Methods of birth control use
  ○ Current stage of reproductive life
  ○ Age with onset of symptoms

- ▪ Occurs at times of "hormonal turbulence"
- Onset duration and severity of symptoms
- Symptom profile
  - ○ Emotional symptoms
    - ▪ Depression
    - ▪ Sadness
    - ▪ Aggression
    - ▪ Mood swings
    - ▪ Potential for harm to self or others
  - ○ Behavioral symptoms
    - ▪ May be related to decreased serotonin activity
    - ▪ Irritability, anger, panic attacks
    - ▪ Alcohol abuse, sweet cravings, binge eating
  - ○ Physical symptoms
    - ▪ Breast tenderness
    - ▪ Migraine
    - ▪ Water retention
    - ▪ Constipation
    - ▪ Joint and muscle pain
    - ▪ Lack of energy
    - ▪ Forgetfulness
    - ▪ Confusion
- Relief measures used and rate of success
- Medical/surgical history
  - ○ Allergies
  - ○ Medications
  - ○ Health conditions
    - ▪ Endocrine disorders
    - ▪ Heart disease, hypertension
    - ▪ Other medical conditions
- Psychosocial history and status
  - ○ Drug/ETOH, tobacco use
  - ○ Usual physical activity
  - ○ Diet review
  - ○ Social and family support
  - ○ Stressors
  - ○ Effect of PMS on daily living
    - ▪ Self-image
    - ▪ Relationships
    - ▪ Employment
- Review of systems (ROS)

Physical Examination: Components of the Physical Exam to Consider

- Age appropriate physical exam
  - ○ If none within previous 6–12 months
  - ○ With new onset of symptoms
  - ○ To update pertinent systems

Clinical Impression: Differential Diagnoses to Consider

- Premenstrual syndrome
- Premenstrual dysphoric disorder (PMDD)
- Perimenopausal changes
- Mood disorder
- Endocrine disorder

Diagnostic Testing: Diagnostic Tests and Procedures to Consider

- Premenstrual symptoms screening tool (PSST) (American Psychiatric Association, 1995)
  - ○ PMMD diagnosis
    - ▪ Symptoms only present during luteal phase
    - ▪ Symptoms occur most cycles
    - ▪ Confirmation of symptoms for at least two consecutive cycles
    - ▪ Five or more symptoms
    - ▪ At least one must be from the first four listed
  - ○ Symptoms
    - ▪ Depressed mood

- Tension
- Mood swings
- Irritability
- Decreased interest in usual activities
- Lack of energy
- Insomnia or hypersomnia
- Physical symptoms such as bloating and breast tenderness
- Difficulty concentrating
- Marked change in appetite
- Feeling overwhelmed

- Laboratory testing is based on age and findings on H & P
  - Thyroid panel
  - TSH
  - LH/FSH
  - Renal function testing
  - Hepatic function testing

Providing Treatment: Therapeutic Measures to Consider

- Combination hormone replacement therapy
  - Hormonal contraceptives
  - Estrogen/progesterone replacement
- Selective serotonin reuptake inhibitors (SSRI)
  - Fluoxetine (Sarafem) (Murphy, 2004)
    - 20 mg daily
    - Pregnancy category C
  - Sertraline (Zoloft)
    - 50 mg daily
    - Pregnancy category C
- Diuretic
  - Aldactone 25–100 mg
  - Use daily during luteal phase
- NSAIDS
  - Prostaglandin inhibitors

- Use during luteal phase
  - Mefenamic acid (Ponstel)
  - Naproxen sodium (Anaprox or Aleve)
- Vitamin and mineral supplementation
  - Calcium 400 mg qid
  - Magnesium 200–400 mg/day
  - Vitamin E 400 IU/day
  - Vitamin B_6

Providing Treatment: Alternative Measures to Consider

- Evening primrose oil 1000 tid mg daily (WholeHealthMD.com, 2000)
- Herbal balancing formula (for additional formulas, see *The Roots of Healing* [Soule, 1996, pp. 124–134])
  - Mix equal parts
    - Chamomile
    - Red raspberry leaf
    - Chasteberries (Vitex)
    - Prepare as tea or tincture
    - Use daily
- Diuretic formula for premenstrual phase of cycle
  - Dandelion leaf or root—2 parts
  - Stinging nettle—2 parts
  - Peppermint—1 part
  - Black cohosh—1 part
  - Mix and prepare as tincture (preferable) or tea
  - Use 10 gtts tincture tid, or tea morning and night
- Premenstrual depression
  - Saint-John's-wort
  - May alter effectiveness of hormonal birth control
- Homeopathic remedies

○ 30x tabs qid for acute symptoms

○ 100x pellets daily as constitutional remedy

○ Calcarea phos—general sense of weakness and fatigue accompanied by breast tenderness, genital sweating, and itching

○ Pulsatilla—for tears and anxiety, nausea, tension; menses are unpredictable

○ Sepia—symptoms of exhaustion, irritability, low back pain, decreased sex drive, anger, and intolerance

Providing Support: Education and Support Measures to Consider

• Reinforce need for

○ Excellent and balanced nutrition

○ Regular daily exercise

○ Personal time

• Discuss potential lifestyle changes

○ Reduce stress

○ Foster self-image and autonomy

○ Encourage family and friends to help

▪ Allow for personal time

▪ Shared responsibility

• Review menstrual cycle and function

• Explore fertility/sexuality issues

Follow-up Care: Follow-up Measures to Consider

• Document

• Client to keep symptom diary x 2+ cycles

○ Review symptoms

○ Plot on menstrual calendar

○ Differentiate between PMMD and depression

• Return for continued care

○ For symptom diary review

○ For persistent or worsening symptoms

○ For medication follow-up

○ For well-woman care

Collaborative Practice: Criteria to Consider for Consultation or Referral

• OB/GYN or medical service

○ For underlying medical or gynecological problem

• Mental health service

○ For mental health issues unrelated to PMS

○ Severe premenstrual dysphoric disorder

○ Client who is a danger to self or others

• Support groups/community resources

○ Music or art therapy

○ Dance

○ Women's groups

○ PMS support group

• For diagnosis or treatment outside the midwife's scope of practice

Syphilis

Key Clinical Information

Syphilis is a complex disorder with the following possible stages: *primary infection* (ulcer or chancre at infection site); *secondary infection* (rash, mucocutaneous lesions, and lymphadenopathy); *latent stage*, and *tertiary infection* (cardiac, neurologic, ophthalmic, auditory, or gummatous lesions). Early latent syphilis is when the illness has been acquired within one year, while late latent syphilis is when the disease was acquired more than one year previously, yet is still in the latent stage. Treatment is most successful when the disease is caught early. Perinatal transmission commonly results in development of congenital syphilis in the newborn (CDC, 2002).

Client History:
Components of the History to Consider

- Age
- Reproductive history
  - LMP, G, P
  - Perinatal losses
  - Last exam, Pap smear, and STI screen
  - Previous diagnosis or treatment of STIs
  - Sexual activity
  - Current method of birth control if not pregnant
  - Duration, onset, and severity of symptoms
- Medical/surgical history
  - Allergies
  - Medications
  - Chronic or acute health conditions
  - HIV status, if known
- Review of systems (ROS)
- Signs and symptoms of syphilis
- Primary syphilis
  - Chancre at site of infection
    - Develops 10–90 days postexposure
    - Single, painless sore
    - Raised edges
    - Lasts 1–5 weeks
    - Infection persists after chancre heals
- Secondary syphilis
  - Symptoms develop 2–28 weeks postexposure
  - Symmetric, macular, papular nonitchy rash
  - Condylomata lata
  - Mucous membrane lesions
  - Alopecia
  - Symptoms of systemic illness
    - Generalized malaise
    - Fever
- Latent phase
  - No clinical manifestations
  - Lasts 2–30 years after infection
  - Testing is essential
- Tertiary syphilis
  - Gumma development
  - Neurologic symptoms
    - Headache
    - Symptoms of CNS involvement
      - Auditory or visual symptoms
      - Paralysis
      - Mental illness
    - Cardiopulmonary symptoms
      - Shortness of breath
      - Hypertension

Physical Examination:
Components of the Physical Exam to Consider

- Vital signs, including BP and temperature
- Observe skin and soft tissue for signs of primary infection (Varney et al., 2004)
  - Alopecia
  - Generalized adenopathy
  - Rash
    - Palms and soles
    - Neck and head
    - Torso
  - Mucous membrane ulcers
- Cardiopulmonary assessment
  - Presence of murmur
  - Lung sounds
- Neurologic assessment
  - Cranial nerve abnormalities
  - Diminished reflexes
  - Change in personality
- Pelvic exam
  - Primary chancre

- Characteristic painless, firm ulcer
- Condylomata lata
  - Evaluation for signs of other STIs
  - Collection of specimens for testing

Clinical Impression:
Differential Diagnoses to Consider

- Syphilis
  - Primary
  - Secondary
  - Latent, (early or late)
  - Tertiary
- Acute bacterial infection
- Viral infections
- Mononucleosis
- Hansen's disease
- HPV-related condyloma

Diagnostic Testing:
Diagnostic Tests and Procedures to Consider

- RPR or VDRL titers
  - Positive 1–4 weeks after chancre
  - Positive VDRL or RPR
    - FTA-ABS or MHA-TP to confirm
      - FTA-ABS = fluorescent treponemal antibody absorbed
      - MHA-TP = microhemagglutination assay for antibody to *T. pallidum*
  - Test with diagnosis of any STI
- Chlamydia and gonorrhea testing
- HCG testing
- Hepatitis screen
- HIV counseling and testing
- Pregnancy RPR or VDRL
  - Initial prenatal visit
  - Repeat for high-risk population at

- 28 weeks gestation
- On admission for delivery
  - With diagnosis of any STI

Providing Treatment:
Therapeutic Measures to Consider

- CDC recommendations (CDC, 2002)
- Parenteral penicillin G is treatment of choice
  - Primary, secondary syphilis and early latent syphilis
    - Benzathine penicillin G
      - 2.4 million units IM as one time dose
      - In pregnancy may repeat dose in 7 days
  - PCN allergy
    - Desensitization to PCN recommended
    - Doxycycline 100 mg po bid x 14 days
      - Pregnancy category D
    - Tetracycline 500 mg po qid x 14 days
      - Pregnancy category D
- Late latent syphilis or syphilis of unknown duration
  - Benzathine penicillin G 7.2 million units total dose
    - Give IM as weekly doses of 2.4 million units
    - 3-week series
  - PCN allergy
    - Doxycycline 100 mg po bid x 28 days
      - Pregnancy category D
    - Tetracycline 500 mg po qid x 28 days
      - Pregnancy category D

Providing Treatment:
Alternative Measures to Consider

- Alternative measures are not a substitute for prompt antibiotic treatment
- General measures to promote healing

Providing Support: Education and Support Measures to Consider

- Reinforce need for sex partners to be tested (ASHA, 1995)
  - Partner exposed within 90 days may be infected yet seronegative
  - Partner exposed > 90 days should be treated presumptively while awaiting serology
- Time periods before treatment used for identifying at-risk partners
  - More than 3 months duration of symptoms for primary syphilis
  - More than 6 months duration of symptoms for secondary syphilis
  - 12 months for early latent syphilis
- Provide written
  - Prevention education information
  - Medication information and instructions
  - Information about STI reporting and contact follow-up
  - Written return visit information

Follow-up Care: Follow-up Measures to Consider

- Document
- Report as required for STIs
  - Disease diagnosis and treatment
  - Sexual contacts
- Return for continued care
  - As indicated during pregnancy
  - Reevaluate and retest
    - Primary or secondary syphilis: 6 and 12 months
    - Latent syphilis: 6, 12, and 24 months
    - HIV positive client: q 3 months x 2 year
  - Retreat for
    - Persistent symptoms

- Failure to have four-fold decline in nontreponemal test titers
  - HIV testing for treatment failures
- Observe for Jarisch-Herxheimer reaction
  - May occur within 24 hours after therapy for syphilis
  - Acute febrile reaction
  - Headache, myalgia, and other symptoms
  - Most common with early syphilis
  - May cause fetal distress or preterm labor

Collaborative Practice: Criteria to Consider for Consultation or Referral

- OB/GYN service
  - For acute illness with primary infection
  - Pregnancy complicated by syphilis
  - Jarisch-Herxheimer reaction
  - Treatment failures
- Medical service
  - For tertiary or neurosyphilis
- Pediatric service
  - Infants at risk for congenital syphilis
- For diagnosis or treatment outside the midwife's scope of practice

References

American Cancer Society [ACS]. (2005). Detailed guide: Endometrial cancer: What are the risk factors for endometrial cancer? Retrieved March 1, 2005, from http://www.cancer.org/docroot/CRI/content/CRI_2_4_2X_What_are_the_risk_factors_for_endo metrial_cancer.asp?sitearea=

American College of Obstetricians and Gynecologists [ACOG]. (1999a). Medical management of endometriosis [Practice bulletin #11]. In 2005 Compendium of selected publications. Washington, DC: Author.

ACOG. (1999b). Surgical alternatives to hysterectomy in the management of leiomyomas [Practice bulletin

#16]. In *2005 Compendium of selected publications.* Washington, DC: Author.

ACOG. (2000). Management of anovulatory bleeding [Practice bulletin #14]. In *2002 Compendium of selected publications.* Washington, DC: Author.

ACOG. (2001). Assessment of risk factors for preterm birth [Practice bulletin #31]. In *2002 Compendium of selected publications.* Washington, DC: Author.

ACOG. (2003). Breast cancer screening. [Practice bulletin #42]. In *2005 Compendium of selected publications.* Washington, DC: Author.

American Psychiatric Association. (1995). *Diagnostic and statistical manual of mental disorders* (4th ed.). Washington, DC: Author.

American Social Health Association [ASHA]. (2005). Learn about STIs/STDs: Syphilis: Questions and answers. Retrieved November 4, 2005, from http://www.ashastd.org/learn/learn_syphilis.cfm

Breast Cancer Care. (2003). Intraductal papilloma. Retrieved March 7, 2005, from http://www.breast-cancercare.org.uk/Breasthealth/Intraductalpapilloma

Burst, H. V. (1998). Sexually transmitted diseases and reproductive health in women. *Journal of Nurse-Midwifery, 43,* 431–444.

Centers for Disease Control and Prevention [CDC] (2000). Tracking the hidden epidemics 2000. Retrieved December 3, 2004, from http://www.cdc.gov/nchstp/od/news/RevBrochure1pdfcloselookHerpes.htm

CDC. (2002). Sexually transmitted diseases treatment guidelines 2002. Retrieved January 26, 2005, from http://www.CDC.gov/std/treatment/TOC2002TG.htm

CDC. (2004a). Increases in fluoroquinolone-resistant *neisseria gonorrhoeae* among men who have sex with men: United States, 2003, and revised recommendations for gonorrhea treatment, 2004. *Morbidity and Mortality Weekly Report, 53,* 335–338.

CDC. (2004b). STD facts: Genital herpes. Retrieved March 5, 2005, from http://www.cdc.gov/std/Herpes/STDFact-Herpes.htm

CDC. (2004c). Genital candidiasis. Retrieved March 5, 2005, from http://www.cdc.gov/ncidod/dbmd/diseaseinfo/candidiasis_gen_g.htm

CDC. (in press). Hepatitis B virus infection: A comprehensive immunization strategy to eliminate transmission in the United States. Retrieved March 3, 2005, from http://www.cdc.gov/ncidid/diseases/hepatitis/b/HBV_ACIP_Recs.pdf

Department of Health and Human Services [DHHS]. (2004). *Guidelines for the use of antiretroviral agents in HIV-1 infected adults and adolescents.* Washington, DC: Author.

Emmons, L., Callahan, P., Gorman, P., & Snyder, M. (1997). Primary care management of common dermatologic disorders in women. *Journal of Nurse-Midwifery, 42,* 228–253.

Ferenci, P., Dragosics, B., Dittrich, H., Frank, H., Benda, L., Lochs, H., et al. (1989) Randomized controlled trial of silymarin treatment in patients with cirrhosis of the liver. *Journal of Hepatology, 9,* 105–113.

Food and Drug Administration [FDA]. (2003). Public health advisory: Safety of topical lindane products for the treatment of scabies and lice. Retrieved March 7, 2005, from http://www.fda.gov/cder/drug/infopage/lindane/lindanePHA.htm

Foster, S. (1996). *Herbs for Your Health.* Loveland, CO: Interweave Press.

Gise, L. H., (1994). The premenstrual syndromes. In J. J. Sciarra (Ed.), *Gynecology and obstetrics* (pp. 1–14). Philadelphia: Lippencott-Raven.

Greenblatt, R. M., & Hessol, N. A. (2001). Epidemiology and natural history of HIV infection in women. In Anderson, J. (Ed.), *A guide to the clinical care with women with AIDS.* Retrieved March 3, 2005, from http://hab.hrsa.gov/publications/womencare.htm

Grube, W., & McCool, W. (2004). Endometrial biopsy. In H. Varney, J. M. Kriebs, & C. L. Gegor (Eds.). *Varney's midwifery* (4th ed.). Sudbury, MA: Jones and Bartlett.

Hepatitis C Technical Advisory Group. (2005). *Alternative therapies for hepatitis C.* National Hepatitis C Program Office. Retrieved March 6, 2005, from http://www.hepatitis.va.gov/vahep?page=tp03-03-07-01#note3

Mercksource.com (2002). Dorland's medical dictionary. W.B. Saunders. Retrieved March 4, 2005, from, http://www.mercksource.com/pp/us/cns/cns_hl_dorlands.jspzQzpgzEzzSzppdocszSzuszSzcommonzSzdorlandszSzdorlandzSzdmd_a-b_00zPzhtm

Mercksource.com (2003). Hepatitis. Retrieved March 4, 2005, from http://www.mercksource.com/pp/us/cns/cns_hl_adam.jspzQzpgzEz/pp/us/cns/content/adam/ency/article/001154.htm

Murphy, J. (1999). Preoperative considerations with herbal medicines. *AORN Journal, 75,* 173–181.

Murphy, J. L. (Ed.). (2004). *Nurse practitioner's prescribing reference.* New York: Prescribing Reference.

National Institutes of Health [NIH]. (2004). Uterine fibroids. Retrieved February 28, 2005, from http://www.nichd.nih.gov/publications/pubs/fibroids/index.htm

Niu, M. T., Stein, D. S., & Schnittman, S. M., (1993). Primary human immunodeficiency virus type 1 infection: Review of pathogenesis and early treatment interventions in humans and animal retrovirus infections. *Journal of Infectious Diseases, 168*, 1490–1501.

Nyirjesy, I., Billingsley, F. S., & Forman, M. R. (1998). Evaluation of atypical and low-grade cervical cytology in private practice. *Obstetrics & Gynecology, 92*, 601–607.

Payne, K. (2003). *Gonorrhea test.* Retrieved March 2, 2005, from http://my.webmd.com/hw/sexual_conditions/hw4905.asp

Saslow, D., Runowicz, C. D., Solomon, D., Moscicki, A. B., Smith, R. A., Eyre, H. J., et al. (2003). American Cancer Society guideline for the early detection of cervical neoplasia and cancer. *Journal of Lower Genital Tract Disease, 7*, 67–86.

Simpson, J., Dressler, L., Cobau, C._D., Falkson, C., Gilchrist, K., et al. (2000). Prognostic value of histologic grade and proliferative activity in axillary node-positive breast cancer: Results from the Eastern Cooperative Oncology Group Companion Study, EST 4189. *Journal of Clinical Oncology, 18*, 2059–2069.

Sinclair, C. (2004). *A midwife's handbook.* St. Louis: Saunders.

Smith, T. (1984). *A woman's guide to homeopathic medicine.* New York: Thorsons.

Soule, D. (1996). *The Roots of Healing.* Secaucus, NJ: Citadel Press.

Thompson, S. R., (2004). Nipple discharge. In *NIH Medline plus medical encyclopedia.* Retrieved March 7, 2005, from http://www.nlm.nih.gov/medlineplus/ency/article/003154.htm

University of Maryland Medical Center. (n.d.). Complementary therapy program herpes simplex. Retrieved March 3, 2005, from http://www. umm.edu/altmed/ConsConditions/HerpesSimplexViruscc.html

Varney, H., Kriebs, J. M., & Gegor, C. L. (Eds.). (2004). *Varney's midwifery* (4th ed.). Sudbury, MA: Jones and Bartlett.

Wang, C., & Celum, C. (2001). Prevention of HIV. In Anderson, J. (Ed.). *A guide to the clinical care of women with AIDS.* Retrieved March 3, 2005, from http://www.hab.hrsa.gov/publications/womencare.htm

WholehealthMD.com. (2000). Evening primrose oil. Retrieved March 15, 2005, from http://www.wholehealthmd.com/refshelf/substances_view/0,1525,779,00.html

Wright, T. C. Jr., Cox, J. T., Massad, L. S., Carlson, J., Twiggs, L. B., Wilkinson, E. J. (2002). 2001 Consensus guidelines for the management of women with cytological abnormalities. *Journal of the American Medical Association, 287*, 2120–2129.

Wright, V. C., & Lickrish, G. M., Eds. (1989). *Basic and advance colposcopy: A practical handbook for diagnosis and treatment.* Houston, TX: Biomedical Communications.

Bibliography

Barger, M. K. (Ed.). (1988). *Protocols for gynecologic and obstetric health care.* Philadelphia: W. B. Saunders.

Barton, S. (Ed.). (2001). *Clinical evidence.* London: BMJ.

Gordon, J. D., Rydfors, J. T., Druzin, M. L., & Tadir, Y. (1995) *Obstetrics, gynecology & infertility* (4th ed.). Glen Cove, NY: Scrub Hill Press.

MacLaren, A., & Imberg, W. (1998). Current issues in the midwifery management of women living with HIV/AIDS. *Journal of Nurse-Midwifery, 43,* 502–521.

Scott, J. R., DiSaia, P. J., Hammond, C. B., Gordon J. D., & Spellacy W. N. (1996). *Danforth's handbook of obstetrics and gynecology.* Philadelphia, PA: Lippincott-Raven.

Speroff, L., Glass, R. H., & Kase, N. G. (1999) *Clinical gynecologic endocrinology and infertility.* Philadelphia: Williams & Wilkins.

Winegardner, M. F. (1998, February 25). The atypical Pap smear: New concerns. *The Clinical Advisor,* 26–31.

Primary Care in Women's Health

9

Many midwives include primary care within their scope of practice. Skill in assessment and diagnosis of common primary care health problems enhances midwifery care, even when the midwife refers the client for treatment.

Women utilize health care services more often than men do. One goal of including primary care within midwifery practice is to increase the opportunities for midwives to provide education and support for women to make positive health choices. Many women only see a women's health provider during their reproductive years and may not have ready access to a primary care practitioner when illness occurs.

The practice guidelines in this section provide a brief overview of select primary care health conditions. The midwife is responsible for caring only for those conditions that are within her or his scope of practice but may opt to expand that scope with continuing education and experience. An experienced colleague with which to consult provides a safe basis for learning and optimal care for the midwifery client. The ability to assess general health problems and make appropriate referrals is valued by clients. Clients who have developed a trusting relationship with the midwife do not expect the midwife to provide comprehensive medical care but rather a problem-oriented referral to the provider that is best able to meet the clients' needs.

Care of the Woman with Cardiovascular Problems

Key Clinical Information

Heart disease is the most common cause of death in women. While most research about the prevention and treatment of heart disease has been performed using male subjects, the latest information from the American Heart Association (AHA) notes that 38% of women who have a heart attack will die within a year (American Heart

Association [AHA], 2004). Midwives, who are often accustomed to caring for essentially healthy women, must keep in mind the risk factors, signs, and symptoms of heart disease, hypertension, and stroke (Madankumar, 2003). Many women may be unaware that they have a problem until significant symptoms develop. Women with diabetes may additionally develop peripheral vascular problems. Clients should be encouraged to participate in a personal review of fixed and modifiable risk factors, and to identify lifestyle changes to decrease personal risk of coronary artery disease. Hypertension guidelines can be downloaded to a handheld device from http://hin.nhlbi.nih.gov/jnc7/jnc7pda.htm.

Client History: Components of the History to Consider

- Age
- Medical/surgical history
  - Allergies
  - Medications
    - Contraceptive hormones
    - Hormone replacement therapy
    - Aspirin
  - Health conditions
    - Diabetes
    - Hypertension
    - Dyslipidemia
    - Kidney disease
    - Cushing's syndrome
    - Thyroid or parathyroid disease
- Family history
  - Coronary artery disease (males < 55, females < 65)
  - Stroke
  - Hypertension
  - Diabetes
- Social history

- CVD rates are higher in (AHA, 2004)
  - African-American women
  - Other minority women
  - Drug and alcohol use
  - Tobacco use (cigarettes, snuff, chewing tobacco)
  - Support systems
  - Stressors
  - Usual coping methods
  - Daily physical activity
  - Usual diet
- Coronary heart disease (CHD) risk assessment (Pearson, et al., 2002; National Heart Lung and Blood Institute, 2003).
  - Begin assessment at age 20
  - Update CHD family history annually
  - Each visit assess
    - Tobacco use
    - Physical activity
    - Nutritional status
    - Alcohol intake
  - Every 2 years (min) assess
    - Blood pressure
    - Pulse
    - BMI
    - Waist circumference
  - Every 2–5 years, based on risk profile assess (National Heart Lung and Blood Institute, 2003)
    - Fasting serum lipids
    - Fasting blood glucose
    - 10-year global CHD risk estimation
      - Calculates risk based on
        - Age
        - Gender
        - Total cholesterol

- HDL cholesterol
    - Tobacco use
    - Systolic BP
  - Available at http://hin.nhlbi.nih.gov/atpiii/calculator.asp?usertype=prof
- Review of systems (ROS)
- Symptoms related to cardiovascular disorders
  - Headache
  - Chest pain
  - Palpitations
  - Shortness of breath with exertion
  - Syncope
  - Numbness or weakness
  - Peripheral and/or dependent edema
  - Nocturnal dyspnea
  - Nocturia

Physical Examination:
Components of the Physical Exam to Consider

- General inspection
  - Obesity, esp. abdominal fat
  - Signs of prior stroke/CVA
- Height, weight, and body mass index
  - BMI = weight lbs/height in^2 x 705
- Vital signs
  - BP goal of 140/90 (National Heart Lung and Blood Institute, 2003; Pearson, et al., 2002).
    - BP 130/85 in renal insufficiency or heart failure
    - BP 130/80 with diabetes
    - Measure supine and standing
    - Diagnosis of hypertension
      - 6–9 elevated BP readings over 2–3 visits
      - Persistent BP of 140/90 on more than one occasion
      - BP 160–170/105–110 on one occasion

- Persistent systolic BP of 140 or above
- Persistent diastolic BP of 90 or above
  - Pulses
    - Rate and rhythm
      - Atrial fibrillation
    - Bruits
    - Decreased pulsed in carotids or extremities
- Fundoscopic exam
- Chest
  - Contour
  - Respiratory rate and effort
    - Auscultate breath sounds
    - Use of accessory muscles
  - Cardiac evaluation
    - Auscultation of heart
    - Rate and rhythm
    - Presence or absence of
      - Murmur
      - Thrills
    - Palpation of heart
  - Percussion of chest
    - Left border cardiac dullness
- Skin and soft tissue
  - Color
    - Pallor
    - Cyanosis
    - Blanching
- Extremities
  - Capillary refill
  - Evaluation for nonhealing wounds/ulcers
  - Edema

Clinical Impression:
Differential Diagnoses to Consider

- Hypertension

- Dyslipidemia
- Coronary artery disease
- Valvular heart disease
- Diabetes mellitus
- Chronic obstructive pulmonary disease

Diagnostic Testing: Diagnostic Tests and Procedures to Consider

- CBC
- Urinalysis for protein, glucose
- Fasting serum lipid profile
  - Cholesterol < 200 mg/dl
  - HDL > 35 mg/dl, LDL < 130 mg/dl
  - Triglycerides < 200 mg/dl
- Chemistry profile
  - Potassium and sodium
  - Creatinine (> 1.3 mg/dl)
  - Fasting glucose (< 110 mg/dl)
  - Serum uric acid
  - Calcium (National Heart Lung and Blood Institute, 2003)
- Liver and renal function profiles
- ECG—12 lead
- Cardiac stress test
- Echocardiogram
- Pulmonary function testing

Providing Treatment: Therapeutic Measures to Consider

- 📞 Initiation of medical therapies
  - By primary care provider or referral specialist
  - As indicated by client condition
  - Per scope of practice/practice setting
- Hypertension (National Heart Lung and Blood Institute, 2003)

- ACE inhibitors
- Angiotensin receptor blockers
- Calcium channel blockers
- ß-blockers
- Thiazide-type diuretics
- Avoid estrogen with hypertension
- Elevated cholesterol
  - Statins
  - Niacin
  - Bile-acid binding resins
  - Fibrates
- Aspirin
  - Avoid with aspirin intolerance
  - Use low-dose 75–160 mg as preventive therapy

Providing Treatment: Alternative Measures to Consider

- 💣 Alternative measures are not a substitute for medical treatment in a client who does not have a favorable response with lifestyle changes
- 💣 Avoid herbs that may increase BP
  - Licorice
  - Ephedra
  - Ma huang
  - Bitter orange
- Measures to promote healing or well-being
  - Adequate rest
  - Nutritional support
    - Well-balanced diet
    - Vegetarian or whole foods diet
    - Fish oils
    - Garlic
    - Sea vegetables for minerals
  - Herbs (Foster, 1996)
    - Atherosclerosis

- Billberry promotes microcirculation
  - Hypertension
    - Garlic
    - Hawthorn
    - Reishi
  - High cholesterol
    - Garlic
    - Psyllium
- Exercise or physical activity
  - At least 10 minutes daily
  - Increase as tolerated to 30+ min/day (National Heart Lung and Blood Institute, 2003)
- Stress-reduction activities
  - Biofeedback
  - Relaxation techniques
  - Meditation or yoga
  - Support groups
  - Schedule personal time
- Review personal life goals

Providing Support:
Education and Support Measures to Consider

- Review AHA recommendations (Pearson, et al., 2002)
  - BP control
  - Weight management
    - BMI greater than 25
    - Waist circumference at iliac crest greater than 35″
  - Physical activity 30 minutes daily
    - Resistance training
    - Flexibility training
    - Aerobic activity
  - Tobacco cessation
  - Dietary recommendations

- Low-fat diet
  - Grains
  - Fruits, vegetables
  - Legumes, nuts
  - Lean meat
  - Low-fat dairy
  - Reduce
    - Saturated fats
    - Cholesterol
    - Trans-fatty acids
  - Limit alcoholic beverages to 1/day
  - Limit salt intake (National Heart Lung and Blood Institute, 2003)
  - Diabetes management
  - Treatment of chronic atrial fibrillation
- Provide information as applicable
  - Personal cardiac risk assessment
  - Potential cardiac risks of hormone use
  - Medication information
    - Correct dosing
    - Side effects
    - Anticipated benefits
  - Need for long-term treatment and follow-up
    - Referral system
    - Signs and symptoms that indicate need for
      - Emergency care
      - Prompt care
      - Referral
    - Return to office

Follow-up Care:
Follow-up Measures to Consider

- Document
- Return for continued care
  - As indicated by lab results
  - For support during

- ■ Smoking cessation (see smoking cessation)
- ■ Dietary and lifestyle changes
- ○ For reproductive health care
- ○ Hypertension
  - ■ For BP monitoring
  - ■ Evaluation of lifestyle changes
  - ■ Significant medication side effects
  - ■ Determination of need for referral for care
- ○ Dyslipidemias
  - ■ Serial evaluation of lipid profile
  - ■ Evaluation of lifestyle changes
  - ■ Medication side effects
  - ■ Determination of need for referral for care

Collaborative Practice:
Criteria to Consider for Consultation or Referral

- • Emergency service
  - ○ BP systolic > 200 or diastolic > 120
  - ○ Signs or symptoms suspicious for stroke or MI
- • Medical service
  - ○ For evaluation and/or treatment
  - ○ Suspected cardiovascular dysfunction
  - ○ Elevated lipid levels consistent with dyslipidemia
  - ○ Hypertension
  - ○ Diabetes
- • For diagnosis or treatment outside the midwife's scope of practice

Care of the Woman with Dermatologic Disorders

Key Clinical Information

Many illnesses and conditions may present with skin changes. Skin lesions may represent a local condition or be a manifestation of a viral infection such as rubella. A good dermatologic text with color photographs can be very handy for the midwife providing primary care. Many dermatologic disorders can be diagnosed by appearance. The exam should include areas inaccessible to self-examination, as this may yield additional information necessary to make an accurate diagnosis.

Client History:
Components of the History to Consider

- • Age
- • Medical/surgical history
  - ○ Allergies and sensitivities
  - ○ Current medications (especially recent onset of use)
  - ○ Chronic and acute conditions
  - ○ Previous surgery
  - ○ Previous skin conditions
- • Family history
  - ○ Melanoma
  - ○ Psoriasis
  - ○ Skin sensitivities
- • Onset, duration, severity of symptoms
  - ○ Location and distribution of lesions
  - ○ Characteristics of skin lesion(s)
  - ○ Associated factors/additional symptoms
    - ■ Fever/chills
    - ■ Nausea/vomiting
    - ■ Pain
    - ■ Swelling
  - ○ Remedies used and their effects
- • Potential exposures
  - ○ Infections
  - ○ Infestations
  - ○ Bites and stings
    - ■ Insects

- Snakes
- Spiders
- Jellyfish
  - Sun exposure
  - Chemicals, toxins
- Review of systems (ROS)

Physical Examination:
Components of the Physical Exam to Consider

- General physical exam, with focus on presenting complaint
- Vital signs, including temperature
- Thyroid
- Lymph nodes
- Systemic signs of disease
- Observation and palpation of the lesion(s) for
  - Location and distribution of lesion(s)
  - Size and number of lesion(s)
  - Symmetry of lesion(s)
  - Surface contour of lesions
    - Flat
    - Raised
    - Macular
    - Papular
    - Bullous
    - Annular
  - Margin characteristics
    - Geographic, irregular
    - Clear, smooth, linear
    - Blended
    - Raised
    - Rolled
    - Varied
  - Coloration of lesion(s)
    - Pigment color(s)
    - Patchy

- Confluent
  - Description of lesion(s)
    - Scaling
    - Crusting
    - Ulceration
    - Erosion
  - Presence of exudate
- Acne
  - Vulgaris and/or nodulocystic: Presents with comedones, inflammatory papules and pustules, erythema and scarring, lesions that are primarily facial, but may spread to back and shoulders
  - Rosacea: Chronic acneform conditions
    - Stage I: Persistent erythema with scattered telangiectases
    - Stage II: Symptoms of Stage I with papules, pustules, and prominent facial pores
    - Stage III: Persistent deep erythema, dense telangiectases, papules, pustules, and plaque-like edema ⇒ peau d'orange texture
  - Ophthalmic rosacea: Photophobia, conjunctivitis, iritis, and chronically inflamed eye margins (Emmons, et al., 1997)
- Bacterial infections
  - Cellulitis: Acute spreading lesion presenting with red, hot, tender skin and subcutaneous tissue, borders are irregular and raised due to edema
  - Impetigo: Acute purulent infection characterized by 1–3 cm denuded weeping area surrounded by honey-colored crust; erythematous halo suggests strep infection; large confluent lesions may occur
  - Abscesses: Such as furuncles, folliculitis, or carbuncles are characterized by local

cellulitis, regional lymphadenopathy, and formation of a fluctuant mass

- Lyme disease: Caused by a spirochete transmitted by minute ticks (Emmons, et al., 1997)
  - Stage I: Hallmark symptom is a "bull's-eye" lesion of 3–15 cm at the site of tick bite; flulike symptoms and lymphadenopathy may develop
  - Stage II: Severe fatigue, malaise as well as dermatologic, cardiovascular, musculoskeletal, and neurologic symptoms may develop
- Dermatitis
  - Contact: Erythema, may progress to scale and plaque formation or desquamation with moist epidermis and lacy border; associated symptoms include puritis, burning, stinging
  - Eczema (Atopic dermatitis): Intensely itching skin lesions characterized by erythema, papules, scaling, excoriations, and crusting; most commonly seen in the crease of elbow and knees, behind the ears, hands, and feet
  - Lichen simplex: Caused by persistent scratching of affected areas resulting in a chronic inflammation of the skin, characterized by itchy dry, scaling, lichenified plaques
- Infestations
  - Scabies: Lesions appear as gray or skin-colored linear or wavy ridges ending in a minute vesicle or papule, associated with severe itching
  - Pediculosis
    - Capitis: Puritis of scalp is primary complaint
    - Corporis: Puritis of shoulders, buttock, and belly is common
    - Pubis: Puritis of pubic area is primary complaint

- Viral infections
  - Rubella: Reddish-pink rash beginning on face and spreads to trunk
  - Herpes
    - *Herpes varicella:* Vesicular lesions that become ulcerated, then crust
    - *Herpes zoster:* Grouped vesicles with erythematous base that are along nerve path; lesions become pustular, then crust
    - *Herpes simplex:* Blisters and ulcerated sores may occur anywhere on body
  - Human papillomavirus
    - Common wart: Flat, flesh-colored papule on elbows, knees, fingers, and palms
    - Flat wart: Smooth, small, grouped lesions on hands, legs, face
    - Plantar wart: Small to large singular or grouped nodules on plantar surfaces of feet
    - Genital warts: Single or clustered flat or pedunculated nodules of the genital region, some varieties are microscopic
  - Mulluscum contagiosum: Dome-shaped papules with umbilicated centers and central waxy core
  - HIV-related skin disorders
    - Thrush: White plaques adherent to mucous membranes of the mouth, tongue, and throat, may cause tenderness
    - Hairy leukoplakia: Painless white plaque on lateral tongue borders
    - *Herpes simplex* and *Herpes zoster:* See above
    - Kaposi sarcoma: Malignant red to purplish macules, papules, and nodules commonly on legs, feet, or mouth; lesions may ulcerate and become painful
- Fungal infections
  - Tinea pedis: Scaling, fissures, and maceration between toes

- Tinea manuum: Scaling, papules and clustered vesicles, usually on dominant hand
- Tinea corporis: Sharply circumscribed annular lesions on trunk or extremities
- Tinea unguium: Brown or yellowish discoloration of nail, spreads under the nail
- Tinea versicolor: Scaly hypo- or hyperpigmented areas on trunk, arms, and neck

- Psoriasis
  - Plaque type: Characterized by deeply erythematous, sharply defined oval plaques; may have overlying silvery scale, puritis
  - Guttate: 1–2 cm papules, primarily seen on the trunk, puritis
  - Erythrodermic: Presents with generalized, intense erythema, puritis
  - Pustular: Sterile pustules 2–3 mm that coalesce then desquamate, puritis

- Skin cancer
  - Basal cell
    - Nodular: Pigmented or translucent nodular growth, may bleed, ulcerate, and appear to heal
    - Superficial: Pink or red scaly patches
  - Squamous cell: Flat red scaly patches that often form a crust
  - Malignant melanoma: Are pigmented lesions that often form from a preexisting mole or freckle; warning signs of melanoma include
    - Asymmetry of lesions shape
    - Border irregularity
    - Color variation: blue, black, brown
    - Diameter larger than 6 mm

Clinical Impression:
Differential Diagnoses to Consider

- Bacterial or viral infections

- Acne
- Psoriasis
- Infestations
- Exposure to irritants or toxins
- Allergic reaction
- Medication reactions
- Skin cancers
- Skin manifestations of systemic disease

Diagnostic Testing:
Diagnostic Tests and Procedures to Consider

- Wet prep of exudate
- Culture of lesions
  - Fungal—Dematophyte test medium
  - Bacterial—Routine culture, consider Gram stain
  - Herpes—Viral culture medium
- Skin biopsy
  - Punch biopsy
  - Excisional biopsy
  - Skin scraping
- Serology and titers
  - Rubella
  - RPR
  - HIV
- Testing for systemic disorders
  - TSH
  - ANA (Lupus)
  - Lyme titer

Providing Treatment:
Therapeutic Measures to Consider

- General relief measures
  - Acetaminophen
  - Ibuprofen

- Benadryl
- Topical aloe vera w/lidocaine
- Acne
  - Topical agents (Murphy, 2004)
    - Tretinoin—0.025 % cream or 0.01% gel, increase strength as tolerated and indicated
    - Benzoyl peroxide—Gel or wash 2.5–10%
    - Clindamycin phosphate—Gel, lotion, and solution
    - Erythromycin—Gel, ointment, or solution
    - Tetracycline (Topocycline)
  - Oral agents
    - Tetracycline 250–500 mg bid
- Acne rosacea
  - Erythromycin—Ointment or solution, apply bid
  - Metronizazole—Gel, apply bid
  - Ketaconazole 2%—Apply 1–2 x daily
  - Clindamycin phosphate
    - Gel, lotion, or solution
    - Apply bid
- Bacterial infections
  - Cellulitis: Requires prompt antibiotic therapy
    - Treat any underlying condition, e.g., tinea
    - Pen V 250–500 mg PO q 6 hours
    - Dicloxacillin 250–500 mg PO q 6 hours
    - Erythromycin 500 mg po q 6 hours
  - Impetigo: Topical *or* systemic antibiotics
    - Scrub with soap and water or Hibiclens
    - Apply topical mupirocin (Bactroban)
    - Oral therapy
      - Dicloxacillin 500 mg po qid
      - Ciprofloxin 500 mg po bid
      - Sulfa-trimethoprim DS 1 po bid

- Lyme disease, early diagnosis (Beers & Berkow, 2005)
    - Amoxicillin 500 mg po tid x 10–21 days (full 21 days for pregnancy)
    - Doxycycline 100 mg po bid x 10–21 days (not for use in pregnancy)
    - Cefuroxime axetil 500 mg BID 10–21 days
    - 📞 Refer for evaluation and treatment when symptomatic
- Dermatitis
  - Topical corticosteroid preparations (many other products are available)
    - Highest potency: Betamethazone dipropionate 0.05 % cream, ointment, or solution (Diprolene AF)
    - High potency: Flucinonide 0.05% cream, gel, ointment, or solution (Lidex)
    - Medium-high potency: Amcinonide 0.1% cream (Cyclocort)
    - Medium potency: Hydrocortisone valerate 0.2% ointment (Wescort)
    - Low potency: Triamcinolone acetonide 0.1% cream or lotion (Aristocort, Kenolog)
    - Mild potency: Desonide 0.05% cream (Tridesilon)
    - Lowest potency: Dexamethasone 0.1% gel (Decadron) (Murphy, 2004; Emmons, et al., 1997)
- Infestations (see Pediculosis)
- Viral infections
  - Herpes
    - Varicella: Symptomatic treatment
    - Zoster: Oral famciclovir, valacyclovir, or acyclovir
      - Immunosuppressed client 📞 IV Acyclovir 10 mg/kg q 8 hour for 7 days (Moon, 2005)
    - Simplex: (See Herpes simplex)

- HPV
  - Nongenital warts: Topical salicylic acid plaster, pad, solution
  - Genital warts: (see Human Papillomavirus)
  - Mulluscum contagiosum: Topical ablative therapy (TCA, BCA)
- Fungal infections
  - Topical agents
    - Allylamine—Apply to affected areas 1–2 x daily; pregnancy category B
    - Ciclopirox olamine—Apply to affected areas bid; pregnancy category B
    - Haloprogin—Apply to affected areas bid; pregnancy category B
    - Imidazole—Apply to affected areas 1–2 x daily; pregnancy category B
    - Tolnaftate—Apply bid; no pregnancy studies
    - Undecyclic acid—Apply to affected areas after bathing; no pregnancy studies
  - Oral antifungals (not recommended for pregnancy)
    - Griseofulvin—250–500 mg bid x 2 weeks–12 months based on indication
    - Ketaconazole—200–400 mg daily for 3–18 months based on indication
    - Itraconazole—200 mg daily for 3 months, or 200 mg bid x 7 days monthly x 2–4 months (Murphy, 2004; Emmons, et al., 1997)

Providing Treatment: Alternative Measures to Consider

- Measures to promote healing and foster immune response
  - Well-balanced diet
  - Avoid alcohol, spicy foods, hot drinks
  - Adequate rest
  - Exposure to light and air (unless contraindicated by medication use)
  - Limit occlusive skin coverings
- Symptomatic relief
  - Itching
    - Cool colloidal oatmeal baths
    - Herbal wash
      - Chamomile
      - Calendula
      - Aloe
      - Lemon balm
- Acne
  - Vitamin and mineral supplements
    - Vitamin B6 50 mg/D
    - Vitamin E 200–400 IU/D
    - Zinc 30–50 mg/D
  - Omega-3 oils: Flaxseed, fish oils
  - Herbal extract of sarsaparilla, yellow dock, burdock, and cleavers (Wong, n.d.)
  - Ti tree oil applied topically
  - Homeopathics (Holisticonline.com, n.d.)
    - Itching with acne: Kali bromatum 6 x tid
    - Pus-filled pimples: Antimonium tartaricum 6 x tid
    - Rough sweaty skin: Sulfur 6 x tid
- Dermatitis
  - Nutritional support
    - Elimination diet to identify contributing factors
    - Vitamin E 200–400 IU/day
    - Zinc 30–50 mg/day
    - Omega-3 oils: Flaxseed, fish oils
  - Stress management
    - Yoga or other planned physical activity
    - Hypnotherapy (Kantor, 1990)
- Tinea (Ledezma, et al., 1996; Tong, et al., 1992)

- Nutritional support
  - Limit simple carbohydrates/sugars
  - Beta-carotene 15,000 IU/D
  - Vitamin C 1000 mg/D
  - Garlic: Orally, or topically applied to affected area
- Vinegar solution soaks
- Ti tree oil applied topically
- Allow ventilation of affected area(s)
- Homeopathics
  - Sepia
  - Graphites

Providing Support:
Education and Support Measures to Consider

- Provide information regarding
  - Working diagnosis
  - Testing recommendations
  - Relief measures
  - Skin care
  - Care of contacts, as applicable
  - Prevention methods
  - Warning signs and symptoms
  - Treatment plan options
  - Medication instructions
- Instructions to return for care
  - As indicated by diagnosis, *or*
  - If condition worsens or recurs

Follow-up Care:
Follow-up Measures to Consider

- Document
- Return for continued care
  - Persistent or worsening symptoms
  - Medication reaction(s)

Collaborative Practice:
Criteria to Consider for Consultation or Referral

- Medical service
  - Skin lesions accompanied by fever, malaise, or other constitutional symptoms
  - Initial diagnosis of HIV infection, or evidence of progressive disease
  - Documented or suspected systemic illness, e.g., Lyme disease, Lupus, etc.
- Dermatologist service
  - Care of chronic dermatologic conditions
  - Treatment of resistant acne with isotretinoin
  - Suspected or biopsy-proven skin cancer
- For diagnosis or treatment outside the midwife's scope of practice

Care of the Woman with Endocrine Disorders

Key Clinical Information

The endocrine system regulates and affects nearly all body systems. Disruption within the endocrine system may cause a multitude of symptoms that often initially appear unrelated. Therefore, during evaluation of women's health problems the impact of the endocrine system on symptom development must be considered. Women are more likely than men to be affected by endocrine disorders. Menstrual dysfunction may be the only presenting complaint or there may be other evidence of an endocrine disorder, such as rapid hair loss, development of a noticeably enlarged thyroid, or the pigment changes associated with adrenal insufficiency.

Client History:
Components of the History to Consider

- Age
- Medical/surgical history
  - Allergies

- Current medications
  - Many drug classes affect thyroid function
- Chronic conditions
- Surgeries
- Previous complaints or problems
- Family history
  - Chronic and acute conditions
  - Endocrine disorders
- Reproductive history
  - LMP, G, P
  - Menstrual history
  - Potential for pregnancy
  - Method of birth control
- Social history
  - Nutrition and activity patterns
  - Sleep patterns
  - Life stresses
    - Living situation
    - Drug or alcohol use
    - Domestic violence
- Recent symptoms
  - Onset, duration, severity
  - Description
  - Contributing or mitigating factors
  - Self-help measures used and results
  - Effect of symptoms on client
- Review of systems (ROS)
- Signs and symptoms of endocrine disorders
  - Hypothyroid
    - Lethargy, malaise
    - Cold intolerance
    - Weight gain
    - Menorrhagia, amenorrhea
    - Depression, irritability, apathy
  - Hyperthyroid

- Nervousness
- Anxiety
- Heat intolerance
- Diplopia
- Shortness of breath
- Weakness
- Oligomenorrhea
- Hyperparathyroid
  - Asymptomatic, or
  - General vague symptoms
    - Fatigue
    - Anorexia
    - Weakness
    - Arthralgia
    - Polyuria
    - Constipation
    - Nausea and vomiting
    - Mental disturbance
- Hypoparathyroid
  - Parasthesias of hands, feet, and circumoral area
  - Mental and emotional status, derangement
  - Lethargy
- Hypopituitary
  - Failure to lactate
  - Symptoms associated with
    - LH and FSH deficiency
    - TSH deficiency
    - ATCH deficiency
- Hyperpituitary
  - Amenorrhea
  - Galactorrhea
  - Infertility, decreased libido, vaginal dryness
  - Hirsutism

- Headache, visual field changes due to tumor impingement
  - Diabetes mellitus
    - Polydipsia
    - Polyuria
    - Polyphagia
    - Weight loss
    - Blurred vision
    - Parasthesias
    - Fatigue
  - Hypofunction of adrenal cortex
    - Fatigue and weakness
    - Anorexia, nausea, and vomiting
    - Cutaneous and mucosal hyperpigmentation
    - Weight loss
    - Hypotension
    - Abdominal pain, constipation, and diarrhea
    - Salt craving
    - Syncope
    - Personality changes and irritability
  - Hyperfunction of adrenal cortex
    - Thick body, thin extremities, round face
    - Cervicodorsal and supraclavicular fat pads
    - Thin fragile skin, easy bruising, poor wound healing
    - Acne, hirsutism
    - Hypertension
    - Hyperglycemia (Payton, et al., 1997)

Physical Examination: Components of the Physical Exam to Consider

- Complete physical exam including vital signs
- Physical findings
  - Hypothyroid
    - Signs may be subtle

- Cool, pale, tough, dry skin
- Hoarse, husky voice
- Bradycardia, cardiomyopathy, pericardial effusion
- Anemia
- Cerebellar ataxia
- Goiter
- Thinning, brittle hair
  - Hyperthyroid
    - Tremors
    - Weight loss
    - Exophthalmos
    - Sweating
    - Palpitations, tachycardia, atrial fibrillation
    - Warm, moist skin
    - Lid lag
    - Goiter, diffuse or nodular
    - Brisk reflexes
    - Thyroid bruit
  - Hyperparathyroid
    - Weakness
    - Arthralgia
    - Polyuria
    - Renal calculi
  - Hypoparathyroid
    - Increased neuromuscular excitability, muscle cramps, tetany
    - Cataract development
    - Abnormalities of skin, hair, teeth, and nails
  - Hypopituitary
    - Evaluation of visual fields
    - Neurologic exam
  - Hyperpituitary
    - Observe for symptoms of hypogonadism
  - Diabetes mellitus
    - Obesity, or recent weight loss

- Signs of fungal vulvovaginitis
- Fruity odor to breath
  - Hypofunction of adrenal cortex
    - Cutaneous and mucosal hyperpigmentation
    - Weight loss
    - Hypotension
    - Syncope
    - Personality changes and irritability
  - Hyperfunction of adrenal cortex
    - Thick body, thin extremities, round face
    - Cervicodorsal and supraclavicular fat pads
    - Thin fragile skin, easy bruising, poor wound healing
    - Acne, hirsutism
    - Hypertension
    - Hyperglycemia (Payton, et al., 1997)

Clinical Impression: Differential Diagnoses to Consider

- Menstrual dysfunction
  - Polycystic ovary syndrome
  - Hypothalamic dysfunction
  - Pituitary dysfunction
- Thyroid disorder
  - Hypothyroid
  - Hyperthyroid
  - Thyroid tumor
- Adrenal dysfunction
- Diabetes mellitus
- Other endocrine disorder

Diagnostic Testing: Diagnostic Tests and Procedures to Consider

- General evaluation
  - Urinalysis
  - Chemistry profile
- Thyroid testing
  - Hypothyroidism TSH $\Downarrow$
  - Hyperthyroid TSH $\Downarrow$, T4 $\Downarrow$, or T3 $\Downarrow$ with normal T4
  - Thyroid antibodies positive in patients with autoimmune disorders of thyroid
- Parathyroid Disorders
  - Abnormal serum calcium, usually found incidentally on chemistry screening
  - Hyperparathyroid
    - Serum calcium $\Downarrow$ (> 10.5 mg/dl)
    - Serum phosphate $\Downarrow$ (< 2.5 mg/dl)
    - Elevated serum parathyroid hormone (PTH) levels confirm diagnosis
  - Hypoparathyroid
    - Serum calcium $\Downarrow$ (< 8.8 mg/dl)
    - Serum phosphate $\Downarrow$ (> 4.5 mg/dl)
    - Low or absent parathyroid hormone (PTH) levels confirm diagnosis
  - Pituitary
    - Hypopituitary
      - ACTH
      - TSH
      - T4
      - FSH and LH
      - Estradiol
      - Prolactin
      - Electrolytes
      - BUN and creatinine
      - CT scan or MRI of sella turcica
  - Hyperpituitary
    - HCG
    - Serum prolactin levels (> 300 mg/ml = prolactinoma [nonpregnant])
- Disorders of glucose metabolism
  - Fasting blood sugar

- > 126 gm/dl diagnostic for DM

- > 110 gm/dl < 126 gm/dl = abnormal glucose metabolism

- 70–110 gm/dl = normal glucose metabolism (Payton, et al., 1997)

- Evaluation of adrenal function

  - Consider referral for testing and evaluation

Providing Treatment:
Therapeutic Measures to Consider

- Initiation of medical therapies by diagnosis

- Maintenance by midwife in consultation with PCP

Providing Treatment:
Alternative Measures to Consider

- Alternative measures may restore balance but are not a substitute medical care

- General measures to promote well-being

  - Emotional support

  - Balanced nutrition

    - Avoid simple carbohydrates

    - Maintain optimal BMI

  - Adequate rest

  - Regular physical activity

    - Balance with nutritional intake

    - Helps regulate blood glucose

  - Stress reduction

- Sea vegetables

  - Trace minerals

  - Iodine

- Blue green algae

- Bilberry

  - Improves microcirculation in diabetes (Foster, 1996)

Providing Support:
Education and Support Measures to Consider

- Provide information regarding diagnosis

  - Potential effects on client, family, reproductive capacity

  - Testing recommendations

  - Signs and symptoms indicating a need to return for care

  - Recommended follow-up

  - Local resources

- Listen to and address client concerns

Follow-up Care:
Follow-up Measures to Consider

- Document

  - Individualized plan in record

    - Follow-up testing—Type and frequency

    - Medications—Type, dose, titration parameters

    - PCP or physician notification parameters

- Work with client's primary care provider to

  - Develop management recommendations

  - Delineate individualized best care parameters

  - Delegate ongoing and follow-up care

- Return for continued care as indicated for

  - Support

  - Reproductive health care

  - Ongoing surveillance of endocrine disorders

  - Care of select problems in medically stable client

Collaborative Practice:
Consider Consultation or Referral

- Medical or endocrinology service

  - Clients with evidence of endocrine dysfunction

- Relevant workup
- Initiation of treatment
- Collaborative care of endocrine disorders
- Ongoing care of endocrine disorders
  - Clients with confusing presentation
- Reproductive endocrinology
  - Endocrine-related infertility
- Social support services
  - Support groups
    - Diabetes
    - Infertility
- For diagnosis or treatment outside the midwife's scope of practice

Care of the Woman with Gastrointestinal Disorders

Key Clinical Information

Problems of the gastrointestinal tract may range from simple nausea to the presence of obstructing colon cancer. Inquiry into usual bowel function is an essential component of the client history. GI symptoms may present as a signal of a GI disorder or as a sign or symptom of an endocrine, reproductive, or nervous system disorder. Many women react to stress with GI symptoms such as nausea, diarrhea, or "butterflies in the stomach." Social history may reveal a psychosocial component to GI disorders.

Client History: Components of the History to Consider

- Age
- Medical/surgical history
  - Allergies
  - Current medications
    - Aspirin
    - NSAID

- Antibiotics
- Laxatives, fiber, stool softeners
- Antidiarrheals
  - Chronic and acute conditions
    - Diverticulitis
    - Gall bladder disease
    - Peptic ulcer disease
  - Past surgical history
    - Cholecystectomy
    - Oopherectomy
    - Appendectomy
- Reproductive history
  - LMP, G, P
  - Menstrual status
  - Potential for pregnancy
  - Method of birth control
  - Last exam, Pap, and STI testing, as applicable
- Current symptoms
  - Description
  - Location, onset, duration
  - Severity
  - Associated symptoms
  - Exacerbating or alleviating factors
  - Self-help measures used and effectiveness
- GI history
  - Usual diet
  - Eating patterns
  - Elimination patterns
  - Pica
- Family history
  - Ulcers
  - Diverticular disease
  - Gastroesophogeal reflux disorder
  - Colon cancer
- Social history

- Living situation
- Travel to or habitation in areas with intestinal parasites
- Stresses
- Drug, ETOH, and tobacco use
- Support systems
- Effect of symptoms on daily living

- Review of systems (ROS)

Physical Examination:
Components of the Physical Exam to Consider

- Vital signs including weight
- General physical exam with focus directed by history
- Observe for evidence of endocrine dysfunction
- HEENT
  - Examination of mouth and throat
    - Presence and condition of teeth
    - Presence and size of tonsils
    - Ability to swallow
  - Palpate thyroid
- Thorax and chest
  - Auscultation of heart and lungs
  - CVAT
- Abdominal exam
  - Inspection for shape, symmetry, pulsations
  - Auscultation for bowel sounds, bruits
  - Percussion
  - Palpation, light and deep
    - Pain
    - Rigidity
    - Guarding
    - Rebound tenderness
    - Masses
- Bimanual abdominopelvic exam
  - Pain
  - Masses
- Rectal exam

Clinical Impression:
Differential Diagnoses to Consider

- Upper GI disorders
  - Lactose intolerance
  - Dyspepsia
  - Hiatal hernia
  - *H. pylori* infection
  - Gastroesophogeal reflux disorder
  - Gastroenteritis
  - Peptic ulcer disease
- Lower GI disorders
  - Irritable bowel syndrome
  - Diverticulitis
  - Chronic constipation
  - Diarrhea related to laxative use
  - Colitis
  - Bowel obstruction
  - Intestinal parasites
  - Hemorrhoids
- OB/GYN disorders
  - PID
  - Pregnancy
  - Ectopic
- Other disorders with GI symptoms
  - Pica
  - Gallbladder disease
  - Cholelithiasis
  - Pancreatitis
  - Hepatitis
  - Endocrine dysfunction
  - Malignancies
- Abdominal pain, unknown etiology

Diagnostic Testing:
Diagnostic Tests and Procedures to Consider

- CBC with peripheral smear
- ESR (erythrocyte sedimentation rate)
- *H. pylori* testing
- Urinalysis or urine culture
- Chlamydia and/or gonorrhea cultures
- Wet prep
- HCG
- Stool testing
  - Occult blood
  - Ova and parasites
  - Culture
- Liver function testing
- Hepatitis screen
- Amylase and lipase levels
- CA-125
- Endoscopy
  - Upper endoscopy
  - Sigmoidoscopy
  - Colonoscopy
- Ultrasound
  - Pelvic
  - Gallbladder and pancreas
- CT of abdomen

Providing Treatment:
Therapeutic Measures to Consider

- Treatment based on differential diagnosis
- H2 receptor antagonists
  - Cimetadine (Tagamet)—400 mg bid or 800 mg qhs
  - Ranitidine (Zantac)—150 mg bid or 300 mg qhs
  - Famotidine (Pepcid)—20 mg bid or 40 mg qhs

- Nizatidine (Axid)—150 mg bid
- Omeprazol (Prilosec)—20 mg daily (Murphy, 2004)
- Antimicrobial treatment for *H. pylori* infection (CDC, 2001)
  - Regimen 1
    - Omeprazole 40 mg QD, plus
    - Clarithromycin 500 mg TID x 2 weeks, then
    - Omeprazole 20 mg QD x 2 weeks
  - Regimen 2
    - Bismuth 15 ml qid x 2 weeks
    - Metronidazole 500 mg tid
    - Tetracycline 500 mg tid
  - Regimen 3
    - Lansoprazole 30 mg BID, plus
    - Amoxicillin 1 g BID, plus
    - Clarithromycin 500 mg TID x 10 days (CDC, 2001)
- Healing agents
  - Sucralfate (Carafate)
    - 1 g tab ac and hs
    - 1–2 g bid to prevent recurrence
  - Misoprostol
    - 100–200 mcg qid w/meals and hs
    - Not for use in pregnancy (Murphy, 2004)
- Laxatives
  - Bulk forming agents: Metamucil, Fiberall, Perdiem
  - Emolients: Docusate products
  - Saline derivatives: Magnesium, sodium, or potassium salts
  - Lubricants: Mineral and olive oil products
  - Hyperosmotics: Glycerin suppositories
  - Stimulants: Aloe, cascara sagrada, danthron, senna
- Antidiarrheal medications

- Opiates: Paregoric, codeine
- Absorbents: Polycarbophil
- Antiperistaltics: Loperamide, diphenoxylate
- Antiemetics
  - Antihistamines: Promethizine, cyclizine, meclizine
  - Phenothiazines: Compazine, sparine, Tigan (Murphy, 2004)

Providing Treatment: Alternative Measures to Consider

- ⚠ Alternative therapies are not a substitute for medical evaluation of acute symptoms
- Diarrhea
  - Increase fiber to regulate fluid balance in stool
  - Bearberry or uva-ursi (not recommended in pregnancy)
  - Bilberry
- Constipation
  - Increase fiber and fluids
  - Cascara sagrada—10 gtts fluid extract, stimulates bowel function
  - Psyllium seed—Increases bulk to stool
  - Senna—Use sparingly, very effective, but may cause cramping
- Reflux
  - Chamomile tea
  - Papaya enzyme tablets with meals and hs
  - Hazelnuts with meals and hs
  - Goldenseal—Pinch of powdered root or tincture 10 gtts tid
  - Licorice tincture or standardized products; use for 4–6 weeks max.

Providing Support: Education and Support Measures to Consider

- Hydration

- Drink ample fluid
- Limit caffeine and alcohol intake
- Lactose intolerance
  - Limit all dairy products
  - Check labels for dairy in packaged products
- Fiber intake; high-fiber foods
  - Peas, beans, and lentils
  - Fresh and dried fruit
  - Uncooked vegetables
  - Whole grain breads and cereals
- Physical activity
  - 20 minutes daily stimulates bowels
- Provide information related to
  - Working diagnosis
  - Testing recommendations
  - Recommended medications and treatment
  - Anticipated results
  - Side effects
  - Warning signs and symptoms
  - Referral criteria and mechanism

Follow-up Care: Follow-up Measures to Consider

- Document
- Return for continued care
  - As indicated by test results
  - 7–14 days if no improvement
  - Follow-up of chronic problems
  - Worsening signs or symptoms

Collaborative Practice: Criteria to Consider for Consultation or Referral

- Emergency service
  - Acute abdomen
  - Intestinal obstruction
- Medical service

- Confirmed or suspected
  - Gall bladder disease
  - Colorectal malignancy
  - GI bleeding
- For GI problem unresponsive to therapy within 7–21 days
- OB/GYN service
  - Ovarian cancer
  - Ectopic pregnancy
  - Hyperemesis gravidarum
  - Hydatidiform mole
- For diagnosis or treatment outside the midwife's scope of practice

Care of the Woman with Mental Health Disorders

Key Clinical Information

While midwifery assessment of mental health conditions may include diagnosis and treatment of mild self-limiting disorders, it is assumed that all women with ongoing psychiatric problems will be referred to a mental health professional for further evaluation and treatment. Active listening is a crucial part of the midwifery assessment process, and it places the midwife in a prime position to evaluate the mental well-being of each woman who comes to her for care. As with other health issues, a strong network of referral options is beneficial in directing women to the type of care that best meets their needs.

Client History: Components of the History to Consider

- Chief complaint, in client's own words
- History of current problem
  - Symptoms
    - Onset, duration
    - Precipitating factors
  - Client's feelings of danger to self or others

- Suicide attempts or ideation
- Expectations for care
- Mental health status
  - Description and theme of mood
    - Effect on daily life
    - Delusions
    - Paranoia
    - Suicidal ideation; thoughts, plans, intent, means
  - General cognitive status
    - Orientation
    - Memory
    - Attention
    - Abstract thinking and reasoning
    - Speech patterns
    - Thought processes; e.g., organization and content
  - Previous diagnosis or treatment
- Reproductive history
  - LMP, current menstrual status
  - G, P, children at home
  - Losses, as applicable
  - Current method of contraception
- Medical and surgical history
  - Allergies
  - Current medications
    - Hormones
    - Antidepressants
    - Analgesics
    - Other meds
  - Medical conditions
    - Viral infection
    - Endocrine problems
    - Chronic pain
    - Chronic fatigue
    - Multiple sclerosis

- Cancer
  - Previous surgery
- Social history
  - Cultural background
    - Effect on primary complaint
    - Social stigma related to seeking help
    - Cultural variations in symptoms presentation
  - Family and community support systems
  - Alcohol, drug, or tobacco abuse
  - Emotional, sexual, or physical abuse
  - Employment or financial status
  - Life stresses
- Related family history
  - Mental illness
  - ETOH or drug abuse/addiction
  - Chronic illness
  - Loss of a loved one
- Review of systems (ROS)

Physical Examination:
Components of the Physical Exam to Consider

- Vital signs, wet
- Mental status assessment
  - Posture
  - Mood
  - Body language and movements
  - Personal hygiene and dress
  - Cooperation, participation, eye contact
  - Affect
- Physical manifestations of mental health issues
  - Tics, agitation
  - Diminished affect
  - Slow speech
  - Obsessive/compulsive behaviors
  - Auditory or visual hallucinations

- Low BMI
- Evaluate for physiologic basis of symptoms
  - Thyroid
  - Cardiopulmonary status
  - Neurologic functioning
  - Reproductive (hormonal) systems

Clinical Impression:
Differential Diagnoses to Consider

- Affective disorders
- Eating disorders
- Personality disorders
- Psychosis or schizophrenia
- Alzheimer's disease
- Endocrine dysfunction, e.g., thyroid, diabetes, adrenal
- Hormonal dysfunction, e.g., PMS, perimenopause, postpartum depression
- Excessive caffeine or stimulant use
- Substance abuse
- Hypoxia due to cardiac, respiratory, or other pathology
- Neurologic disorder, e.g., encephalopathy or seizure disorder

Diagnostic Testing:
Diagnostic Tests and Procedures to Consider

- Evaluate for physical disorder based on
  - History
  - Physical exam
- Labs
  - Electrolytes
  - Toxicology
  - TSH
  - FSH, LH

- Evaluate for symptoms of mental/emotional disorders
  - ⊙ 🔵 Use appropriate screening tools
    - Age appropriate
    - Developmentally appropriate
    - Culturally appropriate
  - Clinician resource: National Institute of Mental Health
    - http://www.nimh.nih.gov/healthinformation/index.cfm
    - Phone: Toll free (866) 615-6464 or (301) 443-4513
- Affective (mood) disorders
  - Depression (NIMH, 2000a)
    - Depressed mood
    - Diminished interest in all activities
    - Weight loss/gain
    - Insomnia/hypersomnia
    - Psychomotor agitation/retardation
    - Fatigue or loss of energy
    - Feelings of worthlessness or guilt
    - Inability to concentrate
    - Recurrent thoughts of death: suicidal ideation, plan, or intent
  - Mania
    - Decreased need for sleep
    - Rapid or "pressured" speech
    - Distractibility
    - Flight of ideas
    - Increased goal-directed activity
    - Inflated self-esteem or grandiosity
    - Engagement in risk-taking behaviors
  - Bipolar disorders
    - Symptoms of depression and mania
    - Symptoms alternate
- Anxiety disorders
  - Generalized anxiety disorder
    - General anxiety about "everything"
  - Panic disorder
    - Subjective symptoms of panic attack
      - Tightness in the chest or throat
      - Difficulty breathing without evidence of obstruction
      - Dry mouth
      - Trembling
      - Palpitations
    - Physical symptoms of panic attack
      - Elevated BP, tachycardia, tachypnea
      - Restlessness, trembling, exaggerated startle response
      - Pallor, sweating, erythema, cold, and clammy hands
      - Vomiting, loss of bowel or bladder control
  - Phobias
    - Irrational fear out of proportion to stimulus
  - Obsessive/compulsive disorder
    - Persistent recurrence of
      - Intrusive thoughts (obsessions)
      - Ritualized behaviors (compulsions)
  - Post-traumatic stress disorder
    - Development of symptoms following a significant traumatic event
    - Symptoms include
      - Flashbacks to the event
      - Emotional numbing to external stimuli
      - Autonomic, cognitive, and dysphoric symptoms
- Eating disorders
  - Bulimia
    - Preoccupation with weight and food intake

- Feelings of being out-of-control related to food intake
- Binge eating
- Purging
- Fasting
- Overexercising
- Laxative or diuretic abuse
  - Anorexia nervosa
    - Preoccupation with weight and food intake
    - Focus on control of food intake
    - Loss of more than 15% of body weight
    - Amenorrhea for at least 3 consecutive cycles
    - Denial
    - Self-repulsion
    - Distortion of body image
- Personality disorders
  - Person with a set of inflexible and maladaptive character traits
  - Ingrained patterns of perceiving and relating to others and environment
  - Classifications
    - Cluster A: Paranoid, schizoid, schizo-typical
    - Cluster B: Histrionic, narcissistic, antisocial, and borderline
    - Cluster C: Avoidant, dependent, obsessive/compulsive, and passive aggressive
- Psychoses (thought disorders)
  - Presence of two or more of the following within a 1 month period
    - Delusions
    - Auditory hallucinations
    - Disorganized speech

- Grossly disorganized or catatonic behavior
- Negative symptoms, e.g., flat affect or psychomotor retardation (NIMH, 2000b)

Providing Treatment: Therapeutic Measures to Consider

- Interactive psychotherapy
  - Individual or group counseling
  - Art therapy
  - Music therapy
  - Expressive therapy
- Consider HRT for new onset mild mental health dysfunction in perimenopausal or menopausal women with no precipitating events (see Hormone Replacement Therapy)
- Commonly prescribed medications by class
  All have potentially serious side effects—check profile before prescribing and against client symptoms/presentation; *When in doubt, consult*
- Antidepressants
  - Selective serotonin reuptake inhibitors (SSRI)—May cause ⇓ libido
    - Prozac 10–60 mg/d
    - Paxil 10–30 mg/d
    - Zoloft 25–150 mg/d
    - Tricyclic—Long history of use
    - Elavil 50–200 mg/d
    - Tofranil 50–150 mg /d
    - Pamelor 50–150 mg/d (Murphy, 2004)
- Monoamine oxidase inhibitors (MAOI) *not recommended for CNM Rx*
  - Nardil 15–90 mg/d
  - Parnate 10–30 mg/d (Murphy, 2004)
- Other antidepressants
  - Wellbutrin 150–450 mg/day

- ○ Desyrel 200–400 mg/day
- ○ Serzone 50–500 mg/d (Murphy, 2004)
- • Anxiolytics and Hypnotics
  - ○ Benzodiazepines
    - ▪ Xanax 0.5–6 mg/d, half life 6–20 hours
    - ▪ Klonapin 0.5–8 mg/d, half life18–50 hours
    - ▪ Valium 2–60 mg/d, half life 30–100 hours (Murphy, 2004)
  - ○ Other
    - ▪ Buspar 10–40 mg/day
    - ▪ Atarax 200–400 mg/day
    - ▪ Ambien 5–10 mg/day (Murphy, 2004)
- • 📞 Mood stabilizers
  - ○ Lithium carbonate 600–1800 mg/day
  - ○ Lithium carbonate slow-release 450–1350 mg/day
  - ○ Lithium citrate 10–30 ml/day (Murphy, 2004)
- • 📞 Anticonvulsants (used as mood stabilizers)
  - ○ Tegretol 400–1200 mg/day
  - ○ Depakene/Depakote 500–1250mg/day (Murphy, 2004)
- • 📞 (Neuroleptics (antipsychotics)
- • 🗝 Medication use by diagnosis
  - ○ Affective (mood) disorders
    - ▪ Depression
      - • Antidepressants for
        - ○ ⇓ mood
        - ○ Sleep dysfunction
        - ○ Obsessive self-flagellation
      - • Anxiolytics if anxiety also present
    - ▪ Bipolar disorders and mania
      - • Mood stabilizers (lithium and anticonvulsants)
  - ○ Anxiety disorders
    - ▪ Anxiolytics for acute and chronic anxiety or panic

- ▪ Antidepressants for panic attacks, phobias, or OCD
- ○ Post-traumatic stress disorder
  - ▪ Antidepressants for depression or obsessive thoughts or behaviors
  - ▪ Anxiolytics for panic, general anxiety, or mild paranoia
  - ▪ Antipsychotics for
    - • Agitation
    - • Anxiety if anxiolytics have poor response or contraindicated
    - • For persistent paranoid thinking
- ○ Eating disorders
  - ▪ Antidepressants for mood disorder and obsessive thinking
  - ▪ Anxiolytics if anxiety present
  - ▪ Antipsychotics if thinking is delusional
- ○ Psychoses (thought disorders)
  - ▪ 📞 Neuroleptics (antipsychotics) referral for Rx

Providing Treatment: Alternative Measures to Consider

- • Warm, loving, safe environment
- • Herbal or homeopathic support for *minor* mood disorders
  - ○ Anxiety
    - ▪ Hops
    - ▪ Kava-kava
    - ▪ Passion flower
    - ▪ Reishi
    - ▪ Valarian
  - ○ Depression
    - ▪ Chamomile
    - ▪ Lemon balm
    - ▪ St.-John's-wort
- • Hormonal effects

- ○ Dong quai
- ○ Black cohosh
- ○ Evening primrose
- Support groups
  - ○ Women's groups
  - ○ Bereavement support
  - ○ Related to other medical diagnosis (e.g., breast cancer support)
  - ○ Religious

Providing Support:
Education and Support Measures to Consider

- Engage client in self-care (NIMH, 2000)
  - ○ Set attainable goals
    - ▪ Set priorities
    - ▪ Break large tasks into small ones
    - ▪ Assume a tolerable amount of responsibility
  - ○ Be with other people when able
  - ○ Participate in activities that may improve mood
    - ▪ Mild exercise
    - ▪ Going to a movie, a ballgame, etc.
    - ▪ Participating in religious, social, or other activities
  - ○ Expect mood to improve gradually
  - ○ Postpone important decisions until improvement occurs
  - ○ Practice positive thinking
  - ○ Let family and friends help
- Provide information related to community resources
  - ○ Health education services
  - ○ Support groups
  - ○ Crisis hotline number(s)
  - ○ Women with abusive partners

- ▪ Safety planning
- ▪ How to access safe-housing
- ▪ Effects of medications on ability to be vigilant
- ○ Women with medical treatment and/or referral
  - ▪ Medication
    - • Name
    - • Dosing instructions
    - • Indication
    - • Desired effects
    - • Potential side effects
    - • Interactions
    - • Pregnancy category (prn)
  - ▪ Referral information and goal of referral
  - ▪ Midwifery plan for continued care
- Signs and/or symptoms indicating need for
  - ○ Return for care
  - ○ Immediate care
  - ○ Emergency care

Follow-up Care:
Follow-up Measures to Consider

- Document
- Verify client compliance with referral(s)
- Provide, as appropriate
  - ○ Support and education related to diagnosis
  - ○ Treatment
    - ▪ Counseling
    - ▪ Continuing medication use
  - ○ Routine women's health care and contraception prn

Collaborative Practice:
Consider Consultation or Referral

- Mental health service

- Psychiatric emergency
  - Suicidal or homicidal ideation
  - Psychosis
  - Need for hospitalization
- Symptoms that suggest a complex psychiatric disorder
- Failure to respond to medication or prescribed treatment
- Formal psychotherapy indicated or requested
- Emergency service
  - Potential life-threatening drug reaction
- Social services
  - Concomitant substance abuse
  - Persistent psychosocial problems
  - Counseling
  - Nontraditional therapy options
- For diagnosis or treatment outside the midwife's scope of practice

Care of the Woman with Musculoskeletal Problems

Key Clinical Information

The midwife may assess for musculoskeletal conditions during a college, sports, or school physical, prior to a client beginning a vigorous exercise program, or as the result of new-onset symptoms. The two most frequently diagnosed musculoskeletal problems diagnosed in women are osteoarthritis and back strain. Rheumatoid arthritis occurs two to three times more often in women than in men. Lupus and fibromyalgia also occur more frequently in women. Lupus is three times more common in African-American women than in Caucasian women.

Client History: Components of the History to Consider

- Primary indication for visit
- Evaluation of symptoms

- Location
  - Unilateral vs. bilateral
  - Symmetric
  - Joint vs. muscle
- Onset
  - Precipitating factors
  - Mechanism of injury
  - Gradual vs. sudden
  - Effect of time of day/weather
- Duration
  - Chronic vs. acute
  - Constant vs. intermittent
- Severity of symptoms
- Relief measures used and their effects
  - OTC or Rx meds
  - Heat/ice
  - Rest
  - Compression
- Symptoms of possible tumor or infection
  - Atypical pain
  - Fever
  - Chills
  - Weight loss
- Medical/surgical history
  - Age (consider client's life stage)
  - Allergies
  - Current medications
  - Last tetanus diptheria immunization
  - History of GI upset, or bleeding with prior NSAID use
  - Osteoporosis risk (see Osteoporosis)
- Family history
  - Osteoarthritis
  - Osteoporosis
- Social history

- ○ ⊛ Ethnic heritage
- ○ Physical activity patterns
- ○ Nutritional status
- ○ Physical abuse/neglect
- ○ Physical exertion/strain related to
  - ▪ Job, child care
  - ▪ Hobby
  - ▪ School
  - ▪ Sports
- ○ Drug or ETOH use
- • Review of systems (ROS)
- • Common symptoms of arthritis (National Institute of Arthritis and Musculoskeletal and Skin Diseases, 2002)
  - ○ Swelling in one or more joints
  - ○ Joint stiffness that lasts over 1 hour on arising
  - ○ Constant or recurring pain or tenderness in a joint
  - ○ Difficulty using or moving a joint normally
  - ○ Warmth and redness in a joint

Physical Examination: Components of the Physical Exam to Consider

- • Vital signs, including temperature
- • Evaluate for neurovascular status of tissues distal to site of injury
- • Evaluate affected area for
  - ○ Heat, redness, or swelling
  - ○ Range of motion, crepitus, clicks
  - ○ Muscle tension or limitation
- • Palpation
  - ○ Tenderness
  - ○ Point tenderness
  - ○ Soft tissue spasm
  - ○ Mass
- • Neurological assessment

- ○ Strength/weakness
- ○ Muscle wasting
- ○ Sensation
- • Vascular assessment
  - ○ Color
  - ○ Pulses
  - ○ Capillary refill
- • Presence or absence of
  - ○ Ecchymosis
  - ○ Hematoma
  - ○ Limb or joint deformity

Clinical Impression: Differential Diagnoses to Consider

- • Osteoarthritis
- • Back strain
- • Physical abuse
- • Joint strain or sprain
- • Malignancy or tumor
- • Infection
- • Systemic disorders (e.g., multiple sclerosis)
- • Vascular disease
- • Peripheral neuropathy and/or radiculopathy
- • Fracture

Diagnostic Testing: Diagnostic Tests and Procedures to Consider

- • Bone mineral density testing
- • Anticipated NSAID administration > 3 months
  - ○ Baseline testing
    - ▪ Liver function
    - ▪ Platelets
- • Inflammatory process vs. infection
  - ○ CBC w/differential
  - ○ Erythrocyte sedimentation rate (ESR)

- ○ C-reactive protein (CRP)
- ○ Creatinine
- Evaluation of mass
  - ○ Ultrasound
  - ○ X-ray
  - ○ CT
- Bony tenderness, with night pain
  - ○ 📞 Referral for diagnostic evaluation

Providing Treatment:
Therapeutic Measures to Consider

- NSAIDs are frequently the first line of therapy
  - ○ Naproxen sodium
  - ○ Ibuprofen (Kriebs & Burgin, 1997)
- Muscle relaxants
  - ○ 💣 Be alert for drug seekers c/o chronic pain
  - ○ Equagesic—Musculoskeletal pain with anxiety
    - ▪ Dose: 1–2 tablets tid or qid
    - ▪ Short-term use only
  - ○ Flexeril—Muscle spasm
    - ▪ Dose: 10 mg tid; max 60 mg daily
    - ▪ Limit use to 21 days or less
  - ○ Robaxin—Painful musculoskeletal conditions
    - ▪ Dose: 1.5 mg qid x 2–3 days m
    - ▪ Maintenance: 4 gm daily in divided doses (Murphy, 2004)
- Sprain or strain
  - ○ Air cast (ankle)
  - ○ Compression bandage
  - ○ Splinting
  - ○ Consider physical therapy
- Fibromyalgia
  - ○ Trial of SSRI antidepressants (see Mental Health Disorders)

Providing Treatment:
Alternative Measures to Consider

- Rest of affected area
- Ice to affected area for first 24 hours followed by heat
- Elevation of affected area when possible
- For soft tissue injury
  - ○ Comfrey leaf compresses
  - ○ Homeopathic arnica montana
  - ○ Massage therapy
  - ○ Hydrotherapy
- Activities to maintain flexibility, balance, and strength
  - ○ Yoga
  - ○ Dance
  - ○ Pilates
  - ○ Resistance training
  - ○ Swimming
- Arthritis
  - ○ Extremely low-fat diet (5 gm day)
    - ▪ May decrease pain, swelling, and progression of disease
  - ○ Planned exercise programs
    - ▪ Range of motion: Swimming, dance
    - ▪ Strengthening: Resistance training, weight lifting
    - ▪ Aerobic and endurance: Walking, bicycling
  - ○ Chondroitin and/or glucosamine
  - ○ Heat and cold therapy
  - ○ Use of assistive devices

Providing Support:
Education and Support Measures to Consider

- Provide information related to diagnosis
  - ○ Review mechanism of injury, as applicable
  - ○ Evaluation and treatment recommendations

○ Provide exercise recommendations

- Limitations and restrictions

- Range of motion

- Strengthening

- Aerobic and endurance

○ Long-term sequelae

- Chronic pain may result in depression

- Changes in ADL, range of motion

- Warning signs

○ Medication information

• Teach/reinforce proper body mechanics

○ Wide base of support

○ Avoid reaching, twisting, hands over head

Follow-up Care:
Follow-up Measures to Consider

• Document

• Return for continued care

○ prn within 7–14 days

○ If problem worsens or persists

○ Depression related to chronic pain syndrome(s)

○ prn for medication management

Collaborative Practice:
Criteria to Consider for Consultation or Referral

• Orthopedic service

○ Following limited results from treatment for

- Bursitis

- Tendonitis

- Carpal tunnel syndrome

- Sprain or strain

- Knee effusion

- Epicondylitis

○ Osteoporotic and other fractures

• Podiatric or orthopedic service

○ Bunion

○ Plantar fasciitis

○ Morton's neuroma

• Rheumatology service

○ Suspected or diagnosed arthritis

○ Suspected fibromyalgia (Kriebs & Burgin, 1997)

• Physical or occupational therapy

○ Evaluation of body mechanics

○ Strength training

○ Ergonomic training

• Mental health service

○ Chronic pain syndromes

○ Depression related to diagnosis

• Neurologic service

○ Herniated disc

○ Suspected multiple sclerosis

• Persistent back pain, without evidence of pathology consider referral to

○ Osteopath

○ Chiropractor

○ Acupuncturist

○ Neurologist

• For diagnosis or treatment outside the midwife's scope of practice

Care of the Woman with Respiratory Disorders

Key Clinical Information

The most common respiratory disorders seen in primary care include sinusitis, bronchitis, asthma, and chronic cough. However, less common problems such as TB, pneumonia, and respiratory malignancies should also be kept in mind. Lung disease affects women of all ages, and is a common cause of illness and death. Lung function may be affected by allergies, air quality, and environmental toxins such as cigarette smoke, chemical fumes, or particulate matter. The primary presenting complaint in the woman with metastatic cancer to the lungs is cough. Women with HIV/AIDS may present with *Pneumocystis carinii*, or drug-resistant tuberculosis.

Client History: Components of the History to Consider

- Primary complaint
  - Symptom review
    - Onset, duration, severity of symptoms
      - Cough
      - Sputum production
      - Color of sputum/nasal discharge
      - Shortness of breath
      - Difficulty with respiration; wheezing
      - Frontal headache
      - Fever and/or chills
    - Other symptoms
      - Weight loss
      - Night sweats
      - Malaise
      - Loss of appetite
      - Weakness
      - Bloody sputum
  - Relief measures used and their effects
- Medical and surgical history
  - Allergies
  - Medications
  - Medical conditions
    - Heart disease
    - Respiratory disease
      - Asthma
      - COPD
      - Emphysema
      - Sinus infection(s)
      - Pneumonia
      - Cystic fibrosis
      - Cancer
    - Exposure to asthma triggers
      - Allergens
      - Irritants
      - Drugs
      - Exercise or cold air
    - HIV status, if known
- Social history
  - Increased risk of lung disease in (American Lung Association, 2004a, 2004b, 2004c, 2004d)
    - African-Americans
      - Asthma
      - Occupational lung disease
      - HIV-related lung disease
    - Hispanic
      - Tuberculosis
      - HIV-related lung disease
    - Native Americans
      - Asthma
      - Cystic fibrosis
      - Tuberculosis
      - Lung cancer
    - Alaskan Natives
      - Tuberculosis
      - Lung cancer
    - Asian Americans
      - Tuberculosis
  - IV drug, alcohol, or tobacco use
  - Exposure to respiratory irritants
  - Living conditions
  - Nutritional status
- Review of systems (ROS)

Physical Examination:
Components of the Physical Exam to Consider

- Vital signs
- Color
  - Pallor
  - Rubor
  - Cyanosis
- Respiratory evaluation
  - Rate and pattern of breathing
  - Depth and symmetry of lung expansion
  - Auscultation
    - Quality and intensity of breath sounds
    - Adventitious breath sounds
      - Pneumonia
        - Crackles
      - Asthma
        - Diffuse wheezes or rhonchi
        - Prolonged expiratory phase
  - Percussion
    - Resonant—Normal, asthma or interstitial lung disease
    - Dull—Consolidation or pleural effusion
    - Hyperresonant—Emphysema or pneumothorax
- Evidence of respiratory distress
  - Nasal flaring
  - Intercostal or supraclavicular retractions
  - Peripheral cyanosis
  - Elevated pulse and respiratory rate
  - Grunting or wheezing

Clinical Impression:
Differential Diagnoses to Consider

- Asthma
- Bronchitis
- Chronic cough, due to
  - Smoking
  - Postnasal drip
- Work-related exposure to inhaled irritants
- Sinusitis
- HIV/AIDS
- Community-acquired pneumonia or bronchitis
- Respiratory malignancies

Diagnostic Testing:
Diagnostic Tests and Procedures to Consider

- Chest X-ray
  - Fever plus abnormal breath sounds
  - Suspicion of tuberculosis
- Gram stain and culture of purulent sputum
  - Suspected pneumonia
- HIV counseling and testing
- Pertussis serology
  - Afebrile client
  - Normal breath sounds
  - Cough > 2 weeks duration
- Pulse oximetry and blood gases
- Peak flow or spirometry to assess
  - Lung function
    - Restrictive
    - Obstructive
  - Progression of disorder
    - Severity
    - Medication effectiveness
- Sinus X-rays
  - Chronic cough
- Tuberculosis testing (American Thoracic Society, 1999)
  - TB Mantoux (PPD)
    - 0.1 ml injected intradermally
    - 2 step procedure indicated for select groups

- PPD interpretation—mm of induration considered positive
  - ≥ 5 mm
    - HIV-infected patients
    - Close contact of newly diagnosed patient with active TB
    - Scars on X-ray suggest prior healed active TB
  - ≥ 10 mm
    - Immigrants from areas with endemic TB prevalence
    - Low-income and/or medically underserved
    - IV drug users
    - Chronic illness or exposure that may increase risk of contracting TB
    - Infants and young children
  - ≥ 15 mm
    - No known risk factors for TB

Providing Treatment: Therapeutic Measures to Consider

- Community-acquired pneumonia or bronchitis
  - Erythromycin 250–500 mg qid x 10 days (pregnancy category B)
  - Azithromycin 500 mg on day 1, then 250 mg q day x 4 additional days (pregnancy category B)
  - Sulfa-trimethoprim 1 DS tablet BID x 10 days (third trimester of pregnancy only)
  - Amoxicillin—Clavulanic acid 250–500 tid x 10 days
  - Cefuroxime 250–500 mg bid x 10 days (Clarke & Paine, 1997)
- Asthma
  - Bronchodilators (fast acting for acute attacks)
    - Albuterol
      - Inhaled β-agonist
      - 2 puffs q 4–6 hours prn
    - Ipratroprium
      - Anticholinergic
      - 3–6 puffs q 6 hours
    - Metaproterenol
      - Inhaled β-agonist
      - 2 puffs q 4–6 hours prn
    - Salmeterol and fluticazone (Advair)
      - Inhaled long-acting β-agonist and steroid
      - 2 puffs q 12 hours
  - Anti-inflammatory medications
    - Decrease airway edema and secretions
    - Beclomethosone
      - Inhaled steroid
      - 2–5 puffs qid
    - Cromolyn sodium
      - Mast-cell stabilizer
      - 2–4 puffs qid
    - Flunisolide
      - Inhaled steroid
      - 2–4 puffs bid
  - Leukotriene modifiers
    - Accolate
    - Singulair
    - Zyflow (Murphy, 2004)
- Bronchitis
  - Cough suppressants
  - Antibiotics generally not indicated, unless pneumonia is suspected
  - Albuterol inhaler (afebrile but diffuse abnormal breath sounds)
    - 2 puffs q 4 hours prn
- Pertussis—Suspected or confirmed

- Erythromycin 1 gm/day in divided doses x 14 days
- Sulfa-trimethoprim DS 1 po bid x 14 days
- Chronic cough
  - Treatment based on definitive diagnosis
- Tuberculosis
  - 📞 See CDC guidelines for treatment of tuberculosis
    - http://www.cdc.gov/nchstp/tb/default.htm

Providing Treatment:
Alternative Measures to Consider

- General measures to promote healing
  - Rest, adequate nutrition
  - Increase fluid intake, especially hot liquids
  - High-protein, high-calorie diet
  - Use positioning to aid drainage of secretions
- Saline nasal irrigation daily (National Jewish Medical and Research Center, 2003)
- Herbal remedies
  - Marshmallow
  - Echinacea (not for use in immunocompromised clients)
  - Licorice
    - Contraindicated with
      - Pregnancy
      - Hypertension
      - Heart or liver disease
- Astragalus (safe for those with immune disorders) (Foster, 1996)

Providing Support:
Education and Support Measures to Consider

- Provide information and recommendations
  - Diagnosis
  - Medication regimen(s)

- Dosage, frequency
- Potential side effects
- Indications for cough suppressants
  - Signs of improvement
    - Symptoms diminish within 1–3 days
    - Afebrile within 2–5 days (pneumonia)
  - Warning signs and symptoms, such as
    - Persistent cough
    - Fever with chills
    - Bloody sputum
    - Shortness of breath
  - Environmental controls
    - Pets/allergens
    - Air conditioning
    - Mask or respirator
  - Limitations, such as
    - Isolation from family
    - Decreased activity

Follow-up Care:
Follow-up Measures to Consider

- Document
- Return for continued care
  - Contact within 7–10 days (phone or visit)
  - As indicated by test results
  - Symptoms persist or worsen in spite of therapy
  - Persistent symptoms at revisit, reevaluate for asthma

Collaborative Practice:
Criteria to Consider for Consultation or Referral

- Medical service
  - Respiratory illness requiring hospitalization
  - Symptoms of respiratory distress
    - Respiratory rate ≥ 30

- Superclavicular or intercostal retractions
- O_2 saturation of < 95%
- Cyanosis
  - Diagnosis of
    - Tuberculosis
    - Pertussis
    - *Pneumocystis carinii*
    - Pneumonia
    - HIV/AIDS
- For diagnosis or treatment outside the midwife's scope of practice

Care of the Woman with Urinary Tract Problems

Key Clinical Information

Urinary tract problems include bladder infections, pylonephritis, renal lithiasis, incontinence issues, and structural problems such as cystocele. Urinary tract problems may create significant discomfort for the woman, whether it be physical, emotional, or social. Many women restrict their activities due to urinary frequency or fear of incontinence. Often women do not address the issue of incontinence with their midwife or health care provider out of embarrassment or the belief that it is an expected consequence of aging. Thoughtfully worded questions during the history may encourage discussion of this problem and exploration of potential solutions.

Client History: Components of the History to Consider

- Urinary history
  - Frequency, volume, and timing of voids
  - Changes in lifestyle related to urinary tract
  - Genital hygiene habits
  - Onset, duration, type, and severity of symptoms
    - Incontinence

- Urgency or frequency
- Flank pain and/or dysuria
- Fever and chills
- Malaise
- Relief measures used and results
  - Previous urinary tract infection or problem
- Risk factors for UTI
  - New sex partner or multiple partners
  - More frequent or intense intercourse
  - Diabetes
  - Pregnancy
  - Use of irritating products
    - Skin cleansers
    - Diaphragms and spermicides
  - Blockage in the urinary tract
  - History of UTIs (Bromberg, 1998)
- Urge incontinence
  - Characterized by involuntary bladder contractions
  - May be neurologic or caused by irritant
- Stress incontinence
  - Occurs when intra-abdominal pressure is greater than urethra's closing pressure
  - May be worsened by
    - Childbearing, regardless of mechanism of birth
    - High-impact activities
    - Heredity
    - Atrophy
- Mixed incontinence
  - Stress and urge incontinence
- Overflow incontinence
  - Obstruction
  - Detruser muscle dysfunction
  - Urethral torsion
- Iatrogenic incontinence

- ○ Surgical scarring or trauma
- ○ Medications (Rovner & Weine, 2000)
- Reproductive history
  - ○ G, P, LMP
  - ○ Vaginal or Cesarean births
  - ○ STIs
  - ○ Sexual activity
    - ■ Anal/vaginal intercourse
    - ■ Lubrication
    - ■ Sex toys
  - ○ Vasomotor symptoms
- Medical/surgical history
  - ○ Allergies
  - ○ Current medications
  - ○ Neurologic disorders
  - ○ Medical conditions, such as
    - ■ Lung disease
    - ■ Elevated BMI
    - ■ Diabetes
  - ○ Genital or pelvic surgery
- Social history
  - ○ Smoking
  - ○ Caffeine and alcohol intake
  - ○ Fluid intake
  - ○ Heavy lifting
- Review of systems (ROS)

Physical Examination:
Components of the Physical Exam to Consider

- Vital signs, including temperature
- Thorax
  - ○ CVA tenderness
  - ○ Flank pain
- Abdominal palpation
  - ○ Suprapubic pain

- Pelvic exam with focus on
  - ○ Urethra
  - ○ Presence of cystocele or rectocele
  - ○ Signs or symptoms of
    - ■ Reproductive tract infection
    - ■ Genital atrophy
    - ■ Genital trauma
  - ○ Evaluation of pelvic floor strength and function

Clinical Impression:
Differential Diagnoses to Consider

- Urinary tract infection
  - ○ Cystitis
  - ○ Urethritis
  - ○ Pylonephritis
- Urinary incontinence
  - ○ Urge
  - ○ Stress
  - ○ Mixed
  - ○ Overflow
  - ○ Iatrogenic
- Interstitial cystitis
- STI affecting the urinary tract
  - ○ Chlamydia/gonorrhea
  - ○ Herpes
- Pregnancy

Diagnostic Testing:
Diagnostic Tests and Procedures to Consider

- Urinary tract infections
  - ○ Urinalysis (dip and/or microscopic)
    - ■ Most common pathogens *E. coli*, *Staph saprophyticus*, proteus, enterococcus
    - ■ Diagnosis considered + if > 100,000 colony count in clean catch specimen

- Culture
  - Recurrent or persistent symptoms
  - Pregnancy
  - Urinary calculi
- HCG
- Ultrasound
  - Renal calculi
  - CVAT +
- Strain urine
  - Renal calculi
- Incontinence
  - 🔊 Urodynamics
  - Postvoid catheterization to determine residual·
- 🔊 Cystoscopy (National Kidney and Urologic Diseases Information Clearing House, 2003)
  - Recurrent urinary tract infections
  - Hematuria
  - Incontinence or overactive bladder
  - Unusual cells in urine sample
  - Painful urination, chronic pelvic pain, or interstitial cystitis
  - Urinary stricture
  - Stone in the urinary tract

Providing Treatment: Therapeutic Measures to Consider

- Urinary tract infection
  - Pyridium for pain relief 200 mg tid x 2 D
  - Appropriate antibiotic therapy
- Pylonephritis
  - IV fluids
  - Pain relief
  - Appropriate antibiotic therapy
- Urge incontinence
  - Detrol 2 mg BID

- Ditropan XL 5 or 10 mg 1 po daily (Murphy, 2004; Czarapata, 1999)
- Stress Incontinence
  - Hormonal treatment for urogenital atrophy
    - Estring
    - Vaginal estrogen cream
  - Medications
    - Pseudoephedrine HCL
    - Phenylpropanolamide
  - Pessary fitting
    - Ring
    - Ring with support
    - Gelhorn
    - Use vaginal cream with pessary
      - Trimo-san
      - Acigel
      - Estrogen cream

Providing Treatment: Alternative Measures to Consider

- Incontinence
  - Scheduled toileting
  - Bladder retraining (biofeedback)
  - Pelvic muscle rehabilitation
- Urinary tract infection
  - Cranberry tablets, capsules, or juice (Avorn, et al., 1994)
  - Flush urinary system
    - Drink water or herbal tea
    - Avoid caffeine, sugar, and alcohol
  - Vitamin C 250–500 mg bid
  - Beta-carotene 25,000–50,000 IU daily
  - Zinc 30–50 mg daily
  - Homeopathic remedies (Jonas & Jacobs, 1996)
    - Aconitum—For early recent infection, with or without flank pain

- Cantharis—Searing lancing pain accompanied by urgency and frequency
  - Herbal teas (Soule, 1996; University of Maryland, 2004)
    - Echinacea
    - Urinary antiseptics
      - Pippsissewa
      - Bearberry (uva-ursi) (not for use in pregnancy)
      - Thyme
    - Soothing inflammation
      - Corn silk
      - Marshmallow root
      - Cleavers
    - Drink ½ cup every hour until symptoms subside
    - Continue 3–5 x daily for 10 days

Providing Support: Education and Support Measures to Consider

- Provide information regarding
  - Diagnosis
  - Treatment options
  - Medication instructions
- UTI recommendations
  - Avoid caffeine, alcohol, and sugar
  - Drink plenty of water
  - Void frequently
  - Void after intercourse
  - Blot from front to back after voiding
- Urge incontinence
  - Void
    - Frequently
    - With initial urge
    - Do not limit fluids
  - Kegel exercises daily
  - Medication instructions
- Stress incontinence
  - Kegel exercises daily
  - Biofeedback plan
  - Pessary use and fitting instructions as indicated

Table 9-1   Medications for Urinary Tract Infections

MEDICATION	DOSE	SIDE EFFECTS
Amoxicillin/Clavulanate	250/125 mg q 8 hours	Rash, GI upset
Cefaclor	250–500 mg q 8 hours	Caution if PCN allergy
Cephalexin	250 q 6 hours or 500 q 8	Caution if PCN allergy
Ciprofloxin	250–500 mg bid	Dizziness, headache, GI upset
Fosfomycin	Single-dose packet	Diarrhea, headache
Lomefloxacin	400 mg once daily	Dizziness, headache, GI upset
Nitrofurantoin	50–100 q 6 hours	Nausea, pulmonitis, neuropathy
Ofloxacin	400 mg bid	Dizziness, headache, GI upset
Sulfa/trimethoprim	800/160 mg bid	Rash, Stevens-Johnson syndrome
Trimethoprim	100 mg q 12 hours	GI upset, delayed rash

Source: Adapted from PDR, 2004.

- Signs and symptoms requiring return for continued care
  - Signs of infection/stones
  - Worsening symptoms
- Option for referral for surgical treatment

Follow-up Care: Follow-up Measures to Consider

- Document
- Plan for continued care
  - UTI
    - Reculture following treatment for
- Acute pylonephritis
- Recurrent symptoms
- Pregnancy
  - Urge/stress incontinence
    - Keep 2–5 day urinary diary
    - Follow-up for
      - Biofeedback
      - Reevaluation of
        - Pelvic floor strength
        - Response to medications
        - Need for pessary
        - Need for surgical consult
  - Pessary use
    - Check q 3 months
    - Clean
    - Evaluate for tissue breakdown

Collaborative Practice: Criteria to Consider for Consultation or Referral

- OB/GYN service
  - Acute pylonephritis
  - Persistent UTI during pregnancy
  - Evaluation of persistent urinary incontinence

  - Pelvic prolapse
  - Pessary fitting
  - Surgical treatment
- Urology service
  - Unresolved, recurrent, or persistent infection
  - Persistent renal calculi
  - Suspected
    - Obstruction
    - Interstitial cystitis
  - Surgical treatment
- For diagnosis or treatment outside the midwife's scope of practice

References

American Heart Association [AHA]. (2004). *Women and coronary heart disease.* Retrieved March 9, 2005, from http://www.americanheart.org/presenter.jhtml?identifier=2859

American Lung Association. (2004a). American Indians/Native Alaskans and lung disease fact sheet. Retrieved March 16, 2005, from http://www.lungusa.org/site/pp.asp?c=dvLUK9O0E&b=36053

American Lung Association. (2004b). African-Americans and lung disease fact sheet. Retrieved March 16, 2005, from http://www.lungusa.org/site/pp.asp?c=dvLUK9O0E&b=35976

American Lung Association. (2004c). Asian Americans/Pacific Islanders and lung disease fact sheet. Retrieved March 16, 2005, from http://www.lungusa.org/site/pp.asp?c=dvLUK9O0E&b=36054

American Lung Association. (2004d). Hispanics and lung disease fact sheet. Retrieved March 16, 2005, from http://www.lungusa.org/site/pp.asp?c=dvLUK9O0E&b=36055

American Thoracic Society. (1999). Diagnostic standards and classification of tuberculosis in adults and children. Retrieved March 4, 2005, from http://www.cdc.gov/nchstp/tb/pubs/mmwrhtml/Maj_guide/List_categories.htm

Avorn, J., Monane, M., Gurwitz, J. H., Glynn, R, J., Choodnovskiy, I., & Lipsitz, L. A. (1994). Reduction of bacteriuria and pyuria after ingestion of cranberry juice. *Journal of the American Medical Association, 271*, 751–754.

Beers, M., & Berkow, R. (Eds.). (1995–2005). Recommendations for antibiotic treatment of adult Lyme disease. In *Merck manual of diagnosis and therapy* [online edition]. Retrieved March 10, 2005, from http://www.merck.com/mrkshared/mmanual/tables/157tb5.jsp

Bromberg, W. D., (1998, August 25). Urinary tract infections: The basics. *The Clinical Advisor*, 60–64.

Brucker, M. C., & Faucher, M. A. (1997). Pharmacologic management of common gastrointestinal health problems in women. *Journal of Nurse-Midwifery, 43*, 145–162.

Centers for Disease Control and Prevention [CDC]. (2001). Helicobacter pylori and peptic ulcer disease. Retrieved March 5, 2005, from http://www.cdc.gov/ulcer/md.htm#fda

Clark, C., & Paine, L. L. (1996). Psychopharmacologic management of women with common mental health problems. *Journal of Nurse-Midwifery, I*, 254–274.

Czarapata, B. J. (1999). Managing urinary incontinence. *Patient care for the nurse practitioner*, April 1999, 37–48.

Emmons, L., Callahan, P., Gorman, P., & Snyder, M. (1997). Primary care management of common dermatologic disorders in women. *Journal of Nurse-Midwifery, 42*, 228–253.

Foster, S. (1996). *Herbs for your health*. Loveland, CO: Interweave Press.

Haas, A. (2004). Prematurity is preventable. *Midwifery Today, 72*, 14-16, 64.

Holisticonline.com. (n.d.). Conventional, holistic, and integrative treatments for acne. Retrieved March 10, 2005, from http://holisticonline.com/Remedies/acne.htm

Jonas, W. B., & Jacobs, J. (1996). *Healing with homeopathy: The doctors' guide*. New York: Warner Books.

Kantor, S. D. (1990). Stress and psoriasis. *Cutis, 46*, 321–322.

Kriebs, J., & Burgin, K. (1997). Pharmacological management of common musculoskeletal disorders in women. *Journal of Nurse-Midwifery, 42*, 207-227.

Ledezma, E., DeSousa, L., Jorquera, A., Sanchez, J., Lander, A., Rodriquez, E., et al. (1996). Efficacy of ajoene, an organosulphur derived from garlic, in the short-term therapy of tinea pedis. *Mycoses, 39*, 393–395.

Madankumar, R. (2003). An overview of hypertensive disorders in women. *Primary Care Update for OB/GYNs, 10*(1), 14–18.

Moon, J. (2005). Herpes Zoster. E-Medicine. Retrieved March 3, 2005, from http://www.emedicine.com/med/topic1007.htm

Murphy, J. L. (Ed.). (2004). *Nurse practitioner's prescribing reference*. New York: Prescribing Reference.

National Heart Lung and Blood Institute. (2003). The seventh report of the joint national committee on prevention, detection, evaluation, and treatment of high blood pressure. Retrieved March 20, 2005 from http://www.nhlbi.nih.gov/guidelines/hypertension/express.pdf

National Institute of Arthritis and Musculoskeletal and Skin Diseases. (2002). Questions and answers about arthritis and rheumatic diseases. Retrieved March 15, 2005 from http://www.niams.nih.gov/hi/topics/arthritis/artrheu.htm

National Institute of Mental Health [NIMH]. (2000a). Depression. Retrieved March 15, 2005, from http://www.nimh.nih.gov/publicat/depression.cfm#ptdep5

NIMH. (2000b). Health information. Retrieved March 15, 2005, from http://www.nimh.nih.gov

National Jewish Medical and Research Center. (2003). Nasal wash. Retrieved March 16, 2005, from http://asthma.nationaljewish.org/treatments/alternative/nasalwash.php

National Kidney and Urologic Diseases Information Clearinghouse. (2003). Cystoscopy and ureteroscopy. Retrieved March 17, 2005, from http://kidney.niddk.nih.gov/kudiseases/pubs/cystoscopy/index.htm

Payton, R. G., Gardner, R., & Reynolds, D. (1997). Pharmacologic considerations and management of common endocrine disorders in women. *Journal of Nurse-Midwifery, 42*, 186–206.

Pearson T. A., Blair, S. N., Daniels, S. R., Eckel, R. H., Fair, J. M., Fortmann, S. P., et al. (2002). AHA guidelines for primary prevention of cardiovascular disease and stroke: 2002 update: Consensus panel guide to comprehensive risk reduction for adult patients without coronary or other atherosclerotic vascular diseases. *Circulation, 106*, 388–391.

Physicians' Desk Reference [PDR] (59th ed.). (2004). Montvale, NJ: Thomson Healthcare.

Rovner, E. S., & Weine, A. J. (2000) Overactive bladder and urge incontinence: Establishing the diagnosis. *Women's Health in Primary Care, 3*, 117–126.

Soule, D. (1996). *The roots of healing*. Secaucus, NJ: Citadel Press.

Tong, M. M., Altman, P. M., & Barnetson, R. S. (1992). Tea tree oil in the treatment of tinea pedis. *Aust J Dermatol, 33*, 145–149.

University of Maryland Medical Center. (2004). Urinary tract infections in women. Retrieved March 17, 2005, from http://www.umm.edu/altmed/ConsConditions/UrinaryTractInfectioninWomencc.html

Wong, C. (n.d.) Natural treatments for acne. Retrieved March 10, 2005, from http://altmedicine.about.com/cs/conditionsatod/a/acne.htm

Bibliography

Alliance for Aging Research. (1997). *Controlling high blood pressure in older women: clinical reference manual.* Washington, DC: National Heart, Lung and Blood Institute.

American Heart Association [AHA]. (1998). Cardiovascular disease in women: A scientific statement from the AHA. *Clinician Reviews, 8,* 145–160.

Benetti, M. C., & Marchese, T. (1996). Primary care for women: Management of common musculoskeletal disorders. *Journal of Nurse-Midwifery, 41,* 173–187.

Davis, L., & Stecy, P. (1997). Pharmacologic management of cardiovascular problems in women. *Journal of Nurse-Midwifery, 42,* 176–185.

Drazen, J. M., & Weinberger, S. E. (1998). Disorders of the respiratory system. In A. S. Fauci, & E. Braunwald, et al. (Eds.). *Harrison's principles of internal medicine* (14th ed., pp. 1407–1410). New York: McGraw-Hill.

Fauci, A. S., & Braunwald, E., et al. (Eds.). (1998). *Harrison's principles of internal medicine* (14th ed.). New York: McGraw-Hill.

Harris, G. D. (1999). Managing hypertension in female patients. *Women's Health in Primary Care, 2,* 395–417.

MacLaren, A., & Imberg, W. (1998). Current issues in the midwifery management of women living with HIV/AIDS. *Journal of Nurse-Midwifery, 43,* 502–521.

Mays, M., & Leiner, S. (1997). Pharmacologic management of common lower respiratory tract disorders in women. *Journal of Nurse-Midwifery, 42,* 163–175.

Mays, M., & Leiner, S. (1996). Primary care for women: Management of common respiratory problems. *Journal of Nurse-Midwifery, 41,* 139–154.

Moser M. (1996). *Clinical management of hypertension.* Caddo, OK: Professional Communications.

National Cholesterol Education Program. (1993). *Second report on the detection, evaluation and treatment of high blood cholesterol in adults.* Washington, DC: National Institutes of Health.

Schmitt, M., (March 1999). Skills workshop: Evaluating the shoulder. *Patient Care for the Nurse-Practitioner,* 42–50.

Shaw, B. (1996). Primary care for women: Management and treatment of gastrointestinal disorders. *Journal of Nurse-Midwifery, 41,* 155–172.

Siris, E. S., & Schussheim, D. H. (1998). Osteoporosis: Assessing your patient's risk. *Women's Health in Primary Care, 1*(1), 99–106.

Smith, T. (1984). *A woman's guide to homeopathic medicine.* New York: Thorsons.

Speroff, L., Glass, R. H., & Kase, N. G. (1994). *Clinical gynecologic endocrinology and infertility* (5th ed.). Philadelphia: Williams & Wilkins.

Swartz, M. H. (1994). *Textbook of physical diagnosis: History and examination* (2nd ed.). Philadelphia: W. B. Saunders.

Weintraub, T. A., Paine, L. L., & Weintraub, D. H. (1996). Primary care for women: Comprehensive assessment and management of common mental health problems. *Journal of Nurse-Midwifery, 41,* 125–138.

Appendix

Table 9-2   Calcium Foods List
Deep green leafy vegetables
Broccoli, turnip, acorn squash, okra
Sea vegetables
Dried beans
Chick peas, hummus
Sesame and sunflower seeds
Almonds, Brazil nuts, pistachios, peanuts
Shellfish, fish with bones (canned salmon)
Fruits: Dried figs, fortified orange juice
Milk, cheese, yogurt
Masa harina or corn tortilla
Blackstrap molasses
Herbal infusions:
Red raspberry leaf, oat straw, borage
Nettle, dandelion greens
Parsley, watercress

Sources: Soule, 1996; Varney, et al., 2004; Haas, 2004; Weed, 1985.

Table 9-3   Magnesium Foods List
Dried beans and peas
Broccoli, cauliflower, kale, cabbage
Beets and beet greens
Whole grains
Tofu
Sweet potato, carrots, turnip
Cashews, almonds, sesame seeds
Summer squash
Parsley, celery
Dandelion, turnip, and mustard greens

Sources: Soule, 1996; Varney, et al., 2004.

Table 9-4   Iron Foods List
Dried peas and beans
Blackstrap molasses
Dried fruit
Sea vegetables
Deep green leafy vegetables
Shellfish
Egg yolk
Fish
Poultry
Meat
Organ meats
Fortified cereals and breads
Herbals:
Yellow dock
Nettle
Alfalfa
Parsley
Dandelion

Sources: Soule, 1996; Varney, et al., 2004.

Index

A

abdominal discomfort
    constipation, 41–43, 48–49. *See also* hemorrhoids
    PMS (premenstrual syndrome), 331–334
    round ligament pain, 55–57
abnormal mammograms, 263–266
abnormal Pap smears, 266–270, 281–284
ABO incompatibility, 88–90
abortion
    emergency contraception, 229–232
    unplanned pregnancies, 241–245
abscess formation (mastitis), 195–197
abstinence, periodic. *See* fertility awareness charting
abused clients. *See* developmental considerations for
    clients
acne, 347
ACNM (American College of Nurse-Midwives), 2
acute pelvic pain, 323–325
adjustment to motherhood. *See* postpartum period
admission forms, 22
adolescents as clients, 8, 270–272
adoptions. *See* unplanned pregnancies
adrenal insufficiency, 352–357
advising clients, 7
    collaborative practice, 3–7, 18–19, 22, 122–125
affective (mood) disorders, 187–190, 361–367
age, client, 8
    adolescent clients, 8, 270–272
    fertility awareness charting, 225–227
    perimenopause, 245–253, 256–259
        bleeding during. *See* endometrial biopsies
AIDS. *See* HIV infections
allergies. *See* PUPPP
alternate health care providers. *See* collaborative practice
alternative treatments, 17
AMA (American Medical Association), 19

amenorrhea, 270–272. *See also* contraceptive
    management; pregnancy
American College of Nurse-Midwives, 2
American Medical Association, 19
amnioinfusion, 120–122
amniotic fluid
    meconium-stained, 139–143
    rupture of the membranes (ROM), 128, 165–169
    size–date discrepancies and, 90–93
anal cancer. *See* human papillomavirus
anemia, 54–55, 62–64. *See also* postpartum hemorrhaging
anesthetics. *See* labor and delivery
annual well woman visits. *See* physical examinations;
    reproductive health
antibiotic prophylaxis. *See* Group B streptococcus
antibodies. *See* HIV infections; Rh isoimmunization
anxiety disorders. *See* mental health disorders
apgar scores. *See* newborns, examination and evaluation of
arrested labor, 130–133
arthritis. *See* musculoskeletal conditions
asphyxia, 197–201
aspiration. *See* meconium
assessment of risk, 3–4, 9–11, 19–20, 34–36. *See also*
    reproductive health
    preconception counseling, 220–222
assessments. *See* evaluation
assisted deliveries
    Cesarean deliveries, 122–128
    shoulder dystocia, 169–172
    vacuum extractors, 172–174
asthma. *See* respiratory conditions
asymptomatic bacteriuria. *See* urinary tract infections
attitude. *See* culturally competent care
augmentation or induction of labor, 136–139
    failure to progress, 130–133
    prolonged latent phase labor, 163–165
autoimmune disorders. *See* infections
avoidance of pregnancy, 229–232

B

babies. *See* fetus; newborns

backaches, 39–41, 55–57. *See also* musculoskeletal conditions

bacterial vaginosis (BV), 272–275

barrier methods (contraception), 227–229

bedrest. *See* preterm labor

belief systems. *See* culturally competent care

benign tumors. *See* fibroids

b-HCG levels, 98–101

billing, 19. *See also* documentation of care

biopsies. *See* screenings and diagnoses

bipolar disorders. *See* mental health disorders

birth control. *See* contraceptive management

Bishop's score, 137

bladder infections. *See* urinary tract infections

bleeding
    dysfunctional uterine bleeding, 284–287
    epistaxis, 46–47
    first-trimester vaginal bleeding, 98–101
    hemorrhoids, 48–49, 193–195
    labor and delivery. *See* third-stage labor
    menstruation. *See also* reproductive health
        amenorrhea, 270–272
        dysfunction, 352–357
        dysmenorrhea, 287–290
        fertility awareness charting, 225–227
        intermenstrual bleeding, 284–287
        premenstrual syndrome, 331–334
    postmenopausal, 292–295. *See also* endometrial biopsies
    postpartum hemorrhaging, 150–153
    uterine, 150–153

blood disorders. *See* Rh isoimmunization

blood pressure
    cardiovascular problems, 57–58, 341–346
    hypertensive disorders, 44–45, 81–85, 156–159. *See also* endocrine disorders

blood sugar
    endocrine disorders, 352–357
    gestational diabetes, 68–72

BMD (bone mineral density). *See* osteoporosis

body lice. *See* pediculosis

bolus amnioinfusion. *See* amniotic fluid

bone mineral density (BMD). *See* osteoporosis

bones. *See* musculoskeletal conditions

bowel disorders. *See* constipation; gastrointestinal disorders

breast-feeding. *See also* postpartum period
    amenorrhea, 270–272
    fertility awareness charting and, 225–227
    mastitis, 195–197
    well-baby care, 210–213

breasts, 195–197, 263–266, 275–278, 318–321

breathing. *See* respiratory conditions

breech. *See also* fetal presentation and position
    Cesarean deliveries, 125–128, 174–177
    meconium, 139–143
        amnioinfusion, 120–122
        resuscitation of newborn, 197–201

bronchitis. *See* respiratory conditions

BV (bacterial vaginosis), 272–275

C

calcium foods list, 381

cancer risks. *See* replacement therapy

cancer screenings. *See also* human papillomavirus (HPV)
    breast, 263–266, 275–278, 318–321
    chronic pelvic pain. *See* chronic pelvic pain
    colposcopies, 281–284
    dermatologic. *See* dermatologic disorders
    endometrial, 290–292
    gastrointestinal. *See* gastrointestinal disorders
    hepatitis. *See* hepatitis
    mammograms, 263–266
    Pap smears, 266–270
    respiratory. *See* respiratory conditions

candidal vulvovaginitis, 316–318

cardiovascular conditions, 57–58, 341–346

care, philosophies of, 1–3, 7–8

care plans. *See* decision making; treatment

CC (chief complaint), 15

cervix
    bleeding. *See* first-trimester vaginal bleeding
    cervical caps. *See* barrier methods
    cervical dysplasia. *See* human papillomavirus
    changes in. *See* labor and delivery; preterm labor
    colposcopy, 281–284
    lacerations of. *See* postpartum hemorrhaging
    Pap smears, 266–270. *See also* human papillomavirus

Cesarean deliveries, 125–128, 174–177

CHD (coronary heart disease), 57–58, 341–346

chief complaint (CC), 15

chlamydia, 278–281. *See also* gonorrhea; pelvic inflammatory disease

chronic hypertension. *See* hypertensive disorders

chronic pelvic pain, 325–328

circumcision, 204–207

clavicle (shoulder dystocia), 169–172

client competency, 8–9, 20–21

client culture, awareness of, 3–4, 8–9, 20, 54–55. *See also* circumcision

client education, 17–18, 20–21, 225–227. *See also* contraceptive management
    advising, 7

client history, 15, 19, 22. *See also* documentation of care

client records, 3–5, 13–28
    fertility awareness charting, 225–227

client rights, 5
clients, socioeconomic challenges of, 8–9
clinical decision making, 4, 19–21. *See also* diagnoses and
    screenings; treatment
        risk management, 3–4, 9–11, 19–20, 34–36. *See also*
            reproductive health
                preconception counseling, 220–222
clinical impressions, 15–16
clinical practice guidelines, 4–5
coagulation. *See* bleeding; postpartum hemorrhaging
coding, 19. *See also* documentation of care
collaborative practice, 3–7, 18–19, 22, 122–125
colposcopies, 281–284. *See also* Pap smears
combination hormone replacement therapy, 249–253. *See
    also* menopause
communication, documentation as, 5, 14–19
competency of client, 8–9, 20–21
complementary therapies, 17. *See also* alternative
    treatments
complications in pregnancy
    newborn variation. *See entries at newborn*
    risk management, 3–4, 9–11, 19–20, 34–36. *See also*
        reproductive health
            preconception counseling, 220–222
conception. *See* fertility; pregnancy
condoms, 227–229
congenital toxoplasmosis infections, 93–95
congential anomalies. *See entries at newborn*
consent, informed, 20–21
constipation, 41–43, 48–49. *See also* hemorrhoids
consultations, 3–7, 18–19, 22. *See also* collaborative
    practice
contraceptive management
    barrier methods, 227–229
    emergency contraception, 229–232
    fertility awareness charting, 225–227
    hormonal contraceptives, 232–236, 239–241
    intrauterine devices, 236–239
    Norplant System, 239–241
contractions. *See* labor and delivery
coping skills of woman in labor, 106–108
Copper-T IUD, 236–239
cord, umbilical
    compression of, 120–122. *See also* fetal presentation
        and position
    prolapsed, 128–130
    as secondary source of oxygen, 197, 200
coronary artery disease, 57–58, 341–346
coughing. *See* respiratory conditions
counseling. *See* client education
CPT (current procedural terminology) handbook, 19
cramps
    leg, 51–52
    menstrual. *See* premenstrual syndrome
    round ligament pain, 55–57

cravings. *See* pica
C-sections. *See* Cesarean deliveries
culturally competent care, 3–4, 8–9, 20, 54–55. *See also*
    circumcision
cultures. *See* screenings and diagnoses
Current Procedural Terminology (CPT) handbook, 19
cyanosis, 197–201
cystic masses. *See* breasts
cystitis. *See* urinary tract infections
cytology, cervical. *See* Pap smears

D
daily fetal kick counts. *See* postterm pregnancy
date-size discrepancies, 90–93
death of fetus, 64–66. *See also* first-trimester vaginal
    bleeding
decision making, 4, 19–21. *See also* treatment
    diagnoses. *See* diagnoses and screenings
    gastrointestinal disorders, 41–43, 48–49, 357–361
        heartburn, 47–48
    risk management, 3–4, 9–11, 19–20, 34–36. *See also*
        reproductive health
            preconception counseling, 220–222
deficiencies, nutrition. *See* diet and nutrition
dehydration. *See* nausea and vomiting
delaying of labor. *See* preterm labor
deliveries. *See* labor and delivery
depression, postpartum, 187–190. *See also* mental health
    disorders
dermatologic disorders, 346–352. *See also* pediculosis
    pediculosis, 321–323
        PUPPP (puritic uticarial papules and plaques of
            pregnancy), 86–88
DES exposure. *See* cervix
developmental considerations for clients, 8–9
diabetes, gestational, 68–72
diabetes mellitus. *See* endocrine disorders
diagnoses and screenings. *See also* decision making;
    primary care for women; reproductive health
    breast, 263–266, 275–278, 318–321
    chronic pelvic pain, 325–328
    colposcopies, 281–284
    dermatologic disorders, 346–352. *See also* pediculosis
        pediculosis, 321–323
            PUPPP, 86–88
    diagnostic impressions, 15–17
    endometrial, 290–292
    for endometriosis, 295–297
    evaluation and management criteria (E/M), 19
    gastrointestinal, 41–43, 48–49, 357–361
        heartburn, 47–48
    hepatitis, 72–74, 307–310
    HPV (human papillomavirus), 310–313. *See also*
        dermatologic disorders; Pap smears

mammograms, 263–266
osteoporosis, 253–256
Pap smears, 266–270
preconception, 220–222
pregnancy confirmation, 30–31
respiratory, 43–44, 139–143, 370–375
working diagnoses, defined, 15
diaphragm (contraception), 227–229
diarrhea. *See* gastrointestinal disorders
diet and nutrition. *See also* gestational diabetes
disorders. *See* mental health disorders
food lists, 381–382
gestational diabetes, 68–72
inadequate weight gain during pregnancy, 79–81
iron deficiency anemia, 54–55, 62–64
nausea and vomiting, 51–52
socioeconomic challenges, 8–9
discharge summaries, 28
distress, fetal. *See* resuscitation of the newborn
diversity. *See* culturally competent care
doctors. *See* physicians
documentation of care, 3–5, 13–28
fertility awareness charting, 225–227
dysfunctional uterine bleeding (DUB), 284–287. *See also*
endometrial biopsies
dysmenorrhea, 287–290
dyspnea, 43–44

E

eating disorders. *See* mental health disorders
eating habits. *See* diet and nutrition
eclampsia, 81–85. *See also* hypertensive disorders
economic challenges to clients, 8–9
ECP (Emergency contraceptive pills), 229–232
ectopic pregnancies. *See* first-trimester vaginal bleeding
edema, 44–45
education, client, 17–18, 20–21, 225–227. *See also*
contraceptive management
E/M (evaluation and management criteria), 19
emergency consultations. *See* collaborative practice
emergency contraception, 229–232
emotional changes following delivery. *See* depression,
postpartum
emotional disorders. *See* mental health disorders
endocrine disorders, 352–357
endometrial biopsies, 290–292. *See also* postmenopausal
bleeding
endometriosis, 295–297. *See also* dysmenorrhea
endometritis, 190–192
endotracheal intubation, 197–201
episiotomies. *See* second-stage labor; third-stage labor
epistaxis, 46–47

ERT (estrogen replacement therapy), 249–253. *See also*
menopause
essential hypertension. *See* hypertensive disorders
estrogen
hormonal contraceptives, 232–236
Norplant System, 239–241
menopause. *See* menopause
replacement therapy, 249–253
ethnically competent care, 3–4, 8–9, 20, 54–55. *See also*
circumcision
evaluation. *See also* screenings and diagnoses
collaborative practice, 3–7, 18–19, 22, 122–125
primary care. *See* primary care for women
risk management, 3–4, 9–11, 19–20, 34–36. *See also*
reproductive health
preconception counseling, 220–222
evaluation and management criteria (E/M), 19
evaluation of care, documentation of, 14
evaluation of woman in labor, 106–108
evidence-based practice, 4
examinations. *See* diagnoses and screenings; evaluation;
physical examinations
exemplary midwifery practice, 1–11
exhaustion
insomnia, 49–51
postpartum depression, 187–190
prolonged latent phase labor, 163–165
external version. *See* fetal presentation and position

F

face presentation. *See* fetal presentation and position
failure to progress in labor, 130–133
family planning. *See* preconception counseling
fatigue
insomnia, 49–51
postpartum depression, 187–190
prolonged latent phase labor, 163–165
feeding newborns. *See* breast-feeding
fertility. *See* contraceptive management; preconception
counseling
fertility awareness charting, 225–227. *See also*
dysmenorrhea
fetal presentation and position, 128, 144–150, 169–172
fetus. *See also* labor and delivery
amnioinfusion, 120–122
congenital anomalies, 207–210
congenital syphilis. *See* syphilis
congenital toxoplasmosis infections, 93–95
fetal demise, 64–66
inadequate weight gain during pregnancy, 79–81
newborn resuscitation, 197–201
perinatal transmission of infections. *See* infections
postterm pregnancy, 153–156

preterm labor. *See also* premature rupture of
    membranes (PROM); vaginitis
  risk management for, 9–10
  second-stage labor, 113–116
  size of
        shoulder dystocia, 169–172
        size–date discrepancies, 90–93
        weight gain during pregnancy, 79–81
  umbilical cord compression, 197–201
  umbilical cord prolapse, 128–130
  weight gain during pregnancy, 79–81
fever, intrapartum. *See* Group B streptococcus
fFN (fetal fibronectin testing). *See* preterm labor
fibrocystic breasts. *See* breasts
fibroids, 297–300. *See also* dysmenorrhea
  size–date discrepancies and, 90–93
fibromyalgia. *See* musculoskeletal conditions
Fifth's disease, 66–68
first-stage labor, 109–113. *See also* labor and delivery
first-trimester vaginal bleeding, 98–101
fluid retention (edema), 44–45
follow-up care, 18
food. *See* diet and nutrition
forceps. *See* vacuum-assisted births
foreskin removal. *See* circumcision
fundus. *See* uterus
fungal infections. *See* dermatologic disorders

G

galactorrhea. *See* nipple discharge
gastroesophageal reflux disease, 47–48
gastrointestinal disorders, 41–43, 48–49, 357–361
  heartburn, 47–48
GBS (Group B streptococcus), 133–136
genetic testing. *See* loss of fetus
genital candidiasis, 316–318
genital tract infections. *See* human papillomavirus
gestation. *See* pregnancy
gestational diabetes, 68–72
gestational hypertension, 81–85. *See also* hypertensive
    disorders
GI (gastrointestinal disorders), 357–361
glands (endocrine disorders), 352–357
glucose levels. *See* gestational diabetes
glucose metabolism disorders, 352–357
goals of midwifery, 1–3
gonorrhea, 300–303. *See also* chlamydia; pelvic
    inflammatory disease
Group B streptococcus (GBS), 133–136
growth of fetus
  shoulder dystocia, 169–172
  size–date discrepancies, 90–93
  weight gain during pregnancy, 79–81

H

H & P. *See* client history; physical examinations
halting labor. *See* preterm labor
handicapped clients, 9
hazard analysis (risk management), 3–4, 9–11, 19–20,
    34–36. *See also* reproductive health
  preconception counseling, 220–222
HBV infections, 307–310
HCG levels, 98–101
head of baby. *See* fetal presentation and position
health care providers. *See* collaborative practice
health risk management, 3–4, 9–11, 19–20, 34–36. *See also*
    reproductive health
  preconception counseling, 220–222
heart disease, 57–58, 341–346
heart rate. *See* vital signs for newborn resuscitation
heartburn, 47–48
HELLP syndrome, 81–85, 156–159
hemoglobin. *See* bleeding
hemorrhaging, postpartum, 150–153. *See also* bleeding
hemorrhoids, 48–49, 193–195. *See also* constipation
hepatitis, 72–74, 307–310
herbal treatments, 17. *See also* alternative treatments
herpes simplex virus, 74–76, 313–316. *See also*
    dermatologic disorders
history, client, 15, 19, 22
  documentation of care, 3–5, 13–28
        fertility awareness charting, 225–227
history of present illness (HPI), 15
HIV infections, 76–79, 303–307
hormonal changes
  amenorrhea, 270–272
  fertility awareness charting, 225–227
  perimenopause, 245–253, 256–259
        bleeding during. *See* endometrial biopsies
hormonal contraceptives, 232–236
  Norplant System, 239–241
hormone replacement therapy, 249–253. *See also*
    menopause
hormones, premenstrual (PMS), 331–334
hospital procedures, 22, 28
HPI (history of present illness), 15
HPV (human papillomavirus), 310–313. *See also*
    dermatologic disorders; Pap smears
HRT (hormone replacement therapy), 249–253. *See also*
    menopause
HSV (herpes simplex virus), 74–76, 313–316. *See also*
    dermatologic disorders
Human Immunodeficiency Virus (HIV), 76–79, 303–307
human papillomavirus (HPV), 310–313. *See also*
    dermatologic disorders; Pap smears
hyperemesis of pregnancy. *See* nausea and vomiting
hyperglycemia (endocrine disorders), 352–357

hypertensive disorders, 44–45, 81–85, 156–159. *See also* endocrine disorders
    cardiovascular problems, 57–58, 341–346
hyperthyroid (endocrine disorders), 352–357
hypoparathyroid (endocrine disorders), 352–357
hypopituitary (endocrine disorders), 352–357
hypothyroid (endocrine disorders), 352–357
hysterectomies. *See* fibroids

I

ICD-9-Diagnosis code book, 19
icons used in this book, 3–4
identification. *See* diagnoses and screenings
illnesses. *See* infections
immigrants as clients, 9
immunizations. *See* reproductive health; well-baby care
implants, contraceptive, 236–241
inadequate weight gain during pregnancy, 79–81
incompetent cervix. *See* preterm labor
incontinence. *See* urinary tract infections
induction or augmentation of labor, 136–139. *See also* postterm pregnancy
    prolonged latent phase labor, 163–165
infants. *See* newborns
infections. *See also* dermatologic disorders
    chlamydia, 278–281
    dysmenorrhea, 287–290
    endometritis, 190–192
    Fifth's disease, 66–68
    GBS (Group B streptococcus), 133–136
    gonorrhea, 300–303
    hepatitis, 72–74, 307–310
    HIV (human immunodeficiency virus), 76–79, 303–307
    HPV (human papillomavirus), 310–313
    HSV (herpes simplex virus), 74–76, 313–316
    mastitis, 195–197
    pediculosis, 321–323
    PID (pelvic inflammatory disease), 328–331
    syphilis, 334–337
    toxoplasmosis, 93–95
    urinary tract infections, 95–98, 375–379
    vaginitis, 316–318
infertility. *See* amenorrhea
infestations. *See* dermatologic disorders
inflammations. *See* musculoskeletal conditions
information. *See* documentation of care
informational consultations. *See* collaborative practice
informed consent, 20–21
inhibition of labor. *See* preterm labor
injectable contraceptives. *See* hormonal contraceptives
injury, risk of. *See* risk management
insomnia, 49–51
instructions to client, 17–18

insulin therapy. *See* gestational diabetes
insurance, liability, 10–11
intercourse
    contraceptive management
        barrier methods, 227–229
        emergency contraception, 229–232
        hormonal contraceptives, 232–236, 239–241
        intrauterine devices, 236–239
        Norplant System, 239–241
    fertility awareness charting, 225–227
    sexually transmitted infections. *See* STIs
intermenstrual bleeding, 284–287
interpreter services, 8, 20. *See also* culturally competent care
interstitial cystitis. *See* urinary tract infections
interventions. *See* treatment
interviews. *See* client history
intestinal disorders. *See* gastrointestinal disorders
intrapartum fever. *See* Group B streptococcus
intrauterine devices, 236–239
intrauterine growth retardation (IUGR), 90–93
intubation of infants at birth, 197–201. *See also* meconium
iron deficiency anemia, 54–55, 62–64
iron foods list, 382
irregular bleeding, 284–287
irregular contractions. *See* labor and delivery
isoimmunization. *See* Rh isoimmunization
itching. *See* infestations; PUPPP
IUDs (intrauterine devices), 236–239
IUGR (intrauterine growth retardation), 90–93

J

Jadelle implants, 239
joint pain. *See* musculoskeletal conditions

K

kyphosis. *See* osteoporosis

L

labor and delivery, 105–177. *See also* postpartum period
    amnioinfusion, 120–122
    Cesarean deliveries, 122–128
    documentation of, 14, 22, 27
    dysmenorrhea, 287–290
    evaluation of woman in, 106–108
    of fetal demise, 65–66
    first-stage labor, 109–113
    Group B streptococcus (GBS), 133–136
    hypertensive disorders, 156–159
    induction and augmentation, 136–139
    meconium-stained amniotic fluid, 139–143
    multiple gestation, 142–146
    postpartum hemorrhage, 193–195
    postterm pregnancy, 153–156

premature rupture of membranes (PROM), 165–169

presentation of fetus, nonvertex, 146–150

preterm, 159–162

prolonged latent phase, 163–165

second-stage, 113–116

shoulder dystocia, 169–172

third-stage, 116–119

vacuum extraction, 172–174

vaginal birth after Cesarean (VBAC), 174–177

lacerations

    postpartum hemorrhage, 150–153

    third-stage labor, 116–119. *See also* postpartum period

    vacuum-assisted births, 172–174

lactation. *See also* postpartum period

    amenorrhea, 270–272

    fertility awareness charting and, 225–227

    mastitis, 195–197

    well-baby care, 210–213

lactose intolerance. *See* gastrointestinal disorders

language interpreters, 8, 20. *See also* culturally competent care

language of documentation, 16

large for gestational age (LGA), 90–93

latent phase of labor, prolonged, 163–165

legal actions, 5, 10, 14

legs, 51–52, 57–58

lesions

    screening for. *See* cancer screenings

    sexually transmitted. *See* STIs

    skin conditions. *See* dermatologic disorders

LGA (large for gestational age), 90–93

liability insurance, 10–11

lice. *See* pediculosis

litigation, 10

liver dysfunction. *See* hepatitis

loss of fetus, 64–66. *See also* first-trimester vaginal bleeding

lung function. *See* respiratory conditions

lupus. *See* musculoskeletal conditions

Lyme disease. *See* dermatologic disorders

lymph nodes. *See* mammograms

M

magnesium foods list, 382

malignancies

    fibroids, 297–300. *See also* dysmenorrhea

        size–date discrepancies and, 90–93

    screening for. *See* cancer screenings

malnutrition. *See* diet and nutrition

malpractice. *See* litigation

mammograms, 263–266

management criteria (E/M), 19

maneuvering baby. *See* fetal presentation and position

mania. *See* mental health disorders

MAS (meconium-aspiration syndrome), 139–143

    amnioinfusion, 120–122

mastitis, 195–197

maternal health. *See* reproductive health

maternal weight gain, 79–81

MDS (minimum data sets), 14

meconium, 139–143

    amnioinfusion, 120–122

    resuscitation of newborn, 197–201

medical abortions. *See* unplanned pregnancies

medical records. *See* documentation of care

medicine vs. midwifery, 13

melanoma. *See* dermatologic disorders

membranes, rupture of, 128, 165–169

menopause

    bleeding during. *See* endometrial biopsies

    fertility awareness charting, 225–227

    hormone replacement therapy, 249–253

    perimenopause, 245–253, 256–259

menstruation. *See also* reproductive health

    amenorrhea, 270–272

    dysfunction (endocrine disorders), 352–357

    dysmenorrhea, 287–290

    fertility awareness charting, 225–227

    intermenstrual bleeding, 284–287

    premenstrual syndrome, 331–334

mental health disorders, 187–190, 361–367

mentally challenged clients, 8

midwifery standards of care, 1–11

minimum data sets (MDS), 14

miscarriage

    first-trimester vaginal bleeding, 98–101

    loss of fetus, 64–66

mohel. *See* circumcision

molar pregnancies. *See* first-trimester vaginal bleeding

monilia. *See* genital candidiasis

mood changes, postpartum, 187–190. *See also* mental health disorders

motherhood, adjustment to. *See* postpartum period

mulluscum contagiosum. *See* dermatologic disorders

multiculturally competent care, 3–4, 8–9, 20, 54–55. *See also* circumcision

multiple gestation, 142–146

muscle pain. *See* backaches

muscle spasms in the leg, 51–52

musculoskeletal conditions, 253–256, 367–370

N

N & V. *See* nausea and vomiting

natural family planning, 225–227

nausea and vomiting, 51–52. *See also* gastrointestinal disorders

neonatal. *See* infants

neonatal GBS infection, 133–136

networking. *See* collaborative practice

newborns. *See also entries at fetus*
    circumcision, 204–207
    delivery. *See* labor and delivery
    examination and evaluation of, 201–204, 207–213
    perinatal transmission of infections. *See* infections
    resuscitation of, 197–201
    risk management for, 9–10
nicotine withdrawal, 222–225
nipple discharge, 318–321
nits. *See* pediculosis
noncyclic bleeding. *See* dysfunctional uterine bleeding
nonpharmacologic methods of birth control, 225–227
nonprogressive labor, 130–133
nonstress tests. *See* postterm pregnancy
nonvertex presentation. *See* fetal presentation and position
Norplant System, 239–241
nosebleeds. *See* epistaxis
notes. *See* documentation of care
nurses vs. midwives, 13
nursing. *See* breast-feeding
nutrition and diet
    disorders. *See* mental health disorders
    food lists, 381–382
    gestational diabetes, 68–72
    inadequate weight gain during pregnancy, 79–81
    iron deficiency anemia, 54–55, 62–64
    nausea and vomiting, 51–52
    socioeconomic challenges, 8–9

O

OB/GYN physicians, 13. *See also* collaborative practice
oblique lie. *See* fetal presentation and position
observation. *See* assessments; evaluation
obsessive/compulsive disorders. *See* mental health disorders
obstetrics and gynecology, 13. *See also* collaborative practice
office visits. *See* physical examinations
older women as clients, 8. *See also* perimenopause
oligohydramnios, 90–93. *See also* meconium
    amnioinfusion, 120–122
opinions, second. *See* collaborative practice
oral contraceptives. *See* hormonal contraceptives
osteoarthritis. *See* musculoskeletal conditions
osteoporosis, 253–256
ovarian cancer. *See* chronic pelvic pain
ovulation. *See* fertility awareness charting
oxygen
    respiratory conditions, 43–44, 139–143, 370–375
    resuscitation of newborn, 197–201

P

panic disorders. *See* mental health disorders
Pap smears, 266–270. *See also* colposcopies; human papillomavirus
parasites. *See* pediculosis
parathyroid disorders (endocrine disorders), 352–357
partners, sexual. *See* sexual activity
parvovirus B19, 66–68
patches for contraception. *See* hormonal contraceptives
patches for smoking cessation, 222–225
pathology. *See* screenings and diagnoses
patients. *See* clients
pediatricians. *See* collaborative practice
pediculosis, 321–323. *See also* dermatologic disorders
pelvic inflammatory disease (PID), 328–331. *See also* chlamydia; gonorrhea
pelvic laparoscopy. *See* endometriosis
pelvic pain, 323–328
pelvimetry, 113
perimenopause, 245–253, 256–259
    bleeding during. *See* endometrial biopsies
    fertility awareness charting, 225–227
perinatal transmission of infections. *See* infections
periodic abstinence. *See* fertility awareness charting
periods. *See* menstruation
personality disorders. *See* mental health disorders
pertussis. *See* respiratory conditions
philosophy of care, 1–3, 7–8
phlebitis (edema). *See* edema
phobias. *See* mental health disorders
physical examinations. *See* primary care for women; screenings and diagnoses
physically handicapped clients, 9
physicians, 13
    collaborative practice, 3–7, 18–19, 22, 122–125
pica, 54–55. *See also* iron deficiency anemia
PID (pelvic inflammatory disease), 328–331. *See also* chlamydia; gonorrhea
PIH (pregnancy-induced hypertension), 81–85, 156–159. *See also* edema
Pill (contraceptive). *See* hormonal contraceptives
pituitary glands. *See* nipple discharge
pituitary glands (endocrine disorders), 352–357
placenta, delivery of, 116–119
placenta, retained. *See* postpartum hemorrhaging
plan of care, defined, 15
PMDD (premenstrual dysphoric disorders). *See* premenstrual syndrome
PMS (premenstrual syndrome), 331–334
pneumonia. *See* respiratory conditions
policies of practice, 10–11
polyhydramnios, 90–93
poor as clients, 8–9
portpartum hemorrhaging, 150–153

position and presentation of fetus, 128, 144–150, 169–172

position of mother during labor. *See* fetal presentation and position; second-stage labor

postmenopausal bleeding, 292–295. *See also* endometrial biopsies

postmenopausal clients, 8

postmenopause. *See* menopause

postpartum hemorrhaging, 150–153. *See also* bleeding

postpartum period, 181–213
  about week 1, 181–184
  about weeks 1 to 6, 184–187
  assessment of the newborn, 201–204, 207–210
  beginning, 116–119
  circumcision of the newborn, 204–207
  depression, 187–190
  documentation of, 22, 27
  endometritis, 190–192
  hemorrhoids, 48–49, 193–195
  mastitis, 195–197
  newborn resuscitation, 197–201
  well-baby care, 210–213

postterm pregnancy, 153–156. *See also* induction or augmentation of labor

post-traumatic stress disorder. *See* mental health disorders

poverty, 8–9

practice guidelines, 4–5, 7, 10

preconception counseling, 220–222
  fertility awareness charting, 225–227
  smoking cessation, 222–225

preeclampsia, 81–85. *See also* edema; hypertensive disorders

pregnancy-induced hypertension (PIH), 81–85, 156–159. *See also* edema

premature deliveries. *See* preterm labor

premature rupture of membranes (PROM), 165–169

premenstrual syndrome, 331–334

prenatal. *See* pregnancy

presentation and position of fetus, 128, 144–150, 169–172

preterm labor, 159–162. *See also* premature rupture of membranes (PROM); vaginitis

Preven. *See* emergency contraception

prevention of pregnancy. *See* contraceptive management

preventive health. *See* primary care for women; reproductive health

primary amenorrhea. *See* amenorrhea

primary care for women, 341–382. *See also* screenings and diagnoses
  cardiovascular problems, 57–58, 341–346
  collaborative practice, 3–7, 18–19, 22, 122–125
  dermatologic disorders, 346–352
  endocrine disorders, 352–357
  gastrointestinal disorders, 357–361
  mental health disorders, 187–190, 361–367
  midwives as providers, 7
  musculoskeletal conditions, 253–256, 367–370

respiratory disorders, 370–375

urinary tract infections, 95–98, 375–379

problem focused visits, 19

problem lists, 20

procedure notes, 21–22

procedures. *See* standards of practice; treatment

procedures of practice, 10–11

professional relationships. *See* collaborative practice

professional standards. *See* standards of practice

progesterone. *See* hormone replacement therapy

progestin. *See* hormonal contraceptives

progress notes, 14, 21

prolapsed cord, 128–130. *See also* premature rupture of membranes (PROM)

prolonged latent phase labor, 163–165

PROM (premature rupture of membranes), 165–169

psoriasis. *See* dermatologic disorders

psychiatric problems. *See* mental health disorders

pulse. *See* vital signs for newborn resuscitation

PUPPP (puritic uticarial papules and plaques of pregnancy), 86–88

pylonephritis. *See* urinary tract infections

R

race. *See* culturally competent care

records of care, 3–5, 13–28
  fertility awareness charting, 225–227

rectal bleeding. *See* hemorrhoids

referrals, 3–4, 22. *See also* consultations

reflux. *See* gastrointestinal disorders

refugees as clients, 9

refusal of treatment, 21

reimbursement for services, 19

renal calculi. *See* urinary tract infections

replacement therapy, hormonal, 249–253. *See also* menopause

reproductive health, 215–259
  amenorrhea, 270–272
  breasts, 195–197, 263–266, 275–278, 318–321
  chlamydia, 278–281
  colposcopy, 281–284
  diagnoses of problems, 263–337
  dysfunctional uterine bleeding, 284–287
  dysmenorrhea, 287–290
  endometrial biopsies, 290–292
  endometriosis, 295–297
  fertility awareness charting, 225–227
  fibroids, 297–300
  genital candidiasis, 316–318
  gonorrhea, 300–303
  hepatitis, 72–74, 307–310
  herpes simplex virus (HSV), 74–76, 313–316
  HIV (human immunodeficiency virus), 76–79, 303–307
  human papillomavirus (HPV), 310–313

mammograms, abnormal, 263–266
nipple discharge, 318–321
pediculosis, 321–323
pelvic inflammatory disease (PID), 328–331
pelvic pain, 323–328
postmenopausal bleeding, 292–295
premenstrual syndrome, 331–334
vaginosis, bacterial, 272–275
reproductive system. *See* fertility awareness charting
research, evaluation of, 4
respiratory conditions, 43–44, 139–143, 370–375
resuscitation of the newborn, 197–201
retained placenta fragments. *See* postpartum hemorrhaging
review of systems (ROS), 15
Rh isoimmunization, 88–90
rheumatoid arthritis. *See* musculoskeletal conditions
rhythm method, 225–227
rights of clients, 5
Ringer's lactate, 120–122
rings (contraceptives). *See* hormonal contraceptives
risk management, 3–4, 9–11, 19–20, 34–36. *See also* reproductive health
preconception counseling, 220–222
STIs. *See* sexual activity
ROM (rupture of membranes), 128, 165–169
ROS (review of systems), 15
round ligament pain, 55–57
routine care of newborns, 210–213
rubella. *See* dermatologic disorders
rupture, membranes (ROM), 128, 165–169
rupture, uterine
postpartum hemorrhage, 150–153
vaginal birth after Cesarean (VBAC), 174–177

S
saline, 120–122
scabies. *See* pediculosis
scar integrity. *See* vaginal birth after Cesarean
scope of practice, defining, 4–5, 7, 10
screenings and diagnoses. *See also* decision making; reproductive health
breast, 263–266, 275–278, 318–321
chronic pelvic pain, 325–328
colposcopies, 281–284
dermatologic disorders, 346–352. *See also* pediculosis
pediculosis, 321–323
PUPPP, 86–88
diagnostic impressions, 15–17
endometrial, 290–292
for endometriosis, 295–297
evaluation and management criteria (E/M), 19
gastrointestinal, 41–43, 48–49, 357–361
heartburn, 47–48

hepatitis, 72–74, 307–310
HPV (human papillomavirus), 310–313. *See also* dermatologic disorders; Pap smears
mammograms, 263–266
osteoporosis, 253–256
Pap smears, 266–270
preconception counseling, 220–222
pregnancy confirmation, 30–31
primary care. *See* primary care
respiratory, 43–44, 139–143, 370–375
working diagnoses, defined, 15
second opinions. *See* collaborative practice
secondary amenorrhea. *See* amenorrhea
second-stage labor, 113–116
self-care. *See* reproductive health
severe hypertension, 81–85. *See also* hypertensive disorders
sexual activity
barrier methods of contraception, 227–229
contraceptive management
barrier methods, 227–229
emergency contraception, 229–232
hormonal contraceptives, 232–236, 239–241
intrauterine devices, 236–239
Norplant System, 239–241
fertility awareness charting, 225–227
STIs (sexually transmitted infections)
chlamydia, 278–281
gonorrhea, 300–303
HIV (human immunodeficiency virus), 76–79, 303–307
HPV (human papillomavirus), 310–313
HSV (herpes simplex virus), 74–76, 313–316
pediculosis, 321–323
PID (pelvic inflammatory disease), 328–331
syphilis, 334–337
SGA (small for gestational age), 90–93
shock. *See* portpartum hemorrhaging
shortness of breath, 43–44
shoulder dystocia, 169–172
Silastic capsules. *See* Norplant System
simple cystitis. *See* urinary tract infections
size of fetus
shoulder dystocia, 169–172
size–date discrepancies, 90–93
weight gain during pregnancy, 79–81
skeletal system. *See* musculoskeletal conditions
skin conditions. *See* dermatologic disorders
sleep deprivation, 49–51
insomnia, 49–51
postpartum depression, 187–190
prolonged latent phase labor, 163–165
small for gestational age (SGA), 90–93
smoking cessation, 222–225
socioeconomic challenges to clients, 8–9

soft tissue injuries. *See* musculoskeletal conditions

specialty care. *See* collaborative practice

spermicides. *See* contraceptive management

spontaneous abortions. *See* first-trimester vaginal bleeding

spontaneous rupture of the membranes. *See* preterm labor

spotting. *See* dysfunctional uterine bleeding

standards of practice, 10–11

standards of terminology, 16

stillbirths, 64–66

stimulation of labor, 136–139. *See also* postterm
    pregnancy
    prolonged latent phase labor, 163–165

STIs (sexually transmitted infections)
    barrier methods of contraception, 227–229
    chlamydia, 278–281
    gonorrhea, 300–303
    HIV (human immunodeficiency virus), 76–79,
        303–307
    HPV (human papillomavirus), 310–313
    HSV (herpes simplex virus), 74–76, 313–316
    pediculosis, 321–323
    PID (pelvic inflammatory disease), 328–331
    syphilis, 334–337

strokes. *See* cardiovascular conditions

suctioning
    amnioinfusion, 120–122
    meconium, 139–143
    resuscitation of newborn, 197–201
    vacuum-assisted births, 172–174

suicide. *See* mental health disorders

supplemental estrogen. *See* hormone replacement therapy

support systems. *See* collaborative practice

surgical procedures
    abortion
        emergency contraception, 229–232
        unplanned pregnancies, 241–245
    Cesarean deliveries, 125–128, 174–177
    circumcision, 204–207
    hysterectomies. *See* fibroids

swelling (edema), 44–45. *See also* musculoskeletal
    conditions

symbols used in this book, 3–4

symptoms. *See* diagnoses and screenings

syphilis, 334–337

T

TB (tuberculosis). *See* respiratory conditions

teamwork. *See* collaborative practice

teens as clients, 8, 270–272

termination of pregnancy, 229–232, 241–245

terminology standards, 16

testing. *See* diagnoses and screenings

therapeutic treatment, 17

third-stage labor, 116–119. *See also* postpartum period

thrombophlebitis (edema), 44–45

thrombosed hemorrhoids, 48–49, 193–195

thyroid (endocrine disorders), 352–357

tobacco addiction, 222–225

tocolysis. *See* preterm labor

toxoplasmosis, 93–95

tracking of clients, 18. *See also* documentation of care

traction-related fetal injury (shoulder dystocia), 169–172

transfer of care. *See* collaborative practice

transient hypertension. *See* hypertensive disorders

transverse lie. *See* fetal presentation and position

treatment, 1–11, 17. *See also* screenings and diagnoses;
    specific condition by name
    documenting, 3–5, 13–28
    philosophy of midwife care, 1–3, 7–8
    refusal of, 21

tuberculosis. *See* respiratory conditions

tumors. *See* cancer screenings

U

ultrasounds. *See* mammograms

umbilical cord
    compression of, 120–122. *See also* fetal presentation
        and position
    prolapsed, 128–130
    as secondary source of oxygen, 197, 200

unborn childr. *See* fetus

unopposed estrogen. *See* hormone replacement therapy

unplanned pregnancies, 241–245

unprotected sex. *See* contraceptive management; sexual
    activity

unwanted pregnancies, 241–245

urinary tract infections, 95–98, 375–379

urticaria. *See* PUPPP

uterine bleeding. *See also* menstruation
    postpartum hemorrhage, 150–153

uterine cancer, 292–295

uterine contractions. *See also* labor and delivery
    prolonged latent phase labor, 163–165

uterine rupture
    postpartum hemorrhage, 150–153
    vaginal birth after Cesarean (VBAC), 174–177

uterus
    bleeding, 284–287
    endometritis, 190–192
    fibroids, 297–300

UTI (urinary tract infections), 95–98, 375–380

V

vaccines. *See* primary care for women; reproductive
    health; well-baby care

vacuum-assisted births, 172–174

vaginal birth after Cesarean (VBAC), 174–177

vaginal bleeding. *See* bleeding

vaginal lacerations. *See* portpartum hemorrhaging

vaginal rings. *See* hormonal contraceptives

vaginitis, 316–318

variations in newborns. *See entries at newborn*

variations in pregnancies. *See* pregnancy

varicosities, 57–58. *See also* edema; hemorrhoids

vascular system, 57–58, 341–346

vasomotor symptoms. *See* hormone replacement therapy

VBAC (vaginal birth after Cesarean), 174–177

veins. *See* varicosities

ventilation, newborn, 197–201

viral illnesses. *See also* dermatologic disorders
    hepatitis, 72–74, 307–310
    herpes simplex virus (HSV), 74–76, 313–316. *See also* dermatologic disorders
    HIV (Human Immunodeficiency Virus), 76–79, 303–307
    HPV (human papillomavirus), 310–313. *See also* dermatologic disorders; Pap smears
    infections. *See* infections
    parvovirus B19, 66–68

vital signs for newborn resuscitation, 197–201

vomiting, 51–52

W

warts. *See* human papillomavirus

watchful waiting. *See* induction or augmentation of labor; postterm pregnancy

weight gain during pregnancy, 79–81

well-baby care, 210–213. *See also* newborns

well-woman care. *See* reproductive health

working diagnoses. *See* diagnoses and screenings

written instructions to client, 17–18. *See also* documentation of care

Y

yeast infections. *See* genital candidiasis; vaginitis